MW00605115

WHAT WENT WRONG

The Truth Behind the Clinical Trial
of the Enzyme Treatment of Cancer

NICHOLAS J. GONZALEZ, M.D.

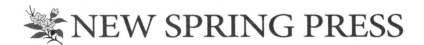 NEW SPRING PRESS

Notice

Foreword Copyright © Sarah Ann Cooper
Foreword Copyright © Paul J. Rosch, M.D.
Copyright © 2012 by Nicholas J. Gonzalez, M.D.

Book design by Anne M. Landgraf, Brooklyn BookWorks LLC.

Cover photograph © roxxephotography.com. Used with permission.

Publisher's Cataloging-in-Publication
(Provided by Quality Books, Inc.)

Gonzalez, Nicholas J., 1947–
    What went wrong : the truth behind the clinical trial
of the enzyme treatment of cancer / Nicholas J.
Gonzalez.
    p. cm.
    Includes bibliographical references.
    LCCN 2012933174
    ISBN 978-0-9821965-3-3
    ISBN 978-0-9821965-4-0
    ISBN 978-0-9821965-5-7

    1. Pancreas—Cancer—Treatment—Evaluation—Case
studies. 2. Clinical trials—United States—Case
studies. 3. Pancreas—Cancer—Diet therapy.
I. Title.

    RC280.P25G66 2012   616.99′4370654′0724
                    QBI12-600047

To My Wife Mary Beth,
Whose Faith in My Mission has Never For a Moment Wavered

Contents

CONTENTS

Foreword

I f I had not been on the Isaacs/Gonzalez protocol for the past 11 years, I would not be here today to tell my story. In December 2000 a mass was found in my pancreas during a CAT scan of my abdomen. In February of 2001, a biopsy by Kaiser and confirmed at the Mayo Clinic diagnosed the 3.2 cm tumor in the head of my pancreas as a carcinoma, better known as pancreatic cancer. I was sent to three surgeons all of whom wanted to perform a surgery called a Whipple operation. After hearing the extent of organs to be removed, I questioned the common sense of having surgery at all. I insisted on a complete explanation of why this was necessary and the prognosis of quality of life and life expectancy, both of which were bleak—so bleak that the prognosis was 3 to 6 months without surgery and only 15 to 18 months with surgery and chemo. I scheduled surgery twice and cancelled each time. I read everything on the Internet from the AMA, the National Cancer Institute and every site involving cancer. I wrote to the AMA and the NCI to receive literature. Bookstores became my friend as I read everything about cancer. I delved into the medical disease publications and books written by medical doctors and alternative medicine practitioners. I felt good and wanted better odds than the surgeons were giving me. I declined surgery.

While researching the cause of cancer and some of the alternative ways of treatment, I started on various herbs, vitamins, minerals and lots of prayer. Then I heard about a clinical trial which did not involve some participants taking a placebo. The trial used only natural methods to treat cancer. On further investigation, I learned the trial was only allowing persons with pancreatic cancer to participate. This was possibly done because of the short life expectancy of a diagnosis of this cancer.

After further checking, I contacted the office of Dr. Linda Isaacs and Dr. Nicholas Gonzalez where I was given the contact information for Columbia-Presbyterian Medical Center, a Dr. Chabot. After a brief phone interview by Dr. Chabot's nurse, she sent me the packet to fill out to see if I qualified for the trial. I also had to get medical records from Kaiser to forward with the packet. After receiving my packet, Columbia called and informed me I qualified for the trial. I was to go to New York and meet with Dr. Chabot and then with Dr. Gonzalez or Dr. Isaacs to discuss the trial protocol. I immediately started securing my finances to make the trip; my sister-in-law gave me a ticket and I made my hotel reservations. I was ecstatic. At last there was hope and a chance to live a quality life. I realized the regimen of 150 plus pills, the coffee enemas, the diet and cleanses would change my life. However at least I would have a chance at life and a quality of life while I fought this battle. We were ready to start. Or so I thought!

Upon arrival in New York City, my first meeting was with Dr. Isaacs. She went over the basic segments of the protocol to be sure I understood it would not be an easy regimen. She was very professional and explained how we would work by phone. Then she asked if I had been able to get my doctor at Kaiser to agree to take periodic blood tests and monitor me. I confirmed my wonderful primary care physician had agreed to do that and send any reports to their office for their perusal. I was scared not because I had chosen this route but because I knew it would be a strict and time-consuming commitment, a commitment I was more than willing to make. The surgery option was not a consideration. I had refused surgery with three surgeons and was on alternative supplements already to try to prolong my life.

My next visit was with Dr. Chabot at Columbia-Presbyterian. The nurse there showed me into a small office. She explained she would go over my paperwork, and then I would be given the final approval by Dr. Chabot. We were zipping along when she asked the fatal question. "Mrs. Cooper, now why are you unable to have surgery?"

I honestly replied, "I can have surgery, however, I have chosen not to."

She immediately stated she would have to discuss this with Dr. Chabot. I waited and soon Dr. Chabot entered the room. Sitting across the desk from me, he said there was no way I could be in the trial since I could have surgery. I was shocked and tried to explain that it was my decision not to have surgery. I would not agree to surgery, chemotherapy, or radiation, now or ever. I was crying when I told him it was my life. I should be able to choose the treatment I felt was best for me. I met all the criteria for the trial and wanted desperately to be in the program. I had completed all the requirements and flown to New York at my expense anticipating starting the program. I tried to explain, I understood the decision I was making since my sister and niece had died of cancer. I left the building not understanding what had just happened and in a state of frozen disbelief. To say I was shocked and upset is an understatement. I was crushed. Hope had been wrung out of me. Nothing remained but darkness.

Returning to my hotel, I fell on the bed and cried. I knew I would not reconsider the Whipple surgery. I feared I would not be able to read and investigate enough alternative ways before becoming bedridden. However, I was convinced that I would pursue that avenue as long as I was able. Just then the phone rang. It was Dr. Isaacs. She had been called by Dr. Chabot's office and was so concerned about me. I felt she was surprised and disappointed in the latest developments also. After I told her I was still not going to go the only route approved by the medical profession, she asked me to come to her office if I was interested in being treated off trial. She explained that it would be at my expense however she would take her fees into consideration for all ongoing consultations.

The cab couldn't get me there fast enough. She spent two hours explaining in detail the procedures, even taping them for my future reference. Instructions were given on my diet, how to obtain the supplements from a supplier in California and sheets on when to take them, and the procedure for the cleanses and the coffee enemas. She informed me to call any time I needed to and she would return the call that day. For 11 years, she has kept that promise and has continued to look over my latest tests from Kaiser. I was blessed with three dedicated doctors, my primary care giver at Kaiser who worked with me in my pursuit of an alternative way to handle my disease, and Dr. Gonzalez and Dr. Isaacs, truly wonderful doctors who stayed with me, always researching any questions or concerns I encountered on my journey. It is a shame that doctors aren't taught in medical school to keep an open mind regarding other options to curing disease. Surgeons and MDs should be open to investigating new alternative treatments with a fair and inquiring mind. Compassion is part of the Hippocratic Oath. When any group takes the attitude that they know what's best for someone else and exert power over that person to get the decision they want, they are tyrants and should reconsider who gave them this right.

I can say without any hesitation that without Dr. Gonzalez and Dr. Isaacs and the protocol they presented to the world, I would not have seen my only granddaughter Sarah, named after me, born or celebrated my 50th wedding anniversary. Neither would I have experienced any of the other joys life has brought me in the last 11 years with my three children, three grandsons and granddaughter. Nor would there have been the joy of family Christmases, eleven birthdays each, for all of us to celebrate and seeing my eldest grandson graduate from high school. My future looks great! I continue to teach a health and wellness class which I started 5 years ago at my church. Also I am writing a book about my journey to give others hope and an inquiring mind. And with God's blessing, I will live to see my great-grandchildren arrive in this wonderful world. Let me not end this without giving thanks to God and the Holy Spirit for leading me with His knowledge and guidance. For without it, I would not be here today.

Dr. Nick Gonzalez and Dr. Linda Isaacs are to be applauded for their courage and perseverance. They are honorable physicians and I hope our world will see more of this kind of dedication and willingness to explore other options in combating cancer.

Sarah Ann Cooper
February 2012

Second Foreword

My interest in the Gonzalez treatment program began after my wife was diagnosed with pancreatic cancer in September 2010. Surgery revealed a small lesion in the head of the pancreas with minimal regional node involvement that the pathology report indicated had been removed with clear margins. Her blood tests returned to normal, imaging studies revealed no abnormalities, and a course of gemcitabine (Gemzar) chemotherapy was unanimously recommended. I was well aware that life expectancy with Gemzar in similar cases averaged less than 15 months, and wanted to see what other options were available. There were numerous websites devoted to unorthodox approaches with anecdotal reports of miraculous results, including with pancreatic cancer, but few had any published scientific studies to support these claims. Dr. Gonzalez was an exception, but in addition to dietary restrictions, his protocol required taking 150–170 supplements and two coffee enemas daily, a combination that I suspected would discourage many prospective patients. What I was interested in were those patients he described with documented pancreatic cancer who were alive and well 5 to 15 or more years after being placed on pancreatic enzyme supplements. Was it possible to prove that such triumphs were due to these enzymes? And if the enzymes were not responsible, was there some other explanation?

Can Stress and Emotions Influence Cancer?

I was aware of the body's innate potential for self-healing and dramatic placebo effects, but was there any way to harness these phenomena? I had spent my professional life studying the role of emotions in health and disease, especially with respect to stress and cancer. My interest in this began during a Fellowship with Hans Selye shortly after the publication of his magnum opus *Stress*,[1] which explained his concept of "Diseases of Adaptation." Selye demonstrated that when laboratory animals were subjected to severe stress, there was a three-phased response he called the "General Adaptation Syndrome." During the course of this syndrome, pathologic changes in organs and tissues developed similar to those seen in patients with peptic ulcers, heart attacks, kidney disease, rheumatoid arthritis and other disorders, which he referred to as "Diseases of Adaptation." We coauthored some book chapters and following my Fellowship, I completed my internship and residency at Johns Hopkins and Walter Reed, after which I entered private practice. Selye and I kept in contact and he called to tell me he was coming to Manhattan and would like to discuss a forthcoming conference his Institute was co-sponsoring with Sloan-Kettering on "Stress, Cancer and Death." We arranged to have dinner, during which he told me that several years earlier he had a histiocytic reticulosarcoma removed from his thigh. This malignancy is usually fatal and he was urged to have chemotherapy and radiation but he refused and attributed his full recovery to an urgent need to complete a very important study. He had collected a number of articles citing similar cases, and many more suggesting that distress could cause cancer or accelerate its downhill course. He asked if I would review these and give a presentation at the conference on "Cancer as a Disease of Adaptation."

It was difficult to refuse any request from Selye, but I felt that proving a stress-cancer link in humans would be impossible. There are many different types of cancer, stress cannot be measured since it is a subjective phenomenon that differs for each of us, establishing a cause-effect temporal relationship is difficult since it is not known how long an asymptomatic malignancy may have been present before its clinical detection, etc., etc. Selye had anticipated all these and other obstacles, but asked if I would at least review the material he had collected before making a final decision. I subsequently became immersed in the large packet of articles he sent, as well as the references they led me to. One recurrent theme was that cancer tended to be more common following the loss of an important relationship, such as the death of a spouse or loved one.

I was also fascinated by the observation that as one descends the phylogenetic scale to lower forms of life, cancer progressively disappears, but the ability to regenerate tissues, and even body parts increases proportionately. Salamanders can grow a replacement limb or tail that has been severed, or even parts of brain, but do not develop cancer. If you inject a chemical that causes cancer in humans into a salamander's leg, it will grow a new accessory limb at that location, and if you remove the lens of an eye and inject the same chemical, it will regenerate a new lens. Thus, the same stimulus that produces purposeful new growth in lower forms of life also resulted in new growth in humans, but this neoplasia is malignant and lethal. I did not think it was too much of a leap to suggest that with man's highly developed cerebral cortex, the death of a loved one might be perceived as a far greater loss than removing part of a limb. Could the body's continued attempts to replace something that was irreplaceable, such as the loss of a spouse, stimulate activities that caused cancer?

I found some medical articles and case reports as well as a few literary works that could be used to support this hypothesis and included these in my presentation. Selye seemed pleased with this and singled it out in his Preface to the publication of the proceedings as follows:

> Perhaps, as Paul Rosch of New York has suggested, cancer might even be an attempt by the human organism to regenerate organs and limbs as lower animals do spontaneously. Going further, one might say that the ultimate health of the organism, like that of society, appears to depend on how well or appropriately its constituents communicate with one another.[2(p xii)]

Enhancing Regeneration and Reversing Cancer with Unorthodox Therapies

I was particularly interested in whether adults retain some vestigial remnants of the remarkable regenerative powers seen in salamanders and other lower forms of life. The liver can regenerate itself even when up to 80 percent is removed, and the spleen has similar but less well developed capabilities. Fetuses can regenerate almost anything that becomes damaged while in the womb. It is also well established that if a fingertip is severed in children up to the age of two, it will always grow back perfectly, nail and all, without any intervention. This ability steadily declines and usually disappears by puberty, but occasional cases have been documented in adults. Could this potential for purposeful regeneration lie dormant in everyone? My interest in this was heightened by Dr.

Robert Becker's studies of the electrical characteristics of tissues following injury and during regeneration. He showed that after he amputated a frog's leg, if he implanted a small battery that sent out a regenerative signal to electrodes at the site of injury, the leg would grow back perfectly. When he attempted the same procedure in rats, he only had partial success, but it was still dramatic to see that nerve, bone, collagen, skin, and hair could be regenerated in a mammal. Was it possible that a stronger or different signal was required in higher life forms to facilitate regeneration?

As previously noted, salamanders have unusual regenerative powers and resistance to cancer-causing chemicals. But Becker showed that if he transplanted a rapidly growing cancer to a salamander's limb, the malignancy would take hold and eventually spread throughout the entire body and cause death. However, if the limb in which the cancer was implanted is amputated through the tumor (so that half of the cancer remains), something very curious happens. A new limb will start to grow back, and as it regenerates, not only does the remaining local cancer disappear, but all the metastases in other parts of the body also revert to normal tissue. Becker reasoned that this resulted from some type of electromagnetic signaling associated with regeneration that was detected by remote cancer cells and stopped them from replicating.

Further research in these areas might have had great potential for treating cancer in humans, but Becker's funding suddenly stopped. He had been one of the first to raise concerns about cancer and other health risks from high power lines, microwave ovens and radar. Since his warnings were ignored, he had become an outspoken enemy of electrical utility companies, the military and others that were polluting the environment with electromagnetic waves. Things intensified when he vigorously opposed building a new high power line facility in New York State and subsequently emphasized his concerns in a highly critical 1997 *60 Minutes* interview. As a result, not only was all government funding cut off, no university, hospital, or company was willing to support his regeneration research, even though it was unrelated to this issue. Becker continued to be blackballed and persecuted by the powerful interests he had offended for the rest of his life.

Could a Cure for Cancer Come from the Pancreas?

Although my wife was doing well on her chemotherapy regimen, I continued to investigate alternative options, particularly pancreatic enzyme therapy, which had been proposed over 100 years ago by John Beard, an English embryologist. Beard had noted that the trophoblastic cells of the primitive placenta surrounding the early embryo resembled and behaved like cancer cells. They constantly divided and as the placenta grew and invaded the uterus, it stimulated the development of new blood vessels to nourish the developing embryo. This was similar to the way cancer cells infiltrated adjacent tissues and metastasized to other structures and organs where they initiate angiogenesis to sustain their continued growth. However, cancer cells continue to divide until the host dies, whereas trophoblasts suddenly stop replicating and become mature placental cells. What caused this sudden cessation of unrestrained growth was a mystery and Beard spent years studying various mammals searching for the solution to this enigma. The only consistent finding was that this cessation always coincided with the development of the fetal pancreas and its ability to secrete enzymes. After birth, these enzymes helped the digestion of food in the duodenum, but Beard showed that in the fetus, where there was no food to digest, pancreatic enzymes also stopped trophoblastic replication, particularly enzymes like trypsin that broke down protein. Since cancer cells behaved like trophoblasts, he reasoned that pancreatic enzymes might also stop cancer cells from dividing. He was able to demonstrate this in a mouse model of adenocarcinoma that had recently been made available. When he injected an extract containing trypsin into these mice, their tumors shrank fairly quickly, while they continued to grow in littermates with the identical transplanted cancers.

Beard, a Sc.D. and not an M.D., could not treat patients directly, but physicians began to treat their own cancer patients with pancreatic enzyme injections under his supervision, with occasional dramatic results. As this practice became increasingly popular, the establishment became furious and Beard was repeatedly vilified in the popular press as well as medical journals. In 1911, he answered these attacks by publishing *The Enzyme Treatment of Cancer and Its Scientific Basis*,[3] which outlined his pancreatic enzyme theory and included documented case reports confirming its efficacy. Despite the fact that he was a distinguished professor, had been nominated for a Nobel Prize for his other achievements, and did not seek notoriety or profit from his discovery, he was continually criticized and condemned. Pancreatic enzyme treatment dwindled with the media frenzy over Madame Curie's new X-ray treatment as a safe and effective cure for cancer, as well as everything from acne and eczema, to lupus and excess hair. By the time Beard died in 1924, pancreatic enzyme therapy had been abandoned and he had been largely forgotten. Krebs, Kelley, and others later revived Beard's treatment with their own embellishments, but they were also viciously attacked in the press and by leading oncologists.

Those Who Don't Learn from the Mistakes of History are Doomed to Repeat Them

I was curious as to why Dr. Gonzalez was resurrecting pancreatic enzyme therapy in view of the negative experience of everyone before him who had attempted to do this. There was little reason to question his results in pancreatic cancer, which were clearly superior to Gemzar. Based on my own experience, I could not help but feel that the patient's faith in this protocol or in those administering it likely played an important role in its success. Why else would people subject themselves to such a seemingly Draconian regimen unless they had absolute and complete faith in its success? My review of well-validated cases of spontaneous remission also showed this phenomenon seemed to be linked to a strong faith in the treatment, the therapist, prayer, a passionate desire to be present for some celebration such as birth of a grandchild, or to accomplish something important, as in Selye's case. I learned from their website that both Dr. Gonzalez and his associate, Dr. Linda Isaacs, were extremely well trained and qualified physicians, and I was particularly impressed with their philosophy as expressed in a quote from one of their patients:

> I imagine the type of patient who does well on this type of approach is a person who takes time to understand health principles; believes in the program; trusts (their practitioner); is willing to make lifestyle changes, perseveres and never gives up; maintains a sense of humor; has support at home; and has a deep belief in God.

In an essay on the site written by Dr. Isaacs, it seemed to me she also felt that the patient's attitude might be as important as the supplements and I wanted to discuss this in a forthcoming Newsletter on "Alternative" cancer therapies that would include a discussion of pancreatic enzymes. I sent Dr. Gonzalez an e-mail asking for his opinion about the role of faith, and also whether any clinical trials were being planned to evaluate his treatment program.

He called me back that evening to say he completely agreed that the patient's faith and attitude were crucial components. Although these could be difficult to assess in an initial interview, both he and Dr. Isaacs routinely refused prospective patients if it was obvious that they could not or would not adhere to the protocol. With respect to clinical trials, he synopsized his experience with the 1998 $1.4 million government grant he had been awarded, which had been such an incredible, insulting and frustrating fiasco, that he was writing a book about it. I thought he might have exaggerated some aspects of what had transpired and since I did not want to misquote him or risk a lawsuit, asked if he would send me some details I might be able to use in a future Newsletter. He agreed, and what I received was even more unbelievable.

I had several questions and we exchanged lengthy e-mails over the following two weeks in which he documented all his claims. I could understand his frustration, since although regulatory authorities and others involved had verified significant deviations from the grant protocol, nothing was done. There was no retraction of the article providing a negative, inaccurate assessment of his treatment program, and none of the parties responsible for the mismanagement were held accountable. Since his reputation had suffered, it seemed to me that he had adequate grounds for a lawsuit. He had discussed this with his attorneys, who advised him that although he would probably prevail, it would be a Pyrrhic victory. Such litigation tended to be protracted, the defendants had high-powered lawyers who could draw it out further, it would consume a great deal of his time, incur huge expenses and take years before any settlement was reached. I had made a few discrete inquiries to individuals and groups that were involved and was stonewalled. Nobody was willing to discuss this even though I had not mentioned Dr. Gonzalez and merely asked how he or she might handle a hypothetical problem similar to his situation.

Has Making More Money Become the Major Motivation for Cancer Research?

The reason this book had to be written is that it is apparently the only way Dr. Gonzalez can hope to achieve some modicum of justice. I believe his present plight is due to the very same reasons the 40-year "War on Cancer" has been a failure—politics, money, greed and corruption. This is largely the result of an unholy alliance between the American Cancer Society (ACS), National Cancer Institute (NCI), Sloan-Kettering and drug companies they have heavily invested in, as well as petrochemical and automotive interests that pollute the environment with potential carcinogens. In 1971, ACS lobbied and aggressively campaigned for President Nixon to promise that cancer could be conquered within five years if NCI funding were increased. The 1972 elections were looming, and ACS, which was closely affiliated with the NCI, was largely responsible for the 1971 National Cancer Act, in which Nixon emphasized, "We need to work out a system that includes a greater emphasis on preventive care." To implement this, he gave the National Cancer Institute unprecedented power and funding. NCI's annual budget went from $233 million in 1971 to $815 million in 1977, and *is now over $5 billion*. Despite this 25-fold increase over the past 40 years and a decline in smoking, we are losing the war on cancer as evidenced by the escalation in rates of many malignancies during this period, including liver (165%), thyroid (145%), non-Hodgkin's lymphoma (82%), testes (60%), childhood (24%), and breast (23%). According to one authority, there has been 50% more cancer in men and 20% percent more cancer in women over the course of just one generation. Pancreatic cancer has markedly increased over the past several decades, and now ranks as the fourth leading cause of cancer death in both men and women. Although we now spend over $2 billion/year on drugs and radiation just for this malignancy alone, pancreatic cancer death rates have not significantly improved since 1971, nor has length of life, which averages little more than six months after diagnosis.

Nixon appointed Benno Schmidt, a former drug and chemical company executive, to head up his "War on Cancer." Schmidt was also Chairman of the Board of Sloan-Kettering, which had thousands of shares in chemotherapy drug companies. Like the ACS, its board also included top executives of drug, tobacco and petroleum companies as well as the automotive industry. That's not surprising since Alfred Sloan was CEO of General Motors and Charles Kettering was their Director of Research. Nixon also appointed Armand Hammer, Chairman of Occidental Petroleum, to the panel that controls NCI policies. Despite this alleged emphasis on prevention, the *Chronicle of Philanthropy* complained that ACS was "more interested in accumulating wealth than saving lives" and described it as "the world's wealthiest non profit organization." It takes in over $700 million/year and has cash reserves over $1 billion, but little if any of this goes to prevention. ACS responds to this criticism by promoting screening, which leads to early diagnosis, but is also very profitable, since it also leads to more tests and surgery that fail to reveal any cause for concern.

ACS indifference to cancer prevention became further embedded in national cancer policy following the appointment of Dr. Andrew von Eschenbach, ACS President-Elect, as NCI Director. There is a revolving door between NCI, ACS and other cancer cartel members. Approximately half of ACS board members are physicians and researchers with close ties to NCI, many of whom receive funding from both organizations, as well as from industries that make gener-ous donations to them. One example is the ACS Breast Cancer Awareness cam-paign, with its exclusive emphasis on mammography while taking no concrete actions to diminish the use of industrial chemicals that have been linked to breast cancer. Five of its past presidents have been radiologists, so it is not surprising that the campaign promotes makers of mammography equipment and film and recommends that every woman should have an annual mammogram starting at age 40, which has recently been shown to do more harm than good. NCI was similarly described by a former director as "a governmental pharmaceutical company." Support comes from a scathing analysis by the National Academy of Sciences requested by Congress, stating, "the leadership of NCI is marked by pervasive conflicts of interest and a revolving door with the cancer drug indus-try."[4] Their focus is on "screening, diagnosis and treatment" rather than preven-tion, and "contrary to the requirements of the 1971 Act, NCI has still failed to inform the public of a wide range of avoidable causes of cancer. This denial of the public's right to know has even been extended to the withholding of readily available scientific information."

There is no question that early detection can save lives, or the benefits of colo-noscopy, especially in those with a family history of colorectal cancer. But ex-cessive screening of healthy people can do more harm than good. Chest X-rays are no longer performed on many annual physical exams or routine hospital admissions, even for heavy smokers at high risk of developing lung cancer. The reason for this surprising change in recommendations is that the available evidence reveals that lung cancer is not detected early enough to affect survival rates. In addition, such routine screening procedures result in unnecessary bi-opsies, chest surgery, disability and other complications and costs. NCI's recent large study also found that no lives were saved from screenings for prostate and ovarian cancers. There are growing concerns about crowds of the worried well flocking to mobile trailers around the country to have their bodies scanned by three dimensional computerized X-rays to make sure there is nothing wrong internally. They don't need a physician's referral and few have any symptoms that would justify an exposure to radiation equivalent to up to 500 X-rays and spending many hundreds of dollars that are not reimbursable. When an abnormality is found, additional tests, biopsies and even surgery are required, which usually reveal that they are harmless lesions or artifacts. Thus, instead of getting peace of mind, many are subjected to weeks of stress wondering if they have a life-threatening condition. As one authority warned, "A negative total body C.T. scan does not provide reason to feel reassured, and a positive scan does not provide information that has been shown to improve life expectancy or quality of life."

Even the inventor of the PSA test for prostate cancer agrees it is worthless as a screening test because it leads to unnecessary surgical procedures, complications, and costs. Yet it is not likely to be abandoned. The chief medical officer of ACS stated that his hospital generated around $5,000 in revenue from each free prostate cancer screening, thanks to ensuing biopsies, treatments and follow-up care. Cancer screening brings in millions of dollars, whereas finding effective preventive measures and treatments would have the reverse effect, which is why the establishment would like to discredit and shut down Dr. Gonzalez. Around the same time ACS instigated the "War on Cancer", Ivan Illich warned in *Medical Nemesis* that it was the nature of most institutions and organizations to eventually end up by performing in a manner opposite to their original purpose because of corruption and greed, and that medicine was a perfect example.[5] Over the ensuing years, the cancer cartel has taken this to a new height. There is nothing legally wrong in investing in and promoting companies and products that have a bright financial future. But when this is done by suppressing competition that might save lives because they threaten profits, it is immoral. The hierarchy of the cancer club is so powerful that even when such transgressions are identified and acknowledged, it is unlikely that responsible parties will be admonished or held accountable, or that any corrective action will be taken, as vividly illustrated in this book. And their tentacles are far reaching. Following his brief stint as NCI director, von Eschenbach became director of the FDA, which in the minds of some has not been open to unconventional therapies. However, eventually "the truth will out," and there are already some chinks in this armor. Last year, the FDA approved cranial electrical stimulation for the treatment of certain brain tumors and there is evidence that this approach will be effective and safer for lung and other malignancies. Another device using different frequencies was recently shown to be superior and safer than standard treatment for cancer of the liver and to reverse breast cancer with metastases. It is essential to denounce the numerous spurious devices and therapies of charlatans, entrepreneurs and misguided zealots who prey on the desperation of cancer victims, but it is equally important not to throw the baby out with the bathwater.

Envoi

During the course of my conversations and correspondence with Dr. Gonzalez, I had never mentioned my wife. She had few side effects from her Gemzar chemotherapy, had gained weight and maintained her usual upbeat attitude. However, follow-up imaging studies now showed liver metastases and she began to have difficulty eating. She was started on a combination of four drugs that had recently been shown to be superior to Gemzar but had a bad reaction that necessitated hospitalization. I knew she could not tolerate taking 150 supplements a day, and I recalled that in Dr. Beard's day pancreatic enzymes were given by intramuscular injection, and even intravenously but such formulations were no longer available. I called Dr. Gonzalez and explained her situation. While he was eager to help in any way he could, it was obvious she would not be able to comply with his protocol, and she passed away a week or so later on October 2, 2011.

I will always wonder if the pancreatic enzyme clinical trial over ten years ago had been conducted in a fair and objective fashion, whether my wife and thousands of others might be alive today. Would a successful outcome have encouraged much needed research into identifying which pancreatic enzymes are indicated and in what amounts for different types of malignancies? Could it have led to the development of injectable enzymes that would be more potent and facilitate patient acceptance and adherence to treatment? I am not qualified to comment on the efficacy of pancreatic enzyme therapy, as I have no personal experience to rely on. But that is not what this book is about. It is about the cancer cartel's focus on raising funds rather than preventing cancer and opposing anything that might threaten the profits of vested interests regardless of adverse health consequences. The sequence of events described here has taken this to a new level, and the real take home message is that there was no punishment, no attempt to correct the mistakes that had been made, and therefore no deterrent to prevent this from happening again and again. As an old saying goes, "The only thing necessary for the triumph of evil is for good men to do nothing."

Paul J. Rosch, M.D., President, The American Institute of Stress
Clinical Professor of Medicine and Psychiatry, New York Medical College
April 2012

References

1. Selye, H. *STRESS: The Physiology and Pathology of Exposure to Stress. A treatise based on the concepts of the General Adaptation Syndrome and the Diseases of Adaptation.* Montreal: Acta Inc.; 1950.

2. Selye, H, Foreword, in *Cancer, Stress, and Death*, Taché, J., Selye, H., and Day, S. B., editors. New York: Plenum Publishing Corp.; 1979.

3. Beard J. *The Enzyme Treatment of Cancer and Its Scientific Basis.* London: Chatto and Windus; 1911.

4. Nass SJ, Moses HL, Mendelsohn JM, editors. *A National Cancer Clinical Trials System for the 21st Century: Reinvigorating the NCI Cooperative Group Program.* Washington: National Academies Press; 2010.

5. Illich, I. *Medical Nemesis: The Expropriation of Health.* New York: Pantheon Press; 1976.

Acknowledgements

M any, many people have helped make this book possible. As a start, my colleague Linda L. Isaacs, M.D., deserves special recognition. Her meticulous concern about proper and complete record-keeping, and her determination that everyone involved in this study abide by its rules, first led us to suspect that this project was not being supervised properly by the Columbia University team in charge. Without giving away the plot, I will say here that without Dr. Isaacs' doggedness this book would never have been possible.

Sarah Ann Cooper, who tells her story in this book's Foreword, deserves enormous thanks for many reasons. She also deserves congratulations for now having survived more than 11 years with a diagnosis of adenocarcinoma of the pancreas, confirmed at the Mayo Clinic and treated only with our regimen. Her victory over the worst of cancers illustrates the potential of our therapy when followed with dedication and with faith.

I owe my friend Suzanne Somers, the actress, best-selling author, and proponent of natural approaches to healing, considerable gratitude—in fact as you will see, she is one of the true heroes of the book and I want to express my deepest thanks to her for standing by me through thick and thin.

Congressman Dan Burton (R-Indiana) supported this study strongly from the beginning and for that I owe him much, even if ultimately it turned out far differently from what we both had hoped. When the project veered terribly off course, Congressman Burton repeatedly intervened on my behalf with a seemingly indifferent government scientific establishment.

Beth Clay, formerly of Congressman Burton's staff and currently a Washington consultant, repeatedly helped me maneuver through the intricate bureaucracy of the federal government that seemed so often unreachable and immovable.

I want to thank my friend and colleague Wayne Jonas, M.D., who while he headed the old Office of Alternative Medicine tried hard to interest the National Cancer Institute in funding a clinical evaluation of my work. I also want to thank Dr. Mary Ann Richardson, formerly of the NIH, who was determined to get this study up and running against all odds and despite much opposition.

JP Jones, Ph.D., retired Vice President for Health Care at Procter & Gamble, was involved with this study in its initial optimistic stages before the NCI offered full funding, and since then has endlessly shared his expertise in clinical trial management with me. At every step during this study's wayward course he was there to offer advice.

Robert Scott Bell, talk show host extraordinaire and staunch defender of health care freedom, plays a pivotal role in my book as you shall see. It was because of information shared by Robert that I first began investigating the background of one of the staff scientists assigned to supervise my study, an effort that proved most illuminating.

My friend Hans Moolenburg, M.D., of the Netherlands, now retired, was a great source of support as the study collapsed. He's been there all the way as a friend, from the hopeful beginnings of this trial in 1997 to its sad end in 2006.

Paul Rosch, M.D., President of the American Institute of Stress, a student and colleague of the great researcher Hans Selye, M.D., and author of our second Foreword, became a friend during the writing of this book when he learned of this clinical trial and suspected it might have been undermined by the conventional scientists assigned to the project. He has written fairly and objectively about my allegations and the study's mismanagement, and I owe him a great debt of gratitude for helping get the truth out.

Julian Hyman, M.D., remains a dear friend and loyal supporter. A conventional oncologist sent by the New York State Medical Board many years ago to look into my practice, he became one of my strongest defenders. My wife and I enjoy our dinners with Dr. Hyman, and look forward to many more in the future.

Jonathan Wright, M.D., a colleague, long-time friend and innovator physician, also rose to my defense early on when the first signs that this study had been mismanaged surfaced. For that, I remain grateful.

I want to thank Joy Butler, Esq., who offered many useful suggestions during the refining of the book. My personal attorney, Rick Edwards, has been a strong supporter and good friend over the years, and I appreciate all he has done for me.

Suzanne Copp, our proofreader, is a consummate professional and stylist, who helped us bring this book into its final form. We recommend her without reservation to any author seeking a top-notch proofreader to review a book.

Pierre Guesry, M.D., former Medical Director of the Pasteur Institute and retired Vice President for Research at Nestlé, convinced that company to finance my first successful pilot study and the animal work that demonstrated the utility of our enzymes against cancer. Dr. Guesry is a true scientist with an open mind, who worked hard to bring our joint projects to a meaningful conclusion.

I also wanted to mention my friend and mentor, the late Ernst Wynder, M.D., who published the first article linking cigarette smoking to lung cancer in 1950 when he was a fourth-year medical student. Dr. Wynder spent much of his life fighting commercial interests who objected to his findings on cigarette smoking and chemical carcinogenesis. In my case he worked very hard behind the scenes to get this study up and running, back in the day when we hoped we might finally have an opportunity to show what this treatment could do.

I owe an enormous debt to Stephen Levine, Ph.D., innovative nutritional researcher and founder of the Allergy Research Group supplement company. Way back in 1987, when I had left the academic world hoping to keep the Beardian enzyme thesis alive, Steve agreed to supply the enzymes I needed for my practice, made the way I wanted. We have remained friends over the years, as my practice grew and as the controversies about what I do have swirled, and his unconditional support has been steady, strong, and always much appreciated.

My wonderful office staff over the years contributed much to getting this book into its final form. Angela Rios-Blumberg and Emily Kintzer both carefully read various drafts, offering many valid and insightful suggestions. They have been an enormous help, in many ways. I also want to thank my current office manager Andrea Sorvillo for keeping our practice running so smoothly.

I wanted to thank the wonderful photographer Roxxe, who took the picture for the cover of this book. She is most accomplished in her field, and I recommend her without reservations for anyone in need of a top-notch professional.

Finally, I want to thank my wife Mary Beth, who endured the endless late nights and long hours on weekends I spent in my office, toiling on this book. She understood the importance that it be done right, and created an environment that allowed me to pursue the work with minimal distraction. For her patience and support in a difficult professional time for me, and through a difficult project, I am deeply grateful.

WHAT WENT WRONG

The Truth Behind the Clinical Trial
of the Enzyme Treatment of Cancer

Introduction

From 1998 to 2005, my colleague Dr. Linda Isaacs and I worked closely with physicians and scientists from Columbia University, the National Cancer Institute (NCI), and the National Center for Complementary and Alternative Medicine (NCCAM), developing and pursuing a formal clinical trial comparing our nutritional treatment to chemotherapy in patients diagnosed with inoperable pancreatic cancer. When the project first began we were excited by, and grateful for, this opportunity to have our regimen tested under what we hoped would be rigorous academic supervision. In a personal sense, the study represented the culmination of nearly 15 long years of our own research efforts and our battles to have our therapy properly evaluated and eventually mainstreamed. We also hoped that in a more global sense, this effort would help usher in a new era of cooperation between mainstream institutions and serious alternative practitioners with promising new treatments. In those long ago days we truly believed that the endless and fruitless war between academic medicine and more unconventional approaches might be coming to an end, to everyone's benefit.

From the outset, the project generated praise and enthusiasm in the alternative medicine press, as well as considerable interest in more traditional venues such as the *New Yorker Magazine*,[1] but also some dismissive attacks. At times, we both felt we were in the middle of a firestorm. Nonetheless, whatever the obstacles we were determined to soldier on, prove to the scientific community the seriousness of our intent, and show once and for all that a treatment developed outside the academic world could come under scrutiny and be vindicated.

Now, some 14 years later, I am sorry to report that despite our early optimism the study collapsed in a morass of poor management and indifference by those assigned to supervise the project. Our enthusiasm long ago died, along with our faith in the academic research world, its concern for such noble ideals as scientific truth and compassion for the seriously ill. In a more practical sense, at this point we strongly believe that any serious-minded alternative cancer practitioner or researcher should avoid working with NCCAM, the NCI, and academic medical centers at all cost, and instead search for other avenues of support, either from industry or private foundations.

So what went wrong?

Chapter 1

Historical Background

I realize that many know, or think they know, the details of my past and the origins of our NCI-NCCAM research project. Nonetheless, since many academicians and media outlets have previously misstated the basic facts, I thought it might be useful to clarify the record and summarize some of the history behind this clinical trial. I believe it also might be of benefit to review the sequence of events that led to formal federal investigations into the management of the study by the Columbia University staff assigned to the project.

In our office, my colleague Dr. Isaacs and I offer an aggressive nutritional program for the treatment of advanced cancer and a variety of other serious illnesses ranging from chronic fatigue to multiple sclerosis. Whatever the underlying problem, our therapy involves three basic components: individualized diets, individualized supplement protocols, and intensive detoxification. The diets we prescribe can range from largely vegetarian to fatty red meat eaten several times each day. The supplement programs also vary considerably, providing vitamins, minerals and trace elements in differing forms and differing doses, as well as glandular and enzyme products chosen to meet each patient's needs. The detoxification routines, an often misunderstood component of our therapy, consist of coffee enemas and other procedures, many taken right from the conventional medical literature.[2-4] These interventions, we believe, help the body neutralize and excrete noxious waste products such as those toxins we

3

take in from our increasingly contaminated environment, as well as the debris released from dying and dead tumors.

We treat many diseases, but we are best known for our work with advanced cancer. In this case, in addition to a prescribed diet, a nutritional supplement routine and the detoxification regimens, we rely on large doses, spread through the day, of orally ingested pancreatic enzymes derived from a pig source. Though we believe the diets, the vitamins, minerals, and trace elements help with tissue and organ repair, we recommend the pancreatic enzymes specifically to attack cancer cells.

Many in the medical world consider my work "alternative," but I come out of a very conventional educational background. I pursued my undergraduate education in literature at Brown University (Phi Beta Kappa, magna cum laude) and subsequently worked as a journalist and writer, first at Time Inc. As a result of several articles I had written dealing with health-related topics, and at the urging of well-known scientists including Linus Pauling, I decided to give up journalism to pursue a career in medicine. After completing my premedical work at Columbia as a postgraduate student, I was subsequently accepted to every major medical school to which I applied, from Stanford to Johns Hopkins. I decided to attend Cornell because of its affiliation with Memorial Sloan-Kettering Cancer Center, and my wish to study under its then President, the controversial but lauded Dr. Robert A. Good. Referred to as the "Founder of Modern Immunology," Dr. Good, now deceased, remains one of the most published authors in the history of medicine, with over 2000 papers to his credit. He also, and perhaps most famously, designed and supervised the first successful bone marrow transplant in history.

I was fortunate that early in my medical school career Dr. Good took on the role of mentor, supervising my first research efforts. After my internship at Vanderbilt, Dr. Good—who by that time had left Sloan-Kettering—invited me to join his group as a full fellow, a unique opportunity that I gladly accepted. I spent a year with Dr. Good as he established a bone marrow transplant unit at the University of Oklahoma, then finished my formal training under him at All Children's Hospital in Florida where he moved to continue his research.

I began investigating the use of aggressive nutritional intervention along with pancreatic enzymes in the treatment of cancer under the direction of Dr. Good while still a medical student at Cornell. I had learned of the rather extraordinary but forgotten scientist Dr. John Beard, a Professor at the University of Edinburgh during the early years of the last century who first suggested an antineoplastic effect for pancreatic enzymes. In a series of articles published in conventional medical journals beginning in 1902, Dr. Beard proposed that the proteolytic (protein-digesting) enzyme trypsin represented the body's main defense against cancer, and might be useful as a treatment for malignant disease.[5-7] Beard's thesis, however odd it appeared in his day, came to fruition during twenty years of meticulous laboratory investigation that began with his own studies of the development of the nervous system of worms.

Beard was neither a physician nor in his early career even vaguely interested in medical research, let alone cancer. His doctoral thesis, for example, described the origins of certain sense organs in an obscure invertebrate parasite.[8] As his interests evolved, he switched his focus to the nervous system of vertebrates, particularly fish. Many of his pioneering findings from this time in his life, now proven correct, are standard fare in the textbooks of our day.

Beard's studies led him through a most convoluted route to consider the formation of the placenta, the tissue anchoring the mammalian fetus to the uterus and serving as the point of connection between the embryo's blood supply carrying the wastes of metabolism and the blood vessels of the mother supplying oxygen and nutrients. He did much to unravel the details of placental development beginning after conception, reporting that in many respects the tissue in its early stages resembled a malignant tumor.

The placenta begins forming as the outer or trophoblastic layer around the early embryo at about its 58-cell stage. Under the microscope, these trophoblasts appear primitive and undifferentiated, that is, without distinguishing characteristics, as do the cells of cancer. Trophoblasts mimic malignant cells not only in looks but in behavior as well, initially replicating without apparent restriction, as cancers were known to do even in Beard's day. The early placenta also quickly and efficiently invades the uterine wall, much as a tumor might infiltrate a tissue or organ. All the while, the proliferating trophoblastic tissues efficiently create a new and dense blood supply to feed itself and the emerging embryo—just as any expanding tumor must, as angiogenesis research today has made clear.

Cancer cells remain undifferentiated and, unless removed or killed off, will continue multiplying, invading, creating new vessels, and metastasizing until death ensues. In contrast, as embryonic development proceeds along its normal pathway, the trophoblastic placenta—though initially resembling a malignancy—at a critical and precise point transforms from an undifferentiated, rapidly dividing, highly invasive, angiogenic tumor-like tissue into the mature non-proliferating, non-aggressive, life-sustaining placenta. In this way the placenta differs from a cancerous tumor, Beard reasoned, because normal trophoblasts know just when to stop replicating and invading, whereas malignant cells do not. Should the signals go awry as they occasionally do, the placental cells can remain primitive and undifferentiated, able to proliferate endlessly, invade, sprout new vessels, and spread to distant organs as the very aggressive choriocarcinoma, the potentially deadly cancer of a misguided pregnancy. Fortunately, most of the time the early trophoblasts change character as expected, in the process losing their malignant potential.

Beard spent years searching for the signal prompting this remarkable shift in appearance and activity, ultimately concluding that the key must be the embryonic pancreas. In every mammalian species he studied, the very day the embryonic pancreas came to life, synthesizing its varied collection of enzymes, the placenta changed its developmental direction, slowing then stopping its cancer-like invasion of the maternal uterus.

Even in Beard's day, more than 100 years ago, the main categories of pancreatic enzymes had been identified: the proteolytic or protein-digesting component; the lipases that break down triglycerides into glycerol and free fatty acids; and the amylases responsible for cleaving complex carbohydrates into simple, easily usable sugars. Physiologists of the time thought all three groups were active only in the duodenum, the first part of the small intestine, where the enzymes continue the reduction of food arriving from the stomach. But Beard effectively provided the data illustrating that above and beyond its role in digestion, trypsin, the main proteolytic enzyme, served to control placental growth, preventing the tissue from invading beyond the uterus as a true cancer might. Beard then proposed that since the early placenta behaves much as a tumor does, since under the microscope its cells look like undifferentiated, primitive neoplastic cells, and since pancreatic enzymes forcefully regulate its growth and development, these very same enzymes could be—in fact, must be—the body's main defense against cancer, and would be useful as a cancer *treatment*.

Dr. Beard presented his trophoblastic theory of cancer in a series of papers published in mainstream medical journals, culminating in a lecture given in

Liverpool in January 1905,[9(p247)] covered extensively in the newspapers of the day both in Europe and in the U.S. Beard then went from the hypothetical to the practical, testing his thesis in an animal model of malignancy available at the time, the Jensen's mouse tumor. He injected an extract of trypsin into two mice growing such cancers, which then promptly regressed, while in the control group of six the tumors continued thriving until the animals died.[5]

Subsequently, during the first decade of the twentieth century, a number of physicians interested in Beard's hypothesis began, under his direction, treating their own human cancer patients with injectable pancreatic enzymes. Reports of their successes appeared in major medical journals of the day, including *The Journal of the American Medical Association*[10] and *The British Medical Journal*.[11] I have tracked down many such documents, which remain to me compelling reports of patients surviving advanced cancer—such as one with a fungating sarcoma of the jaw, well beyond any chance of surgical cure, who with enzyme therapy experienced a total regression of his disease.[9] The patient thereafter lived a normal life. Other articles described patients with metastatic colorectal[12] and uterine cancer,[13] as deadly today as in Beard's time, evidently disease-free after receiving the enzyme treatment—all carefully documented and appropriately presented in the scientific literature.

Despite the evidence from both laboratory experiments and his work with human patients, the enzyme thesis provoked an enormous and angry backlash against Beard and his few loyal supporters. Editorials in medical journals vilified him, speakers at scientific conventions belittled his theory mercilessly, newspapers mocked his treatment. Beard fought back with articles and letters to the editor, and in 1911 published *The Enzyme Treatment of Cancer and Its Scientific Basis,*[9] which presented in some detail his hypothesis, his decades of research, and his promising and compelling results. Despite such efforts, interest in Beard's approach gradually petered out, to the point that when he died in 1924 he died in obscurity, his therapy already considered no more than an historical oddity.

The vitriolic—and irrational—response of so many eminent scientists to Beard's well-documented research, this rejection of the enzyme therapy by the medical establishment 100 years ago, I believe had little to do with science but everything to do with politics, psychology, and popularity. Beard was an ivory tower professor, with little patience for his critics; he didn't court the press, didn't care about fame, and didn't seem at all interested in international acclaim.

Importantly, at the same time Beard intently pursued his own course, others such as Madame Curie, more lauded by the media, extolled the benefits of the newly discovered X-ray as a safe, effective, non-toxic treatment for all cancer.[14] The press of the time and the scientific and medical community at large latched onto radiation as the final solution to the cancer plague—as well as acne and a host of other complaints, major and minor. Of course, radiation hardly warranted such enthusiasm, but only after Beard's death did researchers realize that few cancers responded long-term to the therapy, that it wasn't perfectly safe as originally thought but instead terribly toxic, in fact carcinogenic in and of itself. Ironically, Madame Curie would die from aplastic anemia, a form of bone marrow failure brought on by her years of exposure to radiation.[15]

After Beard's death, periodically a handful of physicians rediscovered his work and kept his ideas alive. During the 1920s and 1930s, a St. Louis doctor, Dr. F.L. Morse, used his version of the enzyme therapy in his practice, with success in some patients diagnosed with poor prognosis malignancies. When he presented his findings in 1934—a proceeding published in the *Weekly Bulletin of the St. Louis Medical Society*—his colleagues attacked him rather viciously, one physician at the session, a Dr. M.G. Seelig, remarking:

> While I heartily agree with Dr. Allen when he strikes the note of encouragement, I recoil at the idea of witlessly spreading the hope of a cancer cure which is implicit in the remarks of Dr. Morse this evening.[16]

During the 1960s, a Dayton, Ohio surgeon, Dr. Frank Shively, learned of Dr. Beard's approach and treated a series of 192 cancer patients with an injectable form of enzymes made available to him by a local pharmaceutical company.[17] Despite some remarkable responses, in 1966 the FDA issued an injunction forbidding the sale or use of injectable pancreatic products, and thereafter Dr. Shively seems to have returned to the more mundane work of general surgery.

Meanwhile, in the mid-1960s the eccentric orthodontist Dr. William Donald Kelley developed his own complex variation of the enzyme treatment, which consisted of large doses of orally ingested—rather than injectable—pancreatic enzymes, individualized diets, individualized supplement protocols, and detoxification routines such as the coffee enemas. Dr. Kelley came to fame at a time of great repression against alternative medicine in general, particularly against anyone foolish enough to suggest a nutritional approach might benefit patients with cancer. As a dentist Kelley was at particular risk because he lacked the legal authority to treat the disease in the first place. The media in all forms, print, radio, and TV, attacked him mercilessly, vilifying him as a "quack," and regulatory agencies at all levels investigated him endlessly. He was thrown in jail as a public menace, had his dental license revoked for five years, spent his earnings defending himself against government assaults, and watched his family life fall apart. But he survived because his successes created an extraordinary word-of-mouth network that brought an endless stream of patients to his Grapevine, Texas, and later his Winthrop, Washington offices.

I met Dr. Kelley by chance during the summer of 1981, following my second year of medical school. At that time, he seemed modest and unassuming, seeking only to have his work properly evaluated so that if the approach had merit, it might become more widely accessible to patients in need. I was fortunate that my research mentor Dr. Good, then President of Sloan-Kettering, encouraged a review of Kelley's cases, believing that even if Dr. Kelley proved to be a charlatan, I would learn much about medicine and research by pursuing a project of my own making. In this regard, I have always thought Dr. Good, often criticized for his management style at Sloan-Kettering, an excellent teacher. During the time I worked under him, I was told that more of his postgraduate fellows had gone on to professorships in U.S. medical schools than from any other research group in history.

With Dr. Good's blessing, I spent the summer of 1981 in Dr. Kelley's Dallas office, reviewing his voluminous patient files. I quickly found evidence of patient after patient with appropriately diagnosed, biopsy-proven, poor prognosis cancer alive five, even ten years since beginning the enzyme therapy. When I subsequently shared my findings with Dr. Good, he suggested I continue the project during my third and fourth years of medical school. What began as a student's summer effort eventually evolved into a full-fledged investigation completed during my fellowship training under Dr. Good at All Children's Hospital in Florida.

For the project, I interviewed and evaluated over 1000 of Kelley's patients, concentrating on some 455 who had done exceptionally well under his care. From this group, I wrote up in detail 50 cases, representing 26 different types of cancer. Even today, 25 years later, Kelley's achievement still impresses, especially considering his lack of academic support and the continual opposition he faced. For example, one of the 50, a woman who ran a gas station with her husband in Wisconsin, had been diagnosed in August 1982 with adenocarcinoma of the pancreas with biopsy-documented metastasis into the liver. At the Mayo Clinic a consulting oncologist suggested no treatment, instead telling her to enjoy her remaining few months. With no viable conventional options available, she then began investigating alternative approaches to cancer, learned about Dr. Kelley, and began his regimen under the direction of a local chiropractor trained in the method. Over the years we've kept in touch by phone, and when she last called in August 2011 she reported to me that she felt well, now some 29 years from her terminal diagnosis. Another patient included in my report, a woman with uterine cancer, had been initially treated with radiation and hysterectomy in 1969. She did well for a time, but in 1975 the disease recurred with a vengeance in the pelvis and throughout both lungs. After undergoing exploratory abdominal surgery and resection of the large pelvic tumor to ward off an impending intestinal obstruction, she subsequently learned of Dr. Kelley and experienced a documented complete reversal of all her many pulmonary lesions under his care. This remarkable lady died in December 2009 at age 95, 34 years after her diagnosis of recurrent terminal metastatic disease.

At Dr. Good's suggestion, I also reviewed all those appropriately diagnosed with pancreatic cancer, one of the most aggressive of malignancies, who consulted with Kelley between 1974 and 1982. I eventually identified 22 such patients, ten of whom, all deceased, had not followed the regimen for a single day. In my interviews with surviving family members I learned that most of these patients decided to pursue some other treatment largely because of the hostility expressed by their doctors or family to this unconventional approach. For them, I determined an average survival of 63 days, quite typical for patients in that era with the inoperable form of the disease. This group, we agreed, could serve as an informal "control."

A second group of seven patients, also all deceased, complied only partially, and for limited periods of time ranging from four weeks to 13 months, before abandoning the therapy. Again, surviving family I interviewed reported strong opposition from the patient's conventional physicians and/or relatives as the most common reason for discontinuing the regimen. For these seven, I calculated a mean and median survival of 302 days, far longer than would be expected.

Five patients, all alive at the time I completed my research, had complied fully. The median and mean survival for this group exceeded eight years, a remarkable statistic in view of the deadly nature of pancreatic cancer, with an average life expectancy reported in the range of three to six months.

By 1986, I had incorporated the results of my five-year investigation into monograph form, which included a history of the treatment going back to Dr. Beard, a discussion of the theory and practice of Kelley's complex nutritional approach, lengthy descriptions of the 50 patients accompanied by copies of the actual medical records, and finally, my evaluation of his success with pancreatic cancer. Despite my findings, despite my careful labors and serious intent, to my disappointment and surprise I could not get the book published, either in its entirety as a monograph or as a summary journal article. The responses from editors ran the gamut from disbelief and accusations of fraud to fear that the book would generate so much controversy their careers might be ruined. No editor, even those who accepted the cases as real, had the courage to take on the project. Even my efforts to place individual case reports of these remarkable patients, either in the medical or popular press, utterly failed.

Our inability to get the study published affected Kelley terribly. It appeared to him that all doors had closed, and that his therapy would never be accepted for what he believed it was, a promising answer to a deadly disease. In 1986 he closed down his office, eventually disappearing from sight, and I last spoke to him in 1987. Subsequently, he spent considerable time writing bizarre and angry e-mails about a variety of subjects before he died in January 2005, alienated from most of his former friends and supporters.

Determined to keep the enzyme therapy alive, I left Dr. Good's group after finishing my fellowship and with his blessing returned to New York in 1987. I parted with Dr. Good not with any animosity, as some later claimed, but because I knew in Florida he lacked the resources to underwrite rigorous testing of a controversial new therapy. Back in New York, my colleague Dr. Isaacs and I began seeing patients, always with the hope of obtaining funding and academic support for our ongoing research efforts.

Though the patients who sought us out during the early days of our practice invariably presented with very advanced disease, we quickly observed firsthand the benefits of the treatment. One woman who consulted with me shortly after I returned to New York in December of 1987 had been diagnosed with inflammatory breast cancer with metastases to the bone that developed while she was receiving aggressive multi-drug chemotherapy. Though given a terminal prognosis, on our regimen she has now survived 24 years, with scans long ago showing total regression of her previously extensive disease. Another patient—Discovery Health Channel would eventually highlight his story—was diagnosed with metastatic adenocarcinoma of the pancreas in September of 1991 with multiple lesions in the liver as well as evidence of cancer in the adrenals, bone and lung. Under our care his disease resolved and he survived 14 years, succumbing only after he was battered in a severe automobile accident.

Once committed to such a non-traditional approach, I had to make serious professional choices: during the late 1980s, as my practice grew, one of my former professors at Cornell offered me a position in his department at Sloan-Kettering, urging me to pursue more acceptable, more mainstream research projects, and give up such flagrantly controversial work. Though I certainly appreciated the opportunity, I turned it down, unwilling to abandon the enzyme treatment.

But as knowledge of our successes spread in the early 1990s, our therapy and our practice did attract some prominent interest. The late Dr. Ernst Wynder, one of the world's premier cancer researchers and epidemiologists of his day, became a close friend and scientific mentor. Dr. Wynder, credited by many for first confirming the link between cigarette smoking and lung cancer, and in whose honor Congress created the annual Children's Health Day, spent considerable time guiding my ongoing research efforts.

In early 1993, officials at the National Cancer Institute first proposed that I come to Bethesda and present summaries of my own patients appropriately diagnosed with poor-prognosis cancer who had enjoyed tumor regression and/ or unusual survival while pursuing my therapy. For the session Dr. Isaacs and I put together 25 case histories, including the two described above, and on July 7, 1993, I spoke for three hours at the NCI before a group of government scientists. Dr. Wynder not only accompanied me to Bethesda, but opened up the meeting with a strong statement urging that my treatment approach be taken seriously.

As a result of that conference, the then Associate Director of the NCI, Dr. Michael Friedman, suggested I pursue as a next step a pilot study under Dr. Wynder's supervision, evaluating my regimen in ten patients diagnosed with advanced adenocarcinoma of the pancreas. In such phase II studies, as they are technically called, an experimental therapy is administered to patients with an aggressive cancer for which no effective standard treatment exists. Though a pilot study frequently involves no control arm—that is, no comparison group given a standard treatment—it can still yield important information about a new approach. And with the prognosis for those diagnosed with inoperable pancreatic cancer so grim, with an average survival in the range of 5–6 months, Dr. Friedman suggested that if three of my patients lived a year he would consider the study a significant success. From my experience with the enzyme therapy I expected to do better, so when asked if I would be willing to take on the challenge, I accepted without hesitation.

Fortunately, around the time of the NCI meeting Dr. Pierre Guesry, an internationally respected scientist, former Medical Director of the Pasteur Institute in Paris, and Vice President for Research at Nestlé (the Swiss-based food company), had already learned of my work and after reviewing a series of case reports in my office suggested Nestlé fund a clinical trial. At his recommendation Nestlé quickly agreed to underwrite the cost of the pilot study proposed by the NCI, with Dr. Guesry, along with Dr. Wynder, supervising the project.

In late 1994, as the pilot study progressed, Dr. J.P. Jones, then Vice President for Research for Health Care at Procter & Gamble (P&G), heard about my regimen and invited me to Cincinnati to lecture his staff. After several subsequent meetings both in New York and in Ohio, P&G agreed to invest several million dollars in basic research support for my therapy. Over a three-year period, with P&G's help we were able to perfect the manufacturing process for the enzymes we currently use. Those were productive years, what I hoped to be the beginnings of a new era of cooperation between government research organizations, industry, and serious alternative researchers.

The pilot study continued without a major hitch, and by mid-1998 Dr. Wynder suggested we had made our point. We eventually included 11 subjects, one more than the NCI suggested, all diagnosed with inoperable, biopsy-proven adenocarcinoma, with eight initially presenting with advanced stage IV disease. A consulting oncologist as well as Dr. Wynder had approved all those entered into the trial. Overall, nine participants lived more than one year, five lived more than two years, four lived more than three years, and two made it beyond four years. The survival statistics for the study, with a median and mean of some 18 months, far exceeded any results previously reported for this malignancy.[18] As a point of reference, in the clinical trial of Gemzar (gemcitabine), the latest agent at the time approved for pancreatic cancer, the median and means were in the range of 5.6 months and of 126 patients treated not one lived longer than 19 months.[19;20] Yet the FDA considered these results so impressive it gave quick approval for the drug.

As a result of the preliminary pilot study data, in 1997 I began meeting with Dr. Karen Antman, a renowned oncologist, the first woman President of the American Society of Clinical Oncology, and at the time director of oncology at Columbia. She agreed to supervise a phase III large-scale trial, comparing chemotherapy to my nutritional regimen, again in patients diagnosed with advanced pancreatic cancer. Initially, P&G agreed to finance the project, but in 1998 Congressman Dan Burton (R-IN) arranged a meeting in his Washington offices with myself, Dr. Richard Klausner, then Director of the National Cancer Institute, and others from the National Institutes of Health (NIH) to explore a possible joint government-Columbia research effort. Shortly thereafter, at Dr. Klausner's direct request the NCI approved funding for a study in which my approach would go up against the best available chemotherapy in the treatment of patients diagnosed with inoperable pancreatic adenocarcinoma. Though the National Cancer Institute agreed to provide full support, as the project took shape administrators from the Office of Alternative Medicine (OAM)—now the National Center for Complementary and Alternative Medicine (NCCAM)—suggested that their group should be involved, both financially and in a supervisory capacity. Since back in 1999 OAM-NCCAM, under the direction of Dr. William Harlan, seemed anxious to work toward a fair and meaningful evaluation of my regimen, I was pleased when the NCI accepted their offer of support.

Dr. Antman, as she had promised, would supervise the project at Columbia, and with Dr. Wynder's help the FDA rapidly gave its IND (Investigational New Drug) approval, required for all government clinical trials of a new treatment. Eventually, Dr. John Chabot, an expert in the surgical treatment of pancreatic cancer at Columbia, joined the study as a co-investigator. With the various institutions on board, the situation seemed perfect for the first major NCI effort to test a non-traditional, nutritional approach to advanced cancer.

As the project geared up, Dr. Isaacs and I published the pilot study results in the June 1999 issue of the peer-reviewed research journal *Nutrition and Cancer.*[18] In an accompanying editorial, Dr. Wynder concluded:

> Gonzalez and Isaacs are to be commended for agreeing to participate in a
> randomized clinical trial to compare their approach with the treatment of pa-

tients with gemcitabine (Gemzar), a trial funded by the National Cancer Institute under the direction of Drs. Karen Antman and John Chabot at Columbia University.[21]

Unfortunately, though carefully conceived and well supervised by prominent scientists, the published pilot data nonetheless generated considerable controversy, even occasional mainstream media attacks. Scientists who had never spoken to me once about the project questioned the methodology in press interviews, though it had been developed in consultation with the NCI and researchers from other institutions. The results were criticized, at times with vitriol. For example, a gastroenterologist from the Dana Farber Institute at Harvard—who never once contacted my office in any way—went on record in the *Washington Post* attacking the study, claiming a number of patients in the trial did not have pancreatic cancer, even though all had been approved by Dr. Wynder and the other supervisors.[22]

But others did take the data seriously. After the publication, Dr. Guesry at Nestlé provided substantial funding to test the enzyme treatment in animal models, to provide supportive information as the human trials continued. A group at the Eppley Cancer Institute at the University of Nebraska, known for their pioneering work decoding the molecular mechanisms of pancreatic cancer, agreed to take on the challenge. Dr. Parviz Pour, the supervisor of the animal work at Eppley, had himself developed mouse models useful in testing promising new treatments for the disease.

In the animal studies, Dr. Pour and his colleagues evaluated the effect of our enzymes administered to nude mice injected with human pancreatic cancer cells of a particularly virulent strain. These inbred, furless animals lack a functional immune system, so transplanted or injected tumors grow rapidly and kill quickly—hence their wide use in the research setting. In the first experiment, designed to measure survival, the mice were divided into two groups, one receiving our enzymes, the other given no therapy. The animals receiving the enzymes survived significantly longer than the control group and appeared to be healthy, happy mice, well into the study—in sharp contrast to the untreated mice, which deteriorated quickly, appearing listless, inactive and bloated as the cancer spread. Two mice in the enzyme group were doing so well they had to be sacrificed so the study could be brought to conclusion. I wonder how long they would have kept going had they been left alone.

In a second experiment, the mice were again divided into two groups, one administered our enzymes, the other again an untreated control. This time around, selected animals were periodically sacrificed and evaluated for tumor growth. The enzymes clearly slowed the spread of the tumors, which in the treated mice remained small and very localized. In addition, overall the enzyme group appeared far healthier than the controls, in which the cancer grew without restraint, invading aggressively until the animals died.

Dr. Pour and his colleagues published the results of these experiments in the May 2004 issue of the peer reviewed journal *Pancreas* with Dr. Guesry and me listed as co-authors.[23] In the "Discussion" section, Dr. Pour wrote:

> In summary, PPE [Porcine Pancreatic Extracts] is the first experimentally and clinically proven agent for the effective treatment of PC [Pancreatic Cancer]. The significant advantages of PPE over any other currently available therapeutic modalities include its effects on physical condition, nutrition, and lack of toxicity.[23]

I believe the results as presented to be particularly significant since Dr. Isaacs and I had not previously conducted animal studies, so in a sense we found ourselves in uncharted territory. We guessed at the appropriate doses to be used, ultimately recommending the amount per kilogram we would normally prescribe for our human patients. Though such an approach might seem reasonable, inbred laboratory mice frequently require much higher doses of drugs than what would be given humans to elicit any effect. In addition, the experiments only evaluated the enzyme component of the treatment, not the additional vitamins, minerals, trace elements, and nutritious food we prescribe for our human patients. The animal chow also contained a fair amount of soy, which, however aggressively it may be pushed as a healthy food, contains a protein, the Bowman-Birk inhibitor, which potently neutralizes trypsin. Had these issues been addressed, we believe the results would have been even more positive.

Chapter 2

Summary of Major Problems Affecting the NCI-NCCAM Study

Working together with a group of dedicated scientists, Dr. Isaacs and I organized and brought to completion the pilot study, including publication of the data, with no great difficulty. And though the animal experiments proceeded smoothly as well, our early optimism about the NCI clinical trial quickly turned to frustration. Numerous problems plagued the effort almost from its inception, and to complicate matters, early on both Dr. Klausner of the NCI and Dr. Harlan of NCCAM went on to other jobs. Midway, Dr. Antman left Columbia, first to go to the NCI as Associate Director, then to Boston University as Dean of the Medical School. Other staff from the NCI and NIH also moved on, so by 2002 most of those who had helped nurture the clinical trial in its beginning stages had been replaced, at times in our opinion by scientists whom we found to be less enthusiastic about the entire effort.

Below, in preparation for the story that follows, I outline the serious issues in design and management that derailed the clinical trial from its original goal, a fair evaluation of my treatment. Note that at times I refer to meetings which Dr. Isaacs and I attended along with the various study supervisors from Columbia,

NCCAM, and the NCI. These sessions, scheduled at regular three-month intervals from the onset of the project in 1997–1998, convened at Columbia in the Milstein Pavilion on 168th Street in Manhattan, home to the offices of both Dr. Antman and Dr. Chabot. Usually, the Washington team flew up, though occasionally they attended via conference call.

In the following discussion, in several places I quote from *Compliance in Healthcare and Research* by Lora Burke, Ph.D., and Ira Ockene, M.D. Though this excellent book was published in 2001, Dr. Isaacs and I did not become aware of its existence until well after the close of our study, when we tried to sort out the various managerial failings we believed had undermined our efforts. In this work the authors discuss at length various factors that can influence, for better or worse, the outcome and validity of a clinical trial.[24] Many of the points raised lend credence to the concerns we expressed over the years, as we tried to guide our project to a meaningful conclusion.

I. Problems with study design: As a start, we believe that flaws in the original design nearly undermined the trial for good. From the beginning, the Columbia team—and later the NCI staff when they came on board—insisted, over our objections, that the study be set up with a randomized format. Simply put, in this model patients who met the predetermined eligibility criteria and who agreed to sign up were to have no say in the treatment they would receive, but instead would be randomly assigned by computer either to the chemotherapy or nutritional arm. In the conventional medical world, experts have long considered this method the ultimate gold standard for clinical trials set up to compare different drugs, based on the assumption that this format creates equivalent groups through the random, unbiased assignment of patients. In this way, the thinking goes, the investigators in charge will be unable, subconsciously or through deliberate attempt, to influence the results by selecting patients with certain characteristics for each group. For example, in a study comparing two drugs, a researcher favoring one therapy might assign earlier stage, healthier patients for the pet treatment while deliberately selecting more advanced, sicker subjects for the competing intervention. In this way, the outcome can be easily skewed.

Dr. Isaacs and I argued against randomization, warning from the outset that in our particular case, such a design most likely would *create* rather than prevent bias. We believed that this unusual study would attract primarily those with a pre-existing interest in alternative medicine and a particular interest in our specific approach. But such patients would undoubtedly only wish to receive our treatment, not chemotherapy. Once such prospective trial candidates—who might otherwise be perfectly suitable—realized that with the randomized design they had a 50% chance of being assigned to the chemotherapy arm, we suspected few if any would proceed further with the admission process. Even if some did pursue entry and met all eligibility criteria, should they be randomized to chemotherapy we predicted none would continue beyond that point. Consequently, the model as proposed would exclude an entire population of patients enthusiastic about our treatment whom we believed by character and inclination would be the most likely to comply and ultimately succeed with our regimen. Not surprisingly, we long ago learned that those with a sincere interest in alternative approaches and our work turn out to be the best, most dedicated patients—and with a lifestyle intervention such as ours, compliance is the key to a positive outcome. But these were exactly the patients who would be reluctant to join the trial faced with the threat of randomization.

It also didn't seem reasonable that more conventional-leaning patients diagnosed with pancreatic cancer and desirous of receiving chemotherapy would have any wish to consider this study as an option, since they might be chosen for our nutrition group. Overall, a randomized design as proposed by Dr. Antman assumed we could draw from some hypothetical population diagnosed with pancreatic cancer who would seek out this particular clinical trial of all the many trials that are available, but who would be completely indifferent to the treatment they might be assigned to receive, that is, either our nutritional regimen or standard chemotherapy. But Dr. Isaacs and I doubted such people existed—it just did not make sense.

For all these reasons, Dr. Isaacs and I argued for a case-control or matched cohort format, in which patients would be allowed to choose the therapy they wanted. Alternatively-oriented patients who met the eligibility criteria could then pursue our regimen if they wished. We suspected the chemotherapy arm could easily be filled with Columbia patients with no interest in alternatives, and already anxious to begin drug treatment. If sufficient numbers expressed interest in the project under these circumstances, with appropriate selection the groups could still be evenly matched by clinical status and disease stage, assuring at the end meaningful data. Dr. Wynder, strongly taking our side, believed that with a disease as virulent as pancreatic cancer, with the known survival rates so dismal, our study hardly required randomization in any event to prove a statistical point about efficacy. Despite our well-founded arguments, the Columbia-NCI staff dismissed our warnings and Dr. Wynder's advice, insisting the study proceed with a randomized design.

As we had expected, once the trial opened accrual proved to be a disaster despite the publicity generated by the project. During the first year of operation, some 260 patients with pancreatic cancer contacted Columbia expressing an initial interest in joining the study. However, after learning of the randomized design a grand total of three patients agreed to proceed, two of whom promptly quit to pursue other options after being assigned to chemotherapy. Unfortunately, all our predictions proved true. Finally, with a full year wasted, the supervisors from Columbia and the NCI agreed to change to a matched cohort approach, our original suggestion, in which patients could select the treatment, either chemotherapy or our nutritional regimen. The switch over took months, but eventually the various regulatory authorities approved the revised format.

Without randomization, it fell to the Columbia team—who for most of the trial's duration supervised the evaluation and approval of prospective study patients—to insure, as much as practically possible, that the nutrition and chemotherapy groups would be more or less equivalent according to various criteria, including total numbers in each, as well as clinical status and stage of disease.

Unfortunately, the specter of the randomized format haunted the study for years, long after the change to matched cohort. Despite the more sensible design, rumors continued to spread within the alternative medicine underground that trial candidates had no choice in terms of therapy. Repeatedly, patients diagnosed with pancreatic cancer called our office, informing my staff they sought our regimen in our private practice, wishing no part of the clinical study because they would not be "forced" to receive chemotherapy. We will never know how many potentially suitable candidates opted not to consider the project because of such perceptions, even after the matched cohort design came into effect. Ultimately, as we warned, the randomized design created a significant bias, the very phenomenon it intended to prevent, by discouraging an entire population of ideal subjects from gravitating to our study.

II. Lack of a lead-in period: The randomized issue proved to be only one of many serious obstacles to the trial's successful completion. In our pilot study we included, at Dr. Wynder's suggestion, a preliminary eight-week "lead-in" or "washout" period. During this test run, we began the treatment process with patients who satisfied the entry criteria, then periodically evaluated each for compliance. If a prospective study candidate could not or would not adhere to the prescribed regimen, he or she would be discounted from further consideration as a study subject. Those that followed through appropriately would then be officially entered. However, if a compliant patient were to die during this time frame—none actually did—we planned to count him or her as a treatment failure. Dr. Wynder, one of the world's preeminent epidemiologists and an expert on clinical trial methodology, particularly for studies involving lifestyle modification, insisted the pilot study include such a lead-in, to help insure that the group of patients ultimately admitted were willing and capable of pursuing the prescribed nutritional regimen.

Burke and Ockene provide a very informative discussion of such "run-ins" as they call this pre-entry observation period:

> a prerandomization "run-in" period is often used to determine whether participants will be good adherers and therefore eligible to be enrolled in the trial. During the "run-in," participants who cannot tolerate the intervention or do not take an acceptable amount of drug or placebo are identified and excluded from enrollment in the trial. Although the advisability of using a "run-in" period as a method of screening out nonadherers has been questioned, it is a widely used strategy for prescreening trial participants to select only those who are motivated or able to adhere in the clinical trial context.[24(p239)]

Clinical trials set up to evaluate lifestyle interventions such as dietary change commonly provide for extensive washout periods, as well as elaborate prescreening to assess each patient's motivation and ability to comply with the regimen under study.[25] The landmark Diabetes Control and Complications Trial helped establish that tight regulation of blood sugar with strict diet and multiple daily insulin doses drastically decreases complications such as blindness and kidney failure. In this major multi-year study, all patients deemed initially eligible underwent roughly 40 hours of screening, including multiple assessments by a psychologist, before formal enrollment.[26]

Many clinical studies in oncology do not include such a lead-in provision, since for the typical chemotherapy regimen the patient need only show up in the doctor's office to receive the medication. In this case, issues of motivation become less important than with a lifestyle approach that needs to be pursued at home on a daily basis. Nonetheless, trials of new cancer drugs do at times provide for such test runs; for example, in 1998, the FDA approved the chemotherapeutic agent Gemzar (gemcitabine) for the treatment of pancreatic cancer based on a clinical trial with an initial one-week observation period for all prospective patients. During this time, the investigators excluded from the study any candidate whose pain could not be controlled.[19] Eventually, 34 potential subjects were so eliminated from further consideration, and of these, we know absolutely nothing. A total of 126 assigned to either of two chemotherapy regimens under investigation eventually qualified as "treated," so after the first week the researchers discounted approximately 21% of those initially considered acceptable, not an insignificant number.

With the somewhat limited resources allocated for our clinical study, we understood extensive pre-screening may not have been possible, but a 1–2 week lead-in would have helped eliminate subjects not able or not willing to follow through with the intensive dietary/nutritional treatment. Dr. Wynder, Dr. Isaacs, and I strongly argued that without such a safeguard, the entire study might be undermined should too many non-compliant patients be entered.

Despite our repeated arguments and regardless of precedent in the scientific literature, the chief investigators of the project refused to allow the lead-in period. To make matters worse, after July 2000, at the insistence of the NCI, Dr. Isaacs and I were removed from any involvement with the patient selection process, supposedly to eliminate the possibility of bias. Subsequently, Dr. Chabot of Columbia, who had no experience whatsoever with our treatment, its intricacies, its demands, and to our knowledge no training in evaluating patients for any type of lifestyle regimen, would alone determine patient eligibility. Unfortunately, the majority of those Dr. Chabot ultimately approved for treatment with us failed in a major way to comply with the therapy. Had a lead-in been in play, even if only a week as in the Gemzar study, we could have discounted, out of the total of 39 eventually admitted into the nutrition arm, 11 patients who never started the therapy or dropped out within the first seven days, all of whom died fairly quickly after their initial consultation with us.

III. Intent-to-Treat Provision: Clinical trials often—though not always—adopt an "intent-to-treat" rule. With such a provision, researchers agree that all patients qualified and entered into the study will be considered as having been treated, whether or not they actually proceed with the prescribed therapy. Though such an approach at first glance might not make much sense, experts justify the intent-to-treat model as necessary to evaluate adequately a new drug. For example, if in a study 100 patients receive some new medication but 50 drop out after a week because of serious side effects and subsequently their disease progresses, it would seem prudent to include these as treatment failures rather than discount them, since they quit *because* of some negative reaction to the therapy. On the other hand, such a design can be disastrous for a lifestyle intervention trial such as ours, since patients who cannot or choose not to proceed with the self-administered dietary/nutritional regimen will be counted as having been fully treated.

In their book, Burke and Ockene discuss in some detail the potential difficulties posed by the "intent-to-treat" approach:

> Nonadherence to treatment regimens is a special problem in clinical trials. Trial data are generally analyzed by the "intent-to-treat" rule, which states that the data from a given participant in a trial should be analyzed as belonging to the treatment group to which that participant was assigned, regardless of whether he or she actually received the assigned treatment. Therefore, even a small amount of nonadherence has a large effect on the sample size needed to detect a difference between groups if one exists.[24(p238)]

In our particular study, the supervisors not only denied our request for a lead-in period, they insisted we abide by the intent-to-treat rule. Unfortunately this requirement allowed Dr. Chabot to count as properly treated the 11 patients assigned to the nutrition arm who did not or could not proceed with the prescribed therapy beyond several days. None of them quit because of side effects attributable to our regimen, but due to choice or their physical inability to follow through. We believe this provision ultimately helped undermine the value and legitimacy of the data by requiring that we count multiple patients who never complied or who did so only briefly as treatment failures.

IV. Attempts to sabotage the clinical study: In standard oncology clinical trials, most of the time everyone involved works together for the benefit of the patient, for knowledge, perhaps even for glory. Having long been subjected to the scorn of conventional researchers and at times the media because of the nature of our treatment, Dr. Isaacs and I did not naively expect enthusiasm from the oncology community about our study. And, as we predicted, shortly after its inception the harassment began. As a rather glaring example, the late Dr. Victor Herbert, a long-time vocal opponent of any form of alternative medicine and my therapy in particular, filed a complaint with the Department of Health and Human Services (DHHS) in Washington in an effort to stop the project. Later, when he attacked my work in the mainstream media and on the Internet, others joined in the fray as well.

Opposition at times took more subtle forms. Despite the backing of the NCI, oncologists nearly universally failed to recommend any of their patients diagnosed with pancreatic cancer to consider this trial, a problem that affected accrual even after the design changed to matched cohort. Over the eight or so years of the study's duration, every patient entered for nutritional treatment was self-referred, having learned about the project on their own through word-of-mouth or the media. Not one sought entry at an oncologist's suggestion.

Unfortunately, the early randomized design had severely affected patient interest, so even the word-of-mouth network wasn't as strong as Dr. Isaacs and I hoped it might be. Consequently, after the change to matched cohort, Dr. Isaacs and I suggested that to help encourage accrual, the NCI with all its power and authority should become more proactively involved. At one point, the lead NCI supervisor assigned to the project promised the Institute would take out ads in the medical journals, as is often done with government studies, requesting oncologists consider our trial for their patients diagnosed with inoperable pancreatic cancer. Though I understand the ads were actually written, none were ever placed, leaving us at the whims of chance to attract patients into the study.

Ultimately, only the oncology team at Columbia cooperated with patient recruitment and only to form the comparison chemotherapy "control" arm. Even for this group, as I will later discuss at length, their involvement proved in my opinion not helpful.

Oncologists not only refused to refer to the trial, but at times actively discouraged those who expressed an interest from seeking admission. A number of suitable candidates who on their own learned about our treatment and the NCI effort informed our office that the local oncologist had strongly argued against considering the project. One physician at a well-known cancer center warned a candidate interested in following up with the trial that I was a "quack" and the study a "fraud."

Frequently, patients who had actually entered the nutritional arm of the study and begun treatment with us were dissuaded by their oncologists from continuing with the prescribed regimen. Unfortunately, a protocol provision required that each patient assigned to our group consult with a physician monthly for an examination and blood studies. On the surface, such visits would hardly seem to be the source of potential catastrophe, since, one might think, how could a visit with a doctor be a problem? Understandably, trials of chemotherapy drugs often require frequent physician assessments to monitor closely the toxic side effects of the medications being tested, such as severe anemia or immune suppression.

For those subjects who lived in the New York area, Dr. Isaacs and I could satisfy this rule by meeting with the patient ourselves monthly. We had no problem with such an arrangement, of course. But as it turned out, only three of the patients ultimately admitted for our treatment lived in the New York area, with the majority residing at a great distance from our office. Consequently, nearly all those assigned to the nutrition arm were followed by a local doctor, most frequently an oncologist completely unfamiliar with our treatment approach and often hostile toward it, with only a few notable exceptions. Repeatedly, we heard from our patients that during the required monthly meetings, their local physicians aggressively encouraged them to discontinue their treatment with us, instead urging them to proceed with some standard approach—despite the fact that the conventional therapies for inoperable pancreatic cancer have proven largely ineffective.

Even in the case of patients who clearly were responding to our treatment, often the local physician tried to persuade them to quit the trial. In several instances, the doctors remarked to the patients how sad it was that they chose to spend the last months of their life following a restricted diet which couldn't possibly help their disease, instead of enjoying themselves with pizza and ice cream.

Should any patient develop a symptom or medical problem—and even our most successful patients with pancreatic cancer will experience periodic difficulties—the local physician usually urged them to stop our regimen in favor of a more conventional approach. In several instances, the discussions deteriorated into heated arguments, with the word "quackery" bandied about. One oncologist told one of our patients that the trial was an elaborate publicity stunt on our part meant to lure in patients for financial gain. This physician held to this story even when told that the patient had paid us no money and that the study was fully funded by the NIH.

25

We are unaware of any clinical trial in oncology or in any other branch of medicine that subjected very ill individuals facing death to such routine and repeated harassment intended to undermine a prescribed treatment. In conventional drug studies evaluating the latest proposed miracle against cancer, the oncologists and researchers involved commonly behave more like cheerleaders, often lauding the potential benefits of the treatment even in the absence of any proof of efficacy.

The Diabetes Control and Complications Trial indicated that patients, to succeed with the prescribed complex dietary regimen, required frequent and repeated positive reinforcement and encouragement.[27] In a more recent trial evaluating the effect of dietary modifications in patients diagnosed with prostate cancer, those assigned to the nutrition arm met in weekly support groups.[28] In great contrast, our patients commonly endured repeated and aggressive monthly discouragement, which not surprisingly influenced patient compliance with the regimen. By our tally, five patients dropped out of the study largely because their local physicians insisted they proceed with a more conventional form of therapy.

As evidence mounted that the local doctors rarely supported the project and might be undermining both the accrual of new patients and compliance of those already admitted, we repeatedly discussed the situation with the study supervisors. We urged that the NCI send out an official mailing to all U.S. oncologists, asking that for the benefit of science, they cooperate with the trial. Though the NCI staff assigned to the project agreed such a letter might prove valuable, and though such a letter was actually written after two years of our prodding, to our great frustration it was never sent.

V. Perpetual delays in the study: Over the years, since my fellowship days under Dr. Good in the mid-1980s, I have observed that when the NCI wants to get a study done, it gets done. I lived through the 1980s miracle of interleukin II, the 1985 cover story in *Newsweek* lauding the treatment, the NCI press conferences and press releases, the tens of millions of dollars assigned to "fast track" what has turned out to be a very toxic, very expensive, and largely ineffective approach. More recently, I, like so many others, witnessed the miracle of angiogenesis, the front page articles in major newspapers, the TV specials, the NCI press conferences and press releases, the millions in funding assigned to research this presumed extraordinary therapy that hasn't proven all that beneficial.

Our study proceeded along a completely different pathway. Most if not all NCI clinical studies must be reviewed and re-approved on a yearly basis, not only in Washington but also at the cooperating academic center, usually a fairly routine business. For clinical trials to run smoothly, this process must be quick and simple. And each year, our clinical trial came up for its regular evaluation at the NCI and at Columbia. In our case, the procedure hardly ran expeditiously; for most of the project's duration, at the onset of each fiscal year we learned that for some reason or another renewal had been delayed, or required some new paperwork, or more commonly, that someone involved with supervising the study had not submitted the appropriate documents in a timely fashion. Not a single delay involved some deficiency or non-compliance on our part.

While we waited for the requested forms to be completed, or located, or submitted, the trial remained suspended so that no new patients could be entered. Due to such bureaucratic delays, during the last three years of its existence, the trial was on hold far more than it was up and running. For example, during the fiscal year beginning June 2004, over a 12-month period, patient accrual was suspended for *11 months*.

No study could possibly run effectively under such conditions, and the serious and chronic delays became well known within the alternative medicine network, the traditional source of our most determined and compliant patients. To many, these repeated suspensions proved government indifference to our nutritional treatment—and to running a fair and honorable trial. We believe these delays, along with the specter of the randomized format, contributed to the widespread distrust among potential study candidates during the last years of the study. By that point, many of the patients diagnosed with pancreatic cancer who called our office anxious to begin our treatment told us they did not want any part of the project, even when open—as it rarely was—for accrual. We found ourselves in the ironic situation of treating patients diagnosed with pancreatic cancer successfully off study in our private practice as the clinical trial stalled into oblivion. Whatever the cause, we believe these repeated and lengthy hold-ups helped jeopardize the integrity of the effort.

VI. Inefficient screening of study candidates at Columbia: Initially, Dr. Antman agreed that Dr. Isaacs and I should participate in the selection of study subjects. But after the trial had been open for some 20 months—and after only four patients had been admitted for treatment with us—in July 2000 the NCI team

27

insisted we be excluded from the entry process to avoid, we were told, the possibility of bias afflicting the project. Thereafter, Dr. Chabot assumed sole responsibility for qualifying patients both for the chemotherapy and nutrition arms. Furthermore, even during the time when we did help supervise—and could veto—patient admission, Dr. Chabot, we were instructed, was to conduct the preliminary evaluation of all candidates. We were also told in no uncertain terms that our staff was to refer all those who might contact our office with a diagnosis of pancreatic cancer expressing an interest in the study to Dr. Chabot to begin the screening process for the clinical trial. The NCI staff even forbade us from discussing the rudiments of our treatment or the trial with any of these trial subjects, until Dr. Chabot had completed his initial assessment.

We believe these stark regulations, which prohibited my staff from talking about our own treatment, must have seemed bizarre to those seeking information from us about the NCI trial. We suspect that these strange rules discouraged many potentially suitable candidates from following up with Dr. Chabot's office.

To make matters worse, the intake process at Columbia hardly proved efficient. After Dr. Chabot assumed sole command of patient entry, many candidates called our office reporting, sometimes angrily, that they had repeatedly left messages for Dr. Chabot expressing an interest in joining the study, but that no one had gotten back to them days or even weeks later. In one case, a patient who had actually sent his records to Columbia for review heard nothing from Dr. Chabot about his status after five weeks, despite phone calls and faxes. At times in such situations, patients asked our office to intervene on their behalf with Dr. Chabot, but he seemed often unresponsive to our calls, faxes, and e-mails. For patients whose lifespan might be measured in months, we believe such delays jeopardized any chance for response to our therapy. We also suspect that many of these study candidates, aware of their dire situation and with no time to waste, simply chose to seek treatment elsewhere. Had I been in their situation, I would certainly have done the same.

VII. Reimbursement delays: At our suggestion, the NCI originally set up the grant for the clinical trial to cover the costs of patient office visits with us, in addition to the supplements and the required equipment such as juicers and water filters. Though expenditures for our treatment invariably represent only a fraction of that spent for a standard course of chemotherapy, nonetheless we thought this financial support for patients a good gesture. After all, insurance companies, which usually reimburse the most expensive drug regimens, rarely if ever cover our alternative approach.

Dr. Isaacs and I were not to be paid for administrative work for the study, only reimbursed for our office visit fees, though at a reduced rate from what we would normally charge. This arrangement seemed fair and simple. However, for reasons never made clear to us, the final version of the protocol omitted coverage for any of our office visits beyond the initial evaluation. Dr. Isaacs and I made no issue of this oversight, since we were grateful for the opportunity to have our work evaluated. Consequently, we essentially treated each patient for free beyond the first consultation.

After approving the $1.4 million budget, for the duration of the trial the NCI and NCCAM funneled all grant monies directly into Columbia's coffers. In turn, our office was to submit to Columbia copies of all bills for patient expenses, including our initial consultation fees and the ongoing supplement expenditures. In terms of these latter costs, Columbia was to pay us and we would then reimburse the company providing the products. As an aside, I think it is important to keep in mind that when an institution such as Columbia agrees to serve as the site for a federally funded study, it receives 10% of the total grant amount as a gift, officially termed "overhead," to use as they wish.

During the last five years of the project, for any variety of reasons that often made no sense to us, payments for the initial office visits as well as the supplements were held up for months. At such times, Dr. Isaacs and I willingly accepted the postponed reimbursement of our office fees, but the supplement costs, which generally ran in the neighborhood of $650 per patient per month, represented a much greater problem. Since those entered into the nutrition arm had been informed the grant subsidized the treatment, we hardly thought it appropriate to announce to them suddenly that they had to start paying for their enzymes and nutrients. Consequently, whenever funds were withheld, Dr. Isaacs, myself and the supplement company began underwriting the nutrition arm out of our own pockets. At one point, the amount we paid out ourselves exceeded $20,000. Only after much effort were we finally repaid, but nonetheless, I have never heard of any NCI study that required an investigator to subsidize for any period of time the costs of the project.

During the fiscal year beginning June 2002, the funding delays had become so pervasive that Dr. Chabot repeatedly warned me the study might be closed down. When I asked why something so simple as the release of approved monies had become such a constant problem, he explained that those within the NCI hierarchy responsible for overseeing the clinical trial simply did not move the proper paperwork through the appropriate channels as needed. The problem was, he said, bureaucratic.

Though the study didn't end at that time, when the funding problems persisted in the spring of 2003 I spoke directly with Dr. Stephen Straus, the then Director of NCCAM, the government group directly responsible for underwriting the project. He assured me that both he and NCCAM stood behind the clinical trial—a claim I would later doubt—and that he, like Dr. Chabot, held the NCI personnel responsible for holding up the release of allocated monies, a charge the NCI later denied. In April of 2003, after Dr. Chabot again advised me that the long suspensions in financial support made it unlikely the clinical trial could continue, I wrote directly to Dr. Andrew von Eschenbach, then NCI director, summarizing the various problems we had faced, including the untimely transfer and release of funds from the NCI:

> When the study has been under threat before, funding is held up, leaving our patients without support to pay for the treatment, which is not covered by insurance. Last year, during a prior hiatus and threat, our office paid out many thousands of dollars to keep the patients on the trial, and fortunately the study continued and the charges were picked up. Now, we simply will not be able to continue to finance the patients on the trial out of our own pocket. If this is not resolved soon, we will have to tell the patients to buy their own supplements. I know in a number of cases, the patients who are currently responding will not themselves be able to pay for the treatment and will die. This prospect has created a nightmare situation for Dr. Isaacs and myself, and I am deeply concerned about this, particularly since as best as I can understand the study may be shut down because paperwork is not moving between offices.

> It has been very difficult to conduct a study under the repeated threat that the study is soon to be closed down, and the patients are on their own. For now, accrual is on hold, so just as potentially good patients are volunteering to enter the study, we have to tell them the study is not open.

> Is there any way to learn from the NCI what the specific problems are? Is there any way the problems can be dealt with in a productive manner, so that patients accepted into the study in good faith are not put at risk?

Instead of responding directly to me, Dr. von Eschenbach referred my concerns back to the very NCI study supervisor both Dr. Straus and Dr. Chabot identified as the source of the problem. Thereafter, the trial continued to struggle along as before, with the various roadblocks, including the endlessly slow release of funds, uncorrected.

Dr. Isaacs and I considered these financial delays extraordinary, whatever the cause. Regardless of the underlying reason, the effect was the same: enormous financial stress on our office. Despite this burden, Dr. Isaacs and I continued onward because we so strongly believed in the importance of clinical trials and the potential benefit of our approach.

VIII. Epidemic non-compliance in the nutrition arm: For a number of reasons, including physical disability, psychiatric instability, lack of social support, poor motivation, and physician harassment, we have calculated that at least 30 of the 39 patients ultimately entered into the nutrition arm followed the prescribed regimen not at all, for only brief periods of time, or incompletely. Such epidemic poor compliance—which ultimately helped render the data meaningless—differed greatly from what we had generally observed among those we see in our private practice. Unfortunately, by the intent-to-treat study design, all patients admitted for treatment with us, even those who never took a supplement, were considered to be fully adherent with the prescribed regimen.

Burke and Ockene point out that non-compliant patients enrolled in a clinical study can obscure a benefit of the therapy being tested:

> Trial results can be affected by nonadherence with the intervention. Nonadherence leads to underestimating possible therapeutic and toxic effects and can undermine even a properly designed study.[24(p238-239)]

IX. Failure to abide by the standards of appropriate clinical trial management: Every legitimate clinical trial must follow certain very precise rules and regulations to help insure a meaningful outcome. I have broken these precepts down into eight distinct categories as follows: accepted patients must meet the entry criteria of the written protocol; the study must have an adequate number of subjects to make a statistically valid point about the therapy or therapies under scrutiny; the numbers in each arm of the study must be more or less, within certain specified limits, equal; the patients in each group must be more or less equivalent in terms of disease stage and clinical status; patients should be admitted into each arm over time in a steady, balanced manner; the supportive care given subjects in each group must be equivalent; the standards for stopping each treatment must be the same; and finally, the Principal Investigator (PI) charged with assessing and approving trial participants must be unbiased toward each therapy being studied, with no financial or intellectual tie to either.

In our opinion, this NCI-NCCAM clinical trial failed on each and every count, as I will now document in summary form.

A. *Entry of unsuitable patients.* From our initial meetings with Drs. Klausner and Antman, Dr. Isaacs and I were willing to put our reputation on the line and put our therapy to the test treating patients diagnosed with inoperable pancreatic adenocarcinoma, one of the deadliest of cancers. However, we knew from our private practice and pilot study experience that many patients with this particular malignancy, if physically able and willing to follow the therapy as prescribed, can do very well. Over the years, we have treated patients diagnosed with inoperable, even stage IV disease who are alive and in good health in excess of five, ten, even fifteen years after beginning treatment with us.

We have limits, of course, to what we can do. Ours is a lifestyle and nutritional regimen that patients pursue daily at home and on their own, unlike chemotherapy which only requires they show up for treatment. With our approach, patients must follow a prescribed diet, ingest some 150 or more supplements (including the enzymes) to be taken at precise times throughout the day, and incorporate the various detoxification procedures, such as the coffee enemas, into their routine. Obviously, patients must be able to swallow normally to succeed, and since the treatment is self-administered they should be able to care for themselves to some degree; those extremely debilitated, bedridden, in the final stages of the disease, or requiring hospitalization, cannot proceed with the therapy. We have no illusions about our approach; we cannot help someone days from death, nor would we ever treat such a patient in our private practice.

By its very nature, the regimen requires, as does any lifestyle intervention, determination, discipline, and above all else, motivation, or, as we learned long ago, patients will simply not follow through with its day-to-day application. And those with obvious mental illness most likely cannot effectively pursue this therapy.

Initially, Dr. Antman, Dr. Wynder, and the others supervising the project agreed that to achieve our stated goal, a fair evaluation of my therapy, we needed to accrue patients into the nutritional arm physically able, psychologically capable, and emotionally willing to adhere to the regimen. Admission of those too ill to pursue the treatment, mentally ill patients, and subjects with little discipline or motivation could lead easily to epidemic poor compliance and useless data.

We were disappointed that Dr. Antman insisted on the randomized format along with the intent-to-treat provision, while disregarding our wish for a lead-in period. However, in the various drafts of the written protocol she did incorporate many of our suggestions pertaining to the formal eligibility criteria, to help ensure that only suitable candidates would be entered. As a start, since pancreatic cancer progresses so rapidly we agreed all patients had to be admitted into the study within eight weeks of biopsy diagnosis. In addition, the protocol required patients be able to eat normally, to increase the likelihood they could comply with our dietary and nutritional therapy.

Candidates seeking entry had to be free of any form of mental disability "preventing informed consent or intensive treatment," to quote the written protocol, and express the motivation to pursue the home-based treatment plan. Furthermore, to be approved for admission, patients needed at least one supportive live-in family member, willing to help with the nuts and bolts of the treatment. We long ago learned that those with advanced cancer need assistance on a daily basis to adhere properly to the regimen. Finally, each trial candidate meeting all these basic criteria was to sign an official statement of informed consent as required for all NCI clinical trials, acknowledging the purposes, risks, and possible benefits associated with both the control chemotherapy and our nutritional approach.

As the study geared up, Dr. Isaacs and I thought, because of our 20-year experience with the therapy, that we should participate with the intake evaluation of patients seeking admission into the nutritional arm, to help cull out inappropriate subjects. Initially, Dr. Antman and the NCI staff agreed we could veto the entry of study candidates whom we believed failed to satisfy any of the eligibility criteria. But as the project proceeded, Dr. Antman and the others in charge expressed an overriding concern that Dr. Isaacs and I needed to be removed from all aspects of the approval process. In this way, we were told, the effort would be protected from any tainting, that is, any potential bias with which we might insidiously infect the project. Despite our protests, after July 2000 we were completely excluded from the selection of trial patients, with full responsibility given to Dr. Chabot at Columbia—who had no experience whatsoever with our treatment. Nonetheless, if Dr. Chabot approved a patient for the nutrition arm, the patient was to be treated by us.

We hoped that the written criteria would protect us, and the trial, from the acceptance of subjects physically, mentally, or emotionally unsuited for our therapy. However, over the years of the project Dr. Chabot repeatedly qualified patients for treatment with us whom we believed failed to fulfill one or more of these objective requirements. At least two, and we believe three, patients assigned to the nutrition group despite our objections had been diagnosed by biopsy well over eight weeks before their entry and should not have been admitted. Many approved patients were in the final terminal stages of their disease, obviously too debilitated to proceed with the therapy (one arrived in our office in a wheelchair barely able to stand). Overall, we identified 11 patients whose appetites were so poor at the time of their admission into the trial they could never follow our rigorous regimen.

Dr. Chabot accepted three patients for the nutrition arm who, because of mental disability, we believe should have been ruled ineligible, and another one with little or no social support. We estimate that ten of the nutrition patients lacked the drive, motivation, or faith in the therapy to stick with it for any length of time. Finally, Dr. Chabot sent three patients for treatment with us who, as it turned out, lacked evidence of the required signed informed consent, which was in violation of the written protocol and federal regulations.

Discounting overlap—several patients should have been excluded for more than one reason—we estimate *conservatively* that 16 of the 39 patients approved for the nutrition arm did not fulfill at least one specific written entry criteria.

B. *Shortfall in total numbers for the study.* As the trial came into being, the Columbia statisticians, working with Dr. Wynder, determined that for the final data to achieve mathematical significance, we must ultimately enter a minimum of 72 total patients, counting both the chemotherapy and nutrition groups together. When our study finally closed to accrual in October of 2005, Dr. Chabot had admitted only 62 patients—80% of the goal. Nonetheless, he and his Columbia colleagues insisted the numbers adequate to "make the point," in this case that my therapy didn't work.

C. *Disparity in numbers between the chemotherapy and nutrition groups and Dr. Chabot's attempts to correct the problem.* In order to generate truly useful data, in any clinical trial the patient groups being compared must be more or less of equal size. Otherwise, the potential benefit of a new therapy under evaluation might be either exaggerated or obscured.

In our case, when the trial finally shut down to accrual Dr. Chabot had accepted only 23 patients for chemotherapy, as opposed to 39 for nutrition. Despite the glaring difference, Dr. Chabot and apparently the Columbia statisticians insisted the groups were comparable. Subsequently, for reasons never explained to us, he first disqualified four nutrition patients, then later—as we shall see—another three, so that on paper the numerical imbalance between the two arms seemed less obvious, though it was still significant.

D. Dr. Chabot's handling of the staging disparity between the chemotherapy and nutrition arms. Oncologists divide pancreatic cancer into four "stages," reflecting the extent of spread. Stage I disease, the earliest and by definition limited only to the pancreas, can at times be cured with surgery. Stage II indicates the cancer has infiltrated locally outside the pancreas, for example into the surrounding fatty tissue or the duodenum, the first part of the small intestine, but not into lymph nodes or distant organs. With stage III, regional lymph nodes adjacent to the pancreas are involved, and in stage IV, the malignancy has spread into organs such as the liver, the lungs, the bone, or distant lymph nodes.

Initially, pancreatic cancer can be largely asymptomatic: for months, patients might complain of mild indigestion, bloating, vague persistent abdominal pain, or reflux after eating. Often unsuspecting doctors prescribe antacids or proton pump inhibitors like Prilosec or Nexium, with no or minimal improvement. Eventually the patient experiences a rapid decline prompting an intense evaluation but by this point, the disease has most often metastasized extensively.

The literature reports only 5% of patients, or even fewer, present at the time of diagnosis with stage I tumors. Of the group categorized as "non-stage I," approximately 25–30% are classified initially as stage II and III, and 70–75% as stage IV, the most advanced and deadly form.[29(p1143)] In the Gemzar study from 1997, which excluded those with potentially operable stage I disease, patients entered into each arm fell into this range, with approximately 28% diagnosed as stage II and III, and 72% as stage IV.[19;20] In our pilot study, which also only accrued patients with non-stage I disease, three, or 27%, had been categorized with inoperable or locally advanced stage II, and eight of the 11 patients, or 73%, were at stage IV, the numbers again conforming to the usual distribution of non-stage I subjects.[18]

It is well documented, and not surprising, that the median and mean survival for earlier stage II and III patients, in the range of 10–14 months, exceeds the 3–6 months average life expectancy for those diagnosed at stage IV—regardless of the conventional therapy offered.[29(p1130, 1143)]

As in the Gemzar trials, our NCI study excluded stage I patients who might be surgical candidates, but permitted inclusion of those with the more advanced stages II, III, and IV. Since the average survival differs significantly between patients with more limited versus those with more advanced disease, the November 1999 version of the protocol, written after the switch to a non-randomized format, required that the chemotherapy and enzyme treatment arms be evenly matched in terms of stage. Such balancing would help prevent an unfair advantage, should, say, one group consist of primarily earlier stage patients, the other primarily late stage IV.

During the group meeting held December 13, 2004 at Dr. Chabot's Columbia office, at which time the clinical trial had been up and running for a full five years, Dr. Isaacs and I first became aware of a very significant difference in both the total number of patients entered into each arm and in their respective staging distribution. By that time, 38 patients had been admitted for our nutrition treatment, and of these, approximately 76% by our accounting had been initially diagnosed with the most advanced stage IV disease, the other 24% with earlier stage II or III. These numbers approximated, as did those of our pilot study, the usual pattern for newly diagnosed pancreatic cancer patients as reported in the literature.

Dr. Isaacs and I were very much familiar with the staging of the nutrition patients, since we had supervised their treatment, but we knew very little until that point about the chemotherapy group. But during that meeting, Dr. Chabot handed out a "data chart" which included the total numbers of patients approved for each of the two arms, with their staging distribution. As I read the sheet, I was surprised that he had tabulated the numbers incorrectly for our group—at least according to our review of the records—reporting 35% at stage II and III and 64.7% at stage IV. I was even more surprised to learn that the chemotherapy arm, created under the direction of the Columbia oncologists, consisted of only 14 patients, 61.5% with earlier stage II and III disease, and 38% with advanced stage IV—a near reversal of the pattern in the nutrition group, and a reversal of the usual distribution described for patients diagnosed with pancreatic cancer.

Though the meager number of chemotherapy subjects enrolled by such a late point in the study's history alone helped make interpretation of the data difficult, the imbalance in the two groups by stage presented an even more serious obstacle. Early stage patients, as we have seen, tend to live much longer than stage IV patients, even if receiving no treatment. Since the majority of nutrition patients at the time of entry had been diagnosed with stage IV cancer, the significant difference between the two arms in this regard precluded any reasonable comparison of treatment effect.

During the session, Dr. Chabot, not surprisingly, reported a survival advantage already evident among the chemotherapy patients. With the significant staging imbalance between the groups so obvious, I expressed my grave concern that the entry of predominantly early stage subjects for chemotherapy, and primarily very advanced patients for nutrition—most of whom weren't able or chose not to stick with the regimen anyway—left us with uninterpretable data.

By March, 2005, Dr. Chabot had, with no explanation to us, disqualified two earlier stage chemotherapy patients, reducing the total number in the group to 12, but adjusting the staging balance so that now 50% were at stage IV, 50% at stages II and III. Thereafter, from April 2005 until the study closed permanently to new patient entry in October 2005, Dr. Chabot admitted only a single patient for nutrition—who like so many others, followed the therapy only briefly—but 11 for chemotherapy, nine at stage IV, during a six-month period when the study was often on hold, bringing the total number in this group to 23. When the trial finally closed for good Dr. Chabot had qualified a total of 39 nutrition patients, with, by our accounting, 23% at earlier stages, 77% at stage IV.

Dr. Chabot did not send us the final data for both groups until late April of 2006, long after the study had closed to accrual; at that time he reported that 34.7% of the 23 patients in the chemotherapy arm had been classified as stage II and III, 65.5% as stage IV. With no explanation Dr. Chabot had also disqualified two stage IV nutrition patients he had previously considered, as far as we knew, as properly entered, and described another five as stage II or III, who—perhaps with one exception—must, by the medical records, be considered at stage IV. With these unexplained revisions, he reported 40.5% of the nutrition group at stages II and III, 59% at stage IV. So six months after the last patient entry, more than six years after the project's start, and long after all participants and their staging had been reported and documented to the supervisory personnel without a challenge, the nutrition patients as a group appeared *less* advanced than those accepted for chemotherapy. Such last minute adjustments, performed by the principal investigator (PI) with no justification for the changes provided to us, did not inspire our confidence in the data.

E. Bunched accrual of patients during the study. Clinical trials can differ in their basic design; some are randomized, some matched cohort, some case-control. Though the details aren't important here, in any clinical effort the PI, in our case Dr. Chabot, should aim to enter patients into each group in a gradual, more or less equivalent fashion over time. That is, for each patient admitted into group A of study XYZ, one should then ideally be approved for group B. Though such a perfect equation can be difficult to sustain in a non-randomized trial, the PI must at least strive for balance in the acceptance of patients.

In our study, patient entry followed a "bunched" pattern, with large groups being approved for each arm at very different times. From the trial's beginning until the end of December 2002, a period of some three years, Dr. Chabot had admitted 32 patients for treatment with us, representing 82% of the 39 that would ultimately be counted. During that same time frame he accepted only two for chemotherapy.

From January 2004 until the project finally closed in late October 2005, a total of 22 months, Dr. Chabot qualified only three patients for the nutrition arm. Yet, from February 22, 2005 until October 2005, a period of eight months, he managed to admit 11 patients for chemotherapy, 48% of the ultimate total, though after July of that year accrual remained frequently suspended. According to our calculations, these subjects gained admission while the trial was open for a grand total of four months. We did not know much about these patients Dr. Chabot approved for the chemotherapy arm: we wondered if they were newly diagnosed, or perhaps recruited from other studies running concurrently at Columbia during the time of our own project.[30]

F. Differences in supportive care between the nutrition and chemotherapy arms. In any clinical trial, the basic supportive medical care provided patients should be equivalent for all. This rule holds true particularly for studies evaluating a treatment for a debilitating and deadly disease such as pancreatic cancer, associated with all manner of serious concurrent medical problems and difficult management issues. In our case, Dr. Robert Fine, director of the Experimental Therapeutics Program at Columbia, directly supervised the treatment of all 23 subjects admitted for chemotherapy. This oncologist has earned admiration within the profession for his aggressive, never-give-up approach, providing the latest advances available at a major medical center for those diagnosed with pancreatic cancer.[31] According to his own published statements, he and his highly motivated team employ all the benefits of modern hospital-based medicine, sparing no intervention, withholding no aid to keep patients alive—even to the point of repeated surgeries, and performing paracentesis (removal of abdominal fluid) two to three times a week, a procedure rarely in the past pursued so determinedly.[32]

Consequently, those subjects in our study destined to receive chemotherapy came under the watchful eye of a very aggressive and determined physician who had at his disposal the resources of Columbia, a team of expert senior physicians, researchers, fellows (oncologists in training), residents, skilled oncology nurses and other support personnel, and all the high tech facilities one could wish for. Patients could not hope to find more intense or sophisticated care, provided by an enthusiastic staff at a major academic institution.

Our group, on the other hand, faced quite a different and often grim scenario at the hands of often indifferent local doctors frequently hostile to our therapy. True, many of the nutrition patients Dr. Chabot approved were too sick even to begin the treatment or to stay with it for any length of time. For these, the attitude of the local physicians hardly mattered, in terms of ultimate outcome. But among those who did try to persevere with the prescribed regimen, the doctors entrusted with their local care seemed most frequently unwilling to address aggressively medical issues that might arise. Instead, they appeared more determined to convince our patients their situation was hopeless and the treatment worthless. The prevailing approach too often was one of non-cooperation with us, coupled with a wish to move patients onto some standard chemotherapy or into hospice.

Of all the nutrition patients, only one—who ultimately survived 3.5 years— received anywhere near the level of supportive care and encouragement given those in the chemotherapy group. In this unique situation, the local doctors coordinated their treatment with me, realizing full well that the patient was sustaining a significant response to our regimen. In no other case did the local doctors encourage aggressive intervention to keep the patient alive and also *on the nutritional therapy*. The general physician approach toward our patients could not contrast more sharply to the enthusiastic team efforts of Dr. Fine's staff, who appeared to have one ultimate, determined goal: to keep patients alive as long as possible and on treatment as long as possible.

At this point, I would like to comment on another aspect of the chemotherapy regimen used with most of the patients in our study, GTX, that makes comparison of the two groups in our clinical trial even more fruitless. Two of the three GTX drugs, Gemzar and Taxotere, must be given intravenously, since no oral form exists. Xeloda was developed for oral ingestion, usually one or two tablets daily for two weeks, followed by a two-week drug vacation, followed by more Xeloda. By the nature of these agents and their route of administration, involving very little intake by mouth, the GTX regimen suits even patients with little or no appetite—unlike our aggressive nutritional/supplement program, involving a carefully prescribed diet and the ingestion of more than 150 capsules a day. With very advanced patients, GTX, as a primarily intravenous regimen, would have an advantage over our intensive dietary treatment approach. Those too sick to eat, those too ill to comply with a therapy such as ours could still be treated with GTX.

Furthermore, whenever Dr. Fine needed to hospitalize a patient at Columbia for any reason, he could continue providing the chemotherapy in the institutional setting with everyone's blessing. In contrast, though every patient assigned to the nutrition arm at some point required in-patient care, not once did the local doctors allow any of them to continue any aspect of our regimen under these circumstances. I believe this additional difference between the two groups allowed for yet another bias in GTX's favor.

G. Different standards for stopping each treatment. In Dr. Fine's worldview, if a patient seems to be worsening, he doesn't discontinue therapy and give up, but instead modifies the doses, changes the scheduling of the drugs, becomes more aggressive.[32] In a sense, Dr. Isaacs and I share a similar attitude: if a patient doesn't appear to be responding, with his or her consent we alter the enzyme dose, adjust the daily and monthly scheduling of the supplements, we might modify the diet or any other number of variables. We, too, ramp up the treatment.

The written protocol for the study permitted Dr. Isaacs and me to change the treatment as needed when scans or other studies showed possible progression of disease. Specifically, section 11.0 (of the November 1999 version) "REMOVAL OF PATIENTS FROM PROTOCOL THERAPY," stated:

11.1 Enzyme-Nutritional Protocol Therapy:

Response or Stable Disease: Continue full treatment with full doses of enzymes and adjunctive nutrients, diet and detoxification routines.

Disease Progression: Modify the doses of enzymes and other nutrients according to the protocol but do not discontinue protocol therapy except at the patients [sic] request. Describe tumor progression including tumor measurements on flow sheets.

The *written* protocol instructions could not have been clearer, giving us the right—assuming the patient agreed—to fine-tune our regimen, just as Dr. Fine does with his chemotherapy.

During the years of our clinical trial, Dr. Chabot seemed quite impressed by the determined efforts of his Columbia colleague. Yet as we came to learn, Dr. Chabot apparently believed our patients required different handling than those of Dr. Fine, as if two standards governed the trial. With any sign of worsening, Dr. Fine expected to continue treatment, but in our case patients were to stop their nutritional regimen and seek other options.

We learned of this double standard late into the study through a very odd series of events. By 2004, as the project moved into its sixth year, we realized the NCI had no intention of intervening to counter the ongoing physician hostility to the project that continued to influence both accrual of new patients and compliance of those entered. To help alleviate the problem of such outside interference, we suggested Dr. Chabot himself begin contacting the local physicians of each patient newly accepted into the nutrition arm, to encourage their support. Dr. Chabot agreed from that point onward either he or one of his staff would call these doctors whenever he approved a subject for treatment with us. As the study progressed into 2005, physician opposition continued, so we suspected that such contacts, if indeed being made, had very little if any effect.

At a meeting of study personnel convened at Columbia on June 20, 2005, Dr. Isaacs and I asked Dr. Chabot if he or someone from his staff had been calling the local physicians of our patients. He said he had, though he was vague about the number, and apparently made the contact only, at least according to what he said, if the patient suggested his or her physician might be hostile toward the study.

After Dr. Wendy Smith of the NCI joined the study in 2000, she began compiling and distributing the official written minutes, usually within a few days after each group meeting, summarizing the issues discussed among the various participants. We had the right to suggest corrections if we noted errors in the document. Though the notes usually arrived in a timely fashion, we did not receive the report of the June 2005 meeting until September 12, 2005, the day before the next regularly scheduled conference. We noticed a number of significant errors in the document, including misstatements about Dr. Chabot's efforts at contacting local doctors. Specifically, Dr. Smith claimed that Dr. Chabot had been contacting the local physicians of our patients "from early on"—a statement completely at odds with our recollection of the situation.

I e-mailed Dr. Smith the following day, September 13, 2005:

> In the second paragraph of this section, you state that Dr. Chabot telephones physicians to confirm that they are indeed supportive and has made these calls from early on. "From early on" is vague, and most readers would assume based on your report that these telephone calls were made to the physicians of the majority of patients. Our recollection is that this policy was only put into place in the last year, and that only after frequent discussions of the hostility of oncologists toward the study were such calls instituted. Frankly, even if calls were made, they had no effect. Patient —, for example, one of the later patients in the trial, reported constant negativity from his oncologist and private physician. If his physicians received a phone call, it certainly didn't make much difference in their attitudes.

However, according to the official record, Dr. Smith did not address the issue of Dr. Chabot's phone calls to local physicians until six months later, during the March 20, 2006 group meeting—which Dr. Isaacs and I did not attend. In a section of the minutes from that day entitled "The PI (Principal Investigator) phone calls to physicians and hostility to the trial," she described Dr. Chabot's response:

> If there was any concern about the supportiveness, that is if the patient mentioned anything to him or if it didn't appear that there was a cooperative physician, he would give them a call to assess whether they were interested in having their patients on this trial, whether they have a problem, and whether they are willing to care for the patient on the trial. *In some situations, Dr. Chabot found that the patient had a physician supportive of their patients' participat-*

ing in the enzyme arm but upon recognition of increased disease, the physician then acted to facilitate the patient moving to other therapy. [Italics mine]

Dr. Chabot's explanation made no sense for a number of reasons. We were of course concerned about the frequent hostility expressed toward the study by physicians of patients already enrolled and actively pursuing our treatment. But in our discussions with Dr. Chabot we had specifically requested he intervene at the time of the patient's entry, not later on. We were unaware that Dr. Chabot made any calls to any physician of a patient already part of the trial whose disease might be progressing under our care.

Even if he did make such contact, the *written* protocol could not be clearer, giving us the right—assuming the patient agreed—to modify our treatment with evidence of worsening disease, just as Dr. Fine could do with his chemotherapy regimen. Consequently, it was neither acceptable nor appropriate for an outside physician who knew nothing about our therapy or the trial requirements to make decisions about stopping the regimen or pushing any of our patients into a different treatment plan—unless again, the patient so requested. However, in his comments, Dr. Chabot wasn't talking about a change of heart on the part of the patient, he was specifically permitting the monitoring physician to make the decision. Such outside interference constituted a violation of the written criteria for the study, and as principal investigator charged with upholding the protocol rules Dr. Chabot should not have justified an obvious breach of its regulations—particularly since he seemed perfectly content with Dr. Fine's never-give-up attitude. Unfortunately, Dr. Chabot's two apparent sets of standards, one for Dr. Fine and one for us, reflected, we believe, a disregard for the study's rules and influenced, as his own statements demonstrated, the treatment course of nutrition patients.

H. Dr. Chabot's conflict of interest. In any legitimate clinical trial, the PI must remain objective and be always neutral, with no tie, either financial or intellectual, to any of the treatments being evaluated. For the first five years of our project, although the chemotherapy patients were being treated at Dr. Chabot's institution, Columbia, and by his colleagues, I did not suspect any conflict of interest on his part.

I first became concerned about a potential problem during the December 13, 2004 group meeting, when Dr. Chabot seemed overly pleased with the unusual survival evident in the chemotherapy group. Dr. Isaacs and I attributed these odd results to the advanced stage and poor compliance among our patients compared to the early stage of those receiving chemotherapy, not to any great benefit of drug treatment. As the study continued throughout 2005, I became only more troubled by Dr. Chabot's growing and obvious enthusiasm for the chemotherapy data, particularly in view of all the management issues which made the results questionable. Subsequently, I was to learn of a significant conflict of interest on Dr. Chabot's part that in our opinion should have disqualified him from serving as principal investigator.

To understand the nature of the conflict, I thought it might be helpful to review just how the drug regimen GTX (Gemzar, Taxotere and Xeloda) became the treatment of choice for the chemotherapy patients accepted into our clinical trial. In 1998, as our study first came into being, the FDA had just approved Gemzar specifically for use with patients diagnosed with pancreatic cancer. The drug, developed by the pharmaceutical giant Eli Lilly, rapidly became the primary tool used by oncologists around the world for treatment of the disease, the new light on the horizon for a very deadly malignancy. Gemzar hadn't been developed at Columbia, so no one there as far as I knew had any special tie to it, either financially or intellectually.

In the original draft of the protocol, we all agreed that the patients assigned to receive chemotherapy should be treated with Gemzar alone, at the time the standard of care for pancreatic cancer. In later versions of the document, Dr. Antman suggested we permit the use of additional chemotherapeutic drugs, since, she and Dr. Chabot argued, oncologists and their patients already realized that Gemzar by itself had proven only marginally effective. Many oncologists around the country, they insisted, already had incorporated multiple drugs into their treatment regimens.

Dr. Antman and her Columbia team then modified the protocol at about the time we changed over to a matched cohort design in early 2000. By that point, Dr. Fine and his colleagues at Columbia had already devised a triple drug regimen, GTX, adding Taxotere and Xeloda to Gemzar for the treatment of pancreatic malignancy. Since Dr. Fine supervised the care of all chemotherapy patients entered into our study, the majority ultimately received the GTX regimen. I want to emphasize that the combination GTX approach was purely a Columbia invention.

When Dr. Antman first suggested we modify the protocol to allow a multiple drug approach, she spoke to us in general terms—not specifying that the che-

motherapy patients in our trial would receive a regimen developed at her institution, Columbia. After she moved on to the NCI and Dr. Chabot assumed the
role of Principal Investigator, we still didn't realize GTX had been developed
at Columbia, so it never occurred to Dr. Isaacs and me that the change might
be inviting a potential conflict of interest in any way. Furthermore, we didn't
believe that Dr. Chabot, a surgeon and not an oncologist, would have much to
do with chemotherapy research under any circumstance, and of course we assumed that if a conflict existed, the trial supervisors would let us know.

But this gradual evolution of the chemotherapy regimen, from simple Gemzar
to complex GTX, altered the landscape of our clinical trial enormously. We
had started with a single drug created by a pharmaceutical company and used
everywhere for treatment of pancreatic adenocarcinoma, then changed over to
a very specific triple agent combination developed by a team of Columbia physicians and scientists. In retrospect, this modification of the allowable treatments
opened up a potential institutional conflict of interest. After all, with the change
in place, my controversial nutritional approach was pitted against an intervention developed at the very medical center serving as home base for the trial.

To make matters worse, it appears that Dr. Fine, the supervisor of the chemotherapy patients admitted into our study, and Dr. Chabot were more than
just Columbia colleagues, two professors at a big medical center who might
occasionally pass each other in the hall. As it turns out for most of the years
of the trial they had worked together very closely on the GTX regimen, as
documented in multiple publications in the medical literature. For example, in
a lengthy *ONCOLOGY NEWS INTERNATIONAL* article dated March 4,
2004, the last paragraph stated:

> "Activation of specific components of the MAP kinase pathway may be a novel
> target for induction of apoptosis in pancreatic cancer," Dr. Fine said. "Further
> study in phase II/III is warranted to ascertain the true clinical benefit of GTX
> and T-GX." His colleagues for the studies were Drs. David Fogelman, John
> Chabot, Ronald Ennis, Stephen Schreibman, James Strauss, and Yin li [sic].[32]

Though this interview came out in early 2004, I actually didn't see it until
2005, when I began to sort out what had really happened during the many
years of this clinical trial. Had I been aware of this connection earlier, I would
have asked that Dr. Chabot disqualify himself from his leadership role on our
project.

Another article linking Dr. Chabot closely to GTX appeared in the October 2004 issue of *Surgical Oncology Clinics of North America*.[31] Entitled "The evolution of adjuvant and neoadjuvant chemotherapy and radiation for advanced pancreatic cancer: from 5-fluorouracil to GTX," this lengthy and technical report put Dr. Chabot right in the middle of the GTX action. The authors, according to the order in which they are listed in the journal, included Fogelman DR, Chen J, Chabot JA, Allendorf JD, Schrope BA, Ennis RD, Schreibman SM, Fine RL. Invariably, publishing etiquette requires that the various contributors to a study be listed in a specified order of importance, so Dr. Chabot's position as third among eight meant he wasn't just a casual bystander, but a major player. It is also important to keep in mind that in recent years, medical and scientific journals have nearly universally required that each author sign a statement acknowledging substantive participation in the research effort.

The very same month of the *Surgical Oncology Clinics of North America* report, the Columbia team published an in-depth description of their laboratory and early clinical findings as they developed GTX in *Current Treatment Options in Gastroenterology*.[33] Once again, Dr. Chabot appeared as an author along with Dr. Fine.

The abstract stated:

> Familiarity with the updated results in genetic screening and work-up presented here is essential to early diagnosis and possible cure. In the metastatic setting, we most frequently begin with the GTX regimen, consisting of Gemcitabine, Taxotere, and Xeloda. The regimen is based on our laboratory data demonstrating a synergistic increase in cell killing of pancreatic cancer cell lines. . . . In our initial experience, we have seen a response rate of 40% at metastatic sites and 31% at the primary site after nine cycles of GTX. . . . In those patients who do not tolerate GTX or progress despite the regimen, we have found that a regimen of the same three drugs, administered on a different schedule, can produce responses.[33]

As an aside, the last sentence above, written with Dr. Chabot as a co-author, confirmed that when patients worsened on GTX, the Columbia team did not refer to hospice but instead adjusted the treatment plan.

We wonder, did not anyone at the NCI, NCCAM, or the NIH see the obvious conflict of interest evident here? The PI of this study should have been a scientist with no personal involvement with either of the regimens being evaluated. In fact, we thought that Dr. Chabot had been chosen to head the study not only because of his expertise, but precisely because he had no involvement with any research related to the chemotherapy regimen selected for our project. But since he was hardly a disinterested third party, he should not have been the man in charge of this clinical trial. I am sure that had the NCI appointed Dr. Isaacs as Principal Investigator, the objections would have been loud and persistent.

I can also now understand why Dr. Chabot seemed so excited during the December 13, 2004 meeting, when he announced an extraordinary survival benefit among the chemotherapy patients—he was part of Dr. Fine's team, of course he was excited. At the time, though I believed his enthusiasm for GTX premature and excessive, I did not put the pieces together until I had reviewed the published literature, including the *ONCOLOGY NEWS INTERNATIONAL* and *Surgical Oncology Clinics* reports.

I believe that had the NCI been on top of this study they would have jumped on this issue, insisting that Dr. Chabot be removed as PI and the trial be transferred to some other institution not so closely entwined with one of the competing treatments.

Chapter 3

Failure in Handling Informed Consent

O ver the years, Dr. Isaacs and I identified significant management lapses on the part of the personnel from the various participating institutions assigned to supervise this trial. Of all the shortcomings, the mishandling by Dr. Chabot of patient informed consent—a crucial component of any government supported clinical trial, the mechanism in place to insure protection of study candidates—was in our opinion the most serious. The strong evidence that Dr. Chabot did not properly obtain the required signed consent forms for three of our patients also helped us prove, amidst a flurry of constant denials that reached right up to the office of the NIH director, that the project had been run improperly.

All U.S. clinical trials involving human subjects, particularly those funded by the NCI and NIH, require that each eligible patient who agrees to participate must *sign* a consent form acknowledging their intent and their understanding of the issues involved. As carefully outlined on the official NCI website, these documents must describe the purpose of the project, possible dangers of the treatment or treatments being tested, potential benefits, options, and responsibilities. And, they must be *signed*:

Sec. 50. 27 Documentation of Informed Consent

(a) . . . informed consent shall be documented by the use of a written consent form approved by the IRB and signed and dated by the subject or the subject's legally authorized representative at the time of the consent. A copy shall be given to the person signing the form.[34]

In addition, the written protocol for our project instructed that each candidate was to sign a consent form as part of the entry process, as stated within sections 3 and 4 (of the November 1999 version):

3.8. Informed Consent. Each patient must be completely aware of the nature of his/her disease process and must willingly give consent for the chosen regimen. The patient must understand the alternatives, potential benefits, side-effects, risks, and discomforts. . . .

4.4 Registration: To register the patient, fax or deliver the completed Eligibility Criteria Form and signed Informed Consent to the Cancer Center Protocol Office, located on MHB 6N-435. . . .

4.5 Required Forms:
Eligibility Criteria Form
Informed Consent

In accordance with the above written regulations, the Columbia team devised a lengthy document for this specific purpose. Though for the first 20 months we could veto entry of trial candidates, from the beginning Dr. Chabot solely supervised the entire consent process, including the signing of the required forms. The completed documents would then be kept in the appropriate patient files at Columbia, not in our charts. We were told that no patient would be officially considered as admitted or even sent to us for treatment as part of the trial unless all the appropriately signed papers were in hand at Dr. Chabot's office.

All this seemed simple enough. However, we first became aware of problems with the consent process early in the study, when in July 2002 Dr. Chabot sent us a patient as appropriately vetted and approved for entry into the nutrition arm. Shortly after her initial consultation with Dr. Isaacs, this patient experienced a series of strokes, discontinued the treatment regimen, and soon died. Some time after her death, Michelle Gabay, Dr. Chabot's physician's assistant, called our office to alert us that Dr. Chabot had disqualified the patient because she never had signed the consent form. Apparently, during her initial meeting with Dr. Chabot, she asked if she could take the paperwork home to "think about it," before signing and mailing the document back. For reasons we do not understand, Dr. Chabot we were told agreed to this arrangement, but then sent the patient to us as if she had been properly enrolled—in complete violation of the written protocol requirements. Dr. Chabot's subsequent decision to exclude the patient didn't and doesn't make right his handling of consent in this case.

At the time we assumed that this episode, as strange as it seemed to us, represented an isolated incident, so we did not make much of it, but in the summer of 2003 the issue resurfaced. Since I was not on staff at Columbia, the administrators there had decided I must sign a subcontract agreement with the University beginning each fiscal year, defining my specific responsibilities for the clinical trial. When Dr. Isaacs and I read the document, we realized we were now required to keep copies of the *signed* consent forms for each patient in our own charts, in addition to the originals which would remain in Dr. Chabot's office files. In order to comply with this regulation, Dr. Isaacs immediately asked Dr. Chabot's staff to send us copies of the documents for all patients entered to that point into the nutritional arm.

Despite repeated requests made over a period of several months, the relevant materials did not arrive. Finally, with the approval of Dr. Chabot's assistant, in October 2003 Dr. Isaacs went in person to Columbia to copy the documents herself. While reviewing the charts, she noticed that in the case of two patients (#9 and #16 by our identifiers), considered as properly admitted into the study, the required, signed papers were missing. I want to emphasize that these two differ from the one (with no identifier number) who had previously been excluded. Both of these later patients, neither of whom had followed the prescribed regimen for any length of time, had died by the summer of 2003.

Dr. Chabot's staff could not locate the forms but assured us some time later that they might be in a second set of charts kept in a different office. However, this proved not to to be the case. In response to our request for an explanation, eventually Dr. Chabot's assistant, Carolyn (Cara) DeRosa, went through the files of Patients #9 and #16. Nearly a year after we first discovered the documents were missing, in an August 19, 2004 e-mail to us she reported the results of her investigation:

Linda/Michelle:

As noted previously, there are no consents in the charts for patients [#9 and #16] seen on 2–7–03 and 2–10–03. There is, however, a note by JC [John Chabot] in the chart that the patient [#16] was given the consent form at the time of the office visit.

But after a year, we still had no idea whether the signed forms existed. Since these two trial subjects had been sent to us as if properly consented—and since we were now required to have copies of the documents in our charts—we continued our efforts to learn their fate, with little success. Finally, with no explanation forthcoming despite repeated attempts over an 18-month period, on February 4, 2005 I e-mailed Dr. Chabot directly about the issue:

We have been trying to get copies of the consent forms for [Patient #9 and Patient #16] for quite some time now, and both Michelle and Cara say that the other person has them. Some intervention here would be appreciated since by the contract requirements, we are expected to keep copies in our charts. The subcontract with Columbia we signed says that we must keep them for all patients on the study.

On February 8, 2005, Dr. Chabot replied:

Last week Michelle went through all the charts to confirm data accuracy. It is loaded loaded [sic] into the system now.

Though we assumed Ms. Gabay's review included a search for the missing consent forms, subsequently we received no explanation as to their whereabouts.

When weeks passed with no resolution of the problem, I began to suspect these two patients, neither of whom followed the prescribed regimen, had not signed the required forms. At the June 29, 2005 group meeting held at Columbia—for a variety of reasons the last we would attend—we briefly discussed the missing documents, but Dr. Chabot seemed unaware of what had happened to them or where they might be. Nonetheless, at that point as far as we could tell Dr. Chabot still counted these two patients as treatment failures in the tabulation of the interim data, despite the absent forms and the significant non-compliance. To me, their inclusion as properly vetted and properly treated made no sense.

On July 26, 2005, I again e-mailed Dr. Chabot about the issue:

The terms of the subcontract require that we have a copy of the consent form that the patient signs. Linda went to Cara's office and copied most of them nearly 2 years ago, but there were two that were not available when she came. . . . She has intermittently tried to get these from either Cara or Michelle ever since. Each said to check with the other, or would say that the consent form must be in a chart that was in another location, or something. Given that both of these patients did not follow through with their protocols, we would like to know if they even signed the consent forms. So we would appreciate either receiving a copy of these consent forms or getting an answer as to whether these patients are data points on this trial.

In his reply the following day, Dr. Chabot wrote:

I will F/U [follow up] with Cara and Jane Lyons on these issues. Thx for the heads-up.

Despite the assurances, Dr. Chabot did not follow up with us about "these issues," leaving us as perplexed as ever about their status.

I finally received the minutes of the June 20, 2005 meeting on Sunday, September 11, 2005, the day before the September 12 session which we did not attend. In response to the many errors in the June 20 record, I subsequently e-mailed the various trial personnel, once again raising the issue of the missing forms:

There are a number of very serious errors in the minutes. Under point 2, you have a question about how many patients are in the enzyme arm. So do we. For quite some time now, we have been trying to get copies of the consent forms of two of the patients on the enzyme arm . . . most recently in an e-mail to Dr. Chabot dated July 27, 2005 [sic: July 26]. We still have not received these, and so we will now bring up the same question we brought up to him at that time. If the patients have consent forms, we want a copy, as the subcontract we were required to sign requires that we keep them. If the patients do not have consent forms, we would like to know if they are included in the clinical trial.

When our questions went unanswered, I began to wonder if Dr. Chabot hoped I would forget about the problem and move on. But I was not going to let the issue drop, so on October 19, 2005, I e-mailed Dr. Chabot yet again, still hoping to get an answer about the fate of the forms:

We are still waiting for an answer about the consent forms for [Patients #16 and #9]. Do they exist, or don't they? If they exist, we would like a copy as is required by the subcontract we signed.. [sic] If they don't exist, we would like to know if the patients are included as data points in the study. We continue to request them because, although your office was entrusted with the job of getting consent forms, as a part of the subcontracts we were required to sign, I am obligated to maintain copies of these consent forms. Linda started trying to get these consent forms in the summer of 2003. She finally came over and photocopied the bulk of them in October of 2003, but has been trying ever since to obtain copies of [#9 and #16]'s forms. We have repeatedly requested copies, or an indication of their status, since we were instructed to treat these patients as if they had met the criteria, including filling out consent forms.

Finally, in an e-mail sent October 26, Dr. Chabot confirmed the documents did not appear to exist for either patient:

The consent forms have not been identified. Both patients were accrued at times when Michelle was away and a research nurse from the cancer center was covering this clinical trial. The IRB was notified of this problem, in writing quite a long time ago and I have no further instructions. . . .

If this was true, and he had indeed notified the IRB (the Columbia Institutional Review Board) "a long time ago," I wondered why Dr. Chabot hadn't shared this information with us months earlier. Despite his explanation, I still did not know if he considered the two patients properly qualified treatment failures. I was also somewhat surprised that a substitute nurse had been assigned any part of the intake process, particularly informed consent, since I had been repeatedly instructed this was Dr. Chabot's, and only Dr. Chabot's, responsibility.

The supervisory staff did not address my many written complaints about the June 2005 minutes and my questions about the consent forms until the March 20, 2006 group meeting, some nine months later. According to the notes of the session—which, as previously mentioned, we did not attend—Dr. Chabot finally provided an explanation for the mysterious missing documents:

1. Number of subjects in the enzyme arm and missing consent forms:

The Columbia staff investigated this issue. Two consent forms from subjects entered in the enzyme arm are missing. Their follow up into this issue revealed that there are notes in both subjects' medical charts indicating that they were consented and in at least one of these cases, it is recalled that the patient requested to take the form with them and planned to return it. It appears that both these patients 'walked off' with their forms. The IRB was informed of this and as both charts note that subjects were consented, the IRB left it up to the investigators to decide about inclusion of this data. The investigators conducted the statistical analyses both with and without these two subjects and there is no effect on the statistical conclusions.

When I first read this paragraph, I was perplexed that Dr. Chabot now reported the medical records of the two patients in question contained written verification that both had been "consented," though in each case the forms were not in the chart. Not once during the 2.5 years we sought some response from Dr. Chabot's office regarding the missing paperwork for Patients #9 and #16 did he or his staff ever inform us in any communication that these two patients had been consented in any way. If this were the case, why had we not been told?

In his February 8, 2005 e-mail, written eighteen months after we first learned of the problem, Dr. Chabot did report, as noted previously, that a staff member "went through all the charts to confirm data accuracy," so by his own statement we know that these two patient files were reviewed at some point. But prior to the official minutes of the March 20, 2006 meeting neither he nor anyone in his office reported that the charts confirmed the patients had been consented.

We have never seen the actual notations referred to by Dr. Chabot for Patients #9 and #16 documenting the consent that may or may not have occurred. However, the August 19, 2004 e-mail sent to us by Dr. Chabot's assistant, Carolyn DeRosa, contradicted Dr. Chabot's claim made at the March 20, 2005 meeting:

Linda/Michelle:

As noted previously, there are no consents in the charts for patients [#9 and #16] seen on 2–7–03 and 2–10–03. There is however, a note by JC [John Chabot] in the chart that the patient [#16] was given the consent form at the time of the office visit.

According to Ms. DeRosa, Dr. Chabot's notation in the case of Patient #16 only indicated the patient "was given the consent form" and not that he signed the document or that he had been consented. Furthermore, Ms. DeRosa said nothing about any written statement in the chart of Patient #9 regarding "consent." One can only assume, since she had searched the records precisely to look for information on this issue, that if a statement actually existed for Patient #9, Ms. DeRosa would have told us, as she did in the case of Patient #16. Since to date no evidence exists to the contrary, I do not believe that the two patients #9 and #16 ever signed the forms.

Regardless of what Dr. Chabot said, the written protocol, as quoted before, required a "signed Informed Consent" be delivered to the Columbia protocol office:

> 4.4 Registration: To register the patient, fax or deliver the completed Eligibility Criteria Form and signed Informed Consent to the Cancer Center Protocol Office, located on MHB 6N-435. . . .

> 4.5 Required Forms:
> Eligibility Criteria Form
> Informed Consent

NCI regulations also instruct that the patient be given a copy of the signed consent, but that the original must remain in the chart:

Sec. 50. 27 Documentation of Informed Consent

(a) . . . informed consent shall be documented by the use of a written consent form approved by the IRB and signed and dated by the subject or the subject's legally authorized representative at the time of the consent. A copy shall be given to the person signing the form.[34]

The rules could not have been simpler. If the forms weren't signed, as I believe to have been the case, Dr. Chabot violated the written protocol, as well as NCI and federal regulations. Even if we assume for the sake of argument that the documents had been signed and misplaced, or that in one case, #16, the patient walked off with the signed forms, or that both walked off with the signed forms, Dr. Chabot still violated the written protocol as well as NCI and federal rules. Nowhere does the NCI allow patients approved for a federally supervised study to "walk off" with the original copy of the consent form, signed or unsigned.

According to the minutes of the March 20, 2006 meeting, Dr. Chabot reported that the Columbia Institutional Review Board (IRB) seemed quite satisfied with his explanation. Not only did the IRB seem unconcerned about the issue, but according to Dr. Chabot they would allow him to qualify or disqualify these two patients from the final tabulation of the data at his discretion—though neither followed the prescribed regimen.

At every academic medical center in this country, an Institutional Review Board helps oversee the safety of patients as well as the ethical management of all scientific investigations conducted at the institution. No clinical trial can begin without IRB consent, regardless of any approval that might already have been granted by a government office, such as the FDA, the NCI or the NIH. The IRB can also stop a study already up and running if its members suspect even minor infractions of the written protocol rules. It was therefore hardly trivial that Dr. Chabot claimed his IRB had given him a free pass on the missing consent forms, even permitting him to decide if these two patients would be considered as appropriately entered and treated.

Assuming the minutes to be accurate, I was nonetheless surprised that the Columbia IRB could be blasé about such a significant oversight. Proper informed consent has become a major issue in academic circles, to the point that even the United Nations' World Health Organization has weighed in on the matter.[35] The National Cancer Institute requires that all candidates *sign* an informed consent document before admission to any clinical trial under its jurisdiction, and that the original be kept in the patient chart. This rule is not optional nor can it be ignored or disregarded at the whim of any IRB. Ironically, the Columbia rules for clinical trials resemble those of the NCI, and the section in our written protocol describing the need for *signed* consent came right from the master template for Columbia oncology studies. And it's helpful to keep in mind that we became aware of the situation when our subcontract with that institution instructed us to keep copies of the signed consent in our files for each patient entered for nutritional treatment.

I could not understand why both Dr. Smith and Dr. White, the NCI representatives at the March 2006 meeting, did not challenge Dr. Chabot's reasoning or his claim of IRB blessing, which amounted to disregard of federal regulations. These NCI personnel, based on what the minutes reported, apparently accepted Dr. Chabot's answers as perfectly legitimate, though his failure to obtain signed consent, or to maintain the documents if they were signed, represented a violation of the written protocol for this study, the regulations of the Columbia IRB, and the rules of their own federal institution.

The evolving story of the missing consent forms ultimately took an even odder twist as the study wound down. Along with a brief April 22, 2006 letter to me in which he defended his handling of the study throughout, Dr. Chabot sent us a chart listing all patients ultimately qualified for both arms of the study. After Dr. Chabot's delay in sharing with us the requested information about the missing forms, after including—as far as we knew—Patients #9 and #16 as valid data points, neither appeared as approved trial subjects.

In our clinical trial, involving a major lifestyle modification, the screening of potential candidates for the nutrition arm should have been a meticulous process, involving in-depth assessment of each patient's ability to eat and care for themselves, their home and social environment, their mental and cognitive state, their willingness to follow through with the prescribed regimen, etc. Obtaining informed consent, in comparison, is quite a simple affair, a basic tenet of every clinical trial. The physician in charge hands the form to the patient, tells him or her what it means, and they either sign it or they don't. The completed form goes into the chart, or if the patient refuses to sign, then the patient is not enrolled. If Dr. Chabot did not effectively manage this basic, straightforward and absolutely critical step in the entry process properly, we wonder why we should assume he better handled its more difficult aspects?

Chapter 4

The December 13, 2004 Group Meeting

Over a period of many years, we expressed our concerns about the design, management, and direction of this study multiple times via e-mail, in lengthy letters, and verbally at the regularly scheduled group conferences. Despite many promises, the institutional supervisors, including Dr. Chabot, took no significant corrective action as far as we could see. The situation reached a critical point during the December 13, 2004 session held at Dr. Chabot's office, attended by the various Columbia, NCCAM, and NCI personnel assigned to the project. There, Dr. Isaacs and I first met Dr. Jack Killen, introduced to us as a career NIH oncologist who had recently transferred to NCCAM, where he now served as their lead investigator on our study. Dr. Killen had come up from Washington accompanied by Dr. Linda Engel, a staff scientist at NCCAM whom we already knew from previous meetings. We were surprised to discover that though he was at least partly in charge, Dr. Killen seemed unfamiliar with the serious issues that had plagued the study from its inception.

At that time, Dr. Isaacs and I first became aware of the pronounced disparity between the nutrition and chemotherapy arms of the study in terms of the total number of subjects entered into each group and their staging distribution. It was also during that meeting that I first suspected Dr. Chabot might be more of a partisan advocate rooting for chemotherapy, instead of a dispassionately objective referee as required in his role of principal investigator. By the afternoon's ending I had become convinced that NCCAM no longer supported the clinical trial the way I once thought it had.

Early in the discussion that day, Dr. Chabot provided a graph depicting the status of the two groups, which clearly showed rather disappointing median and mean survival in the range of 7 and 9 months for the nutrition arm, far less than what we had observed for the patients we had followed for the pilot study. I wasn't surprised by the poor outcome since so many of those accepted for treatment with us had failed, for whatever reason, to follow the regimen properly. Somewhat unexpectedly, Dr. Chabot seemed pleased as he reviewed the data for the chemotherapy patients, showing what appeared to be unusual longevity for the group with a median and mean survival in excess of a year. These figures not only surpassed the numbers for the nutrition patients in our trial, but clearly exceeded any survival statistics ever described previously for any drug regimen used in those diagnosed with inoperable pancreatic cancer. Dr. Chabot referred to the findings rather enthusiastically as a "sea change" in the treatment of the disease. At that point, Dr. Killen—whom we had just met that day—suggested rather firmly that the project should be ended at once, with the results announced in a press release "as quickly as possible to counter the positive data of the pilot study."

To say the least, I found his comment unsettling, though not completely surprising. For years I had suspected that under its director at the time, Dr. Stephen Straus, NCCAM was increasingly unenthusiastic about this study or my treatment regimen. I had met Straus at a conference in Washington years earlier, shortly after he had taken over NCCAM's helm in 1999, and his behavior toward me verged on rudeness. And in several press interviews with major media outlets, Straus had been less than flattering toward me and the trial.

As for Dr. Chabot, I was not yet aware, in December 2004, of any possible conflict of interest on his part. But as Dr. Chabot and Dr. Killen lauded the advantage shown by the GTX chemotherapy, I continued reading through the various documents Dr. Chabot had distributed to us that day, trying to sort out the meaning of the data. I noticed quickly that in addition to the survival information, Dr. Chabot had provided a breakdown of the two groups by total numbers indicating that only 14 patients had been entered for chemotherapy, now five years into the study, compared with 38 for treatment with us. That disparity alone, with the chemotherapy arm only 37% the size of our nutrition group, obscured any legitimate comparison. In any clinical trial, the two arms being studied should be more or less equivalent in terms of overall numbers.

On his chart Dr. Chabot had also broken down the two groups by stage, the first time we had seen such information. According to the information before me, the two arms differed substantially in this regard, with far more advanced patients, that is, far sicker patients admitted for our treatment than for chemotherapy. I well knew that at the time of diagnosis about 75% of all pancreatic cancer patients showed evidence of advanced stage IV disease. In our particular case, of the 38 patients approved for nutrition therapy, by our review of the records approximately 76% had initially presented with stage IV cancer, the other 24% with earlier stage II or III. But the Chabot chart showed a very different pattern for the 14 chemotherapy patients, with 61.5% at earlier stage II and III and 38% at stage IV, a near reversal of the usual distribution reported among patients diagnosed with pancreatic cancer.

I thought this disparity quite significant, since patients diagnosed with earlier stage disease, as deadly as it might be, still live longer even without treatment than those initially classified at stage IV. As I looked at this data during that meeting, I realized this staging imbalance gave the chemotherapy arm a clear survival advantage over our group, consisting as it did of mostly stage IV patients.

Speaking to the assembled study supervisors, I pointed out that the poor survival data for those receiving our treatment meant nothing since so few had complied with treatment—a statement no one at the meeting disputed. I then said rather firmly that even discounting the compliance issue, the two groups could not be compared because they differed so fundamentally in total numbers admitted, and in their staging distribution. Dr. Killen, ignoring the numbers issue entirely, responded by insisting that the discrepancy between the groups by stage meant nothing, since all non-stage I pancreatic patients have the same life expectancy. Dumbfounded that a government oncologist could make such a statement, I argued the point. But Dr. Killen, with Dr. Chabot backing him up, did not relent even when I pointed out that the literature clearly showed that patients with earlier stage II and III pancreatic cancer live longer that those presenting initially at late stage IV. As the debate continued I thought to myself that Dr. Chabot, a national expert on pancreatic cancer, should know this.

When the meeting ended some time later, Dr. Isaacs and I felt frustrated, unhappy with the tone and direction of the conversation. On the long cab ride back to our office, we discussed what we perceived as a newly evident attitude among the study personnel to be done with this study once and for all and as quickly as possible—and show chemotherapy to be superior. Though discouraged, we were determined not to let Dr. Killen's behavior, and his suggestion to stop the trial, go unchallenged.

Over the next three weeks I composed a 29-page letter to Dr. Killen in which I described in great detail on a fact-by-fact, case-by-case and issue-by-issue basis, the flaws in both design and management of the project that I believed made valid assessment of my treatment impossible to that point. I specifically addressed the attempts by oncologists to undermine the project: the perpetual accrual delays, the entry of unsuitable patients, the effect of non-compliance among the nutrition patients, and the disparity in total numbers and in the staging distribution between the two groups that had just become evident. I also addressed Dr. Killen's assumption that survival had no correlation with stage for patients diagnosed with non-stage I pancreatic adenocarcinoma.

Below I excerpt the introduction along with several pertinent summary paragraphs. Note that I deliberately avoided placing blame on anyone, wishing to give Dr. Chabot and the NCI-NCCAM team the benefit of the doubt, hoping we might still work together toward a productive conclusion to the study. I was also at the time quite unaware of any conflict of interest among any of the supervisory personnel:

> Dear Dr. Killen:
>
> After the meeting at Columbia on December 13, I felt it important to follow up with a letter, to document my response to a number of points you raised.
>
> First I want to emphasize that those of us involved with the current study over the past five years—Dr. Isaacs and myself in our office, Dr. Antman, now at the NCI, Dr. Chabot, Dr. Grann, and Ms. Michelle Gabay at Columbia, Dr. Smith and Dr. White at the NCI have worked very hard to get this study off the ground and continue despite very unique problems, extraordinary bureaucratic demands and very intense opposition. We've had to deal with desperate patients, who at times will do anything to get into the nutritional arm of the trial, even if they aren't suitable subjects. Then, the hostility of oncologists toward our work and toward the study has led to difficulty with accrual to the

control group, and epidemic problems with patient compliance among those receiving our therapy. The IRB at Columbia has created, and continues to create, delay after delay so that over the past two years the study has been on hold more than it's been up and running. Dr. Chabot alone has invested days of his life dealing with the bureaucratic demands from the IRB as well as those from Washington agencies.

I believe, after many meetings and conversations about the trial we have all kept working toward a fair and reasonable study because we accept the prior evidence indicating there might be something useful in our treatment, as non-traditional as it might be, that warrants appropriate objective investigation. I thought it unfortunate that you arrived at the December 13 meeting apparently with a completely different agenda.

By my counting, on three separate occasions you remarked rather forcefully the importance of "getting the negative data" out quickly. At one point, you emphasized that this was particularly crucial because at this time, the only information "out there"—to use your terms—is the positive documentation in the pilot study. I assume from your manner you believe that the positive data is some unfortunate anomaly that requires an urgent counter-response. Not once did you ask any of us why there might be a discrepancy between the two sets of data, nor did you seem interested when I attempted to offer a reasoned, carefully thought out explanation.

Your implication is that somehow the pilot study data can't be legitimate. One would think that by this point, that issue would have been laid to rest, but I suspect some physicians hope for this to be the case since it would be the easiest and least annoying answer for them, even if it isn't true. Of course, if the first study is real, one must consider that the discrepancy represents not a problem with the pilot study data, but with some aspect, either in design or execution, of the current study. Frankly, I don't look at the disparity as a terrible problem, but rather an interesting scientific issue that needs to be carefully, calmly and unemotionally dissected so we can all learn from it. I certainly don't see it as a situation requiring the rapid discrediting of good data that may be unsettling.

At the risk of being tedious, I feel you've put me in the position where I must repeat once again the basics about the pilot study. This effort developed at the suggestion of the NCI, with the late Dr. Ernst Wynder serving as the New York supervisor. Dr. Wynder, who many consider the premier cancer epidemiologist of his day, had—in addition to his 700 plus publications—designed, implemented and pursued hundreds of research studies, ranging from laboratory investigations to expansive epidemiological trials. Most cancer epidemiologists consider his *JAMA* paper from 1950, the report that essentially jumpstarted his research career, the first convincing documentation linking cigarette smoking to lung cancer. Dr. Wynder was an expert in clinical trial development and implementation, and from the time he first began to mentor me in my own work in the late 1980s, I spent enormous amounts of time with him discussing research methodology.

As we all know, Nestlé funded the pilot study under the supervision of their Chief of Research (now retired) Pierre Guesry, M.D. Dr. Guesry, though not an oncologist, trained in pediatrics and immunology, and at a young age became Medical Director of the Pasteur Institute in Paris. Both at Pasteur and at Nestlé, Dr. Guesry directly supervised hundreds of research studies, again ranging from laboratory animal investigations to human clinical trials. Both Dr. Wynder and Dr. Guesry were involved, in a very hands on way, with the pilot study from the beginning.

Every patient entered was approved by both Dr. Wynder and by Dr. Julian Hyman, an experienced oncologist in New York whose son, Dr. Steve Hyman, incidentally, was head of the National Institutes of Mental Health and is currently Provost of Harvard University.

Inclusion criteria were very straightforward, and in each case the diagnosis of inoperable pancreatic adenocarcinoma had to be confirmed by Dr. Wynder and Dr. Hyman. Patients were also assessed for compliance during an initial lead-in period of eight weeks. Patients who did not follow through with the treatment, or did it briefly or incompletely during this time, would be removed from the study, though subjects who died within eight weeks of entry while actively pursuing the therapy would be considered treatment failures. These criteria were Dr. Wynder's suggestion, not mine. He felt a washout period was important in the pilot study, so that we would end up with a group of patients who actually did the treatment. As he said and as Dr. Guesry confirmed, there is little point studying patients with inoperable pancreatic cancer who don't do the therapy, since we already know what happens to them. Dr. Wynder emphasized that lead-in periods are used in oncology studies of chemotherapy agents, and in fact, were to be later used in the premier Gemzar study published in 1997 (Burris, et al: Improvements in Survival and Clinical Benefit With Gemcitabine as First-Line Therapy for Patients With Advanced Pancreas Cancer: A Randomized Trial. *Journal of Clinical Oncology* 1403–2413, 1997).

Quite deliberately, we did not require or even suggest that trial patients see an oncologist regularly, since our experience to that date had taught us oncologists in general were not supportive of our work and were more often quite hostile, frequently launching into personal attacks against me when my name came up. Certain well-known physicians at the time were actually trying to generate lawsuits against me, one even offering to help provide a lawyer to any patient who had seen me. Such behavior, though it might make for an interesting study of scientific bias, is not helpful to patients facing life-threatening illnesses.

Dr. Wynder, Dr. Hyman and Dr. Guesry assessed and corroborated the data, so there could be no doubt as to its validity. To provide full disclosure, in the final published report we included the statistics and survival information on every single pancreatic patient who had entered our office during the period of the study, whether they were included in the trial or not and whether they pursued the treatment or not.

Since several times you referenced the pilot study as a source of what apparently you perceive as unfortunate positive data, I think it important to remind you of the results of animal studies published earlier this year in the peer-reviewed research journal *Pancreas* (Saruc, et al: Pancreatic Enzyme Extract Improves Survival in Murine Pancreatic Cancer. *Pancreas* 28:4. 401–412, May 2004.) This report rather strongly lends credence to the idea proteolytic pancreatic enzymes have an anti-neoplastic effect. Nestlé also financed this animal work, conducted at the Eppley Cancer Center at the University of Nebraska under the direction of Dr. Parviz Pour, the scientist who developed the gold standard animal model for the disease. Dr. Guesry selected Dr. Pour to run the tests because of his international reputation and great expertise in the molecular biology of pancreatic cancer. Though this was my first effort designing treatment protocols for animals and we guessed at dosing for the inbred mice, the results were significantly positive in an experimental system Dr. Pour has told me was resistant to any prior intervention.

Then, there are also numerous anecdotal reports in the mainstream medical literature dating from 1902 confirming an anti-cancer effect of certain pancreatic enzymes, and the results of my own intensive investigation of Kelley's cases, pursued and completed during my immunology research training with Dr. Robert Good.

So much for the historical groundwork. Basically, we are left with a problem, because we have a study today that does not correlate or mimic the pilot study or the animal work. Again, I don't look at this as something terrible, but an interesting scientific conundrum that deserves a reasoned explanation. I would like to offer mine.

Of greatest significance, only a handful of patients, we estimate—even being liberal in analysis—no more than eight did the program fully and stayed with it. The most notable example of a compliant patient remains Patient 1 who is now three years from his biopsy diagnosis of pancreatic adenocarcinoma, and has enjoyed near total regression of his once widely metastatic disease.

So of a total population of 38 patients in the nutrition arm (discounting a patient who never did any of the treatment and disappeared essentially without a trace), 30 were incompletely, poorly, or totally non-compliant. Such widespread non-compliance, whatever the reason for it, is not typical of our private practice, and was certainly not evident in the pilot study. In that investigation, one patient did quit after some six months of good compliance, but the others stuck to the therapy well.

Dr. Isaacs and I have carefully analyzed the reasons for patient non-compliance in the current study, and certain trends emerge. At the meeting of December 13, we provided an updated survival chart that lists outcomes for all patients entered into the nutritional arm. In the column on the far right we summarize both medical and non-medical problems that contributed to poor adherence to the regimen. We also distributed a list of 15 patients who demonstrated significant non-compliance during the first month after being approved for the study. I would like to discuss this group first.

Of these 15 patients the great majority, we estimate 13, were simply too sick to adhere to the treatment plan. We estimate nine could barely eat at the time they began treatment with us. One of these, Patient 2, developed projectile vomiting before taking a single supplement because of a gastric outlet obstruction. Despite duodenal stenting, he could never subsequently follow the protocol.

Another seven who could hardly eat at the time of entry had already, from our perspective, deteriorated into the terminal spiral of the disease, when appetite precipitously declines. For example, Patient 3, after only three days on the supplements, required hospitalization for management of severe pain and vomiting, then quickly began radiation and chemotherapy. She never resumed her nutritional protocol. Patient 4, who at the time of entry had been diagnosed with pleural effusions, followed the therapy only intermittently after the first eight days because of poor appetite and repeated hospitalizations necessitated by pulmonary distress. Patient 5 reported very poor appetite within 13 days of entry into the trial, was hospitalized and discharged on hospice. He never continued the treatment. Patient 6, who had difficulty eating from day one on the regimen, developed a biliary obstruction within six weeks and never thereafter pursued the therapy. During the first appointment with Dr. Isaacs, Patient 7 reported severe nausea that never relented, and precluded any significant compliance with the supplement program. After being diagnosed with a gastric outlet obstruction, she underwent bypass surgery, but afterwards did not pursue the therapy. Patient 8 arrived in our office already on Megace because of very poor oral intake. Once home, he never could follow the diet, instead relying on Ensure for nourishment. I estimate he never got more than half the pills down, and deteriorated very quickly. Patient 9 had lost more than twenty pounds because of poor appetite over a several-week period before acceptance into the study. During my initial consultation with him, I never thought he would be able to do the treatment because of his severe anorexia and general weakness. He went home, began Megace, and quit the therapy within four weeks.

Patient 10, with extensive carcinomatosis, tried hard to do the program, but had so much difficulty eating I doubt he did the therapy for more than two weeks. He ended up doing his "own version" of the treatment, to use his wife's words, before pursuing the GemTax chemotherapy regimen at Columbia. He died very quickly, far faster than any patients described in the GemTax arm of our study. Nonethe-less he will be considered a Gonzalez failure.

Two patients could eat somewhat normally but never could follow the treatment because of significant concurrent medical problems related to their pancreatic cancer. At the time of entry, Patient 11 had a history of pulmonary emboli, and was so debilitated he arrived in our office for his first appointment in a wheelchair, with a resting pulse of 120. He appeared to us to be in the terminal phase of his illness, and did his therapy fully for less than a month. In our private practice we don't accept pancreatic patients this fragile, because we know they are too weak to do it.

Patient 12 also seemed to be in an end stage condition when first seen by Dr. Isaacs. Visibly cachectic, with a BMI of 19, he was so weak during the initial interview he could barely hold up his head. When asked about his appetite, his wife prompted him, "You're eating three meals a day, right, honey?" Within six days of his initial visit he was hospitalized for treatment of dehydration, and after discharge was promptly re-admitted because of coffee-ground emesis and biliary stent blockage. Then, while undergoing evaluation for PEG tube placement less than a month later, he was found to be completely obstructed. He never could follow the therapy.

One patient, Patient 13, could not begin his protocol in a timely fashion because of life-threatening medical problems unrelated to his pancreatic cancer diagnosis. Though presenting with multiple liver lesions, I thought, during my first session with him and his family that he would make an ideal candidate. He seemed very enthusiastic about our treatment, appeared determined to follow through, and his family, including his surgeon brother, supported his choice 100%. However, upon returning home, literally within a day or two, before he had even ordered his supplements, he suffered an intestinal obstruction, the result of adhesions from a laparotomy and nephrectomy performed for kidney cancer twenty years earlier. After emergency surgery for lysis of adhesions, he had a prolonged and tenuous recovery, complicated by postoperative pulmonary emboli. Because of such problems, he remained hospitalized for five weeks, during which time he could not adhere to the diet, nor take any of the prescribed supplements. After his discharge, he then valiantly began the program, some six weeks after I had seen him, but his window of opportunity for effect was long gone. I was amazed he lasted as long as he did, considering the long delay before he actually got started.

Patient 14's course was uniquely peculiar. Because of a long history of severe depression and suicidal ideation, Dr. Chabot did not immediately approve her for the trial, but instead requested she be seen by a psychiatrist for further evaluation since active mental illness is grounds for exclusion. Nonetheless, Dr. Isaacs did agree to see her and begin the treatment process before a final decision about eligibility had been made, so the patient could get started with the program. Unfortunately, the psychiatric work-up dragged on for a month, and though seen by us 12/20/02, she was not officially accepted into the trial until 1/24/03, **a full five weeks later**. During this period, the patient did not begin any aspect of the therapy because, as she told us, she didn't want to follow the regimen if she wasn't going to be a part of the study, and therefore had to pay for the supplements herself. Her husband also inquired if the supplements would stimulate her rapidly deteriorating appetite (they don't). Though quite debilitated, she thereafter struggled to follow the treatment plan and did survive 40.6 weeks from the time of her initial biopsy. In this case, her lack of urgency about the situation caused a critical loss of valuable time.

In the case of two patients, Patients 15 and 16, we attribute their disastrous non-compliance within the first month to psychosocial issues. Patient 15 misrepresented her family situation, had in fact no family support whatsoever, and quit after trying for two weeks. Patient 16, a problem from day one, appeared attracted to the study primarily because it offered, as he said, "free benefits." During the first session with me, he asked repeatedly for me to explain what expenses would be covered. I think he had hoped the grant would subsidize his rent! Though he never took a single supplement, he will be considered a Gonzalez failure. Patient 16 would never have come to us as a private patient, if he had to pay for it. I also believe a patient like this would not have been interested in joining the pilot study, which required the patient pay out themselves for the treatment during the first two months, until we were sure they were going to do it, and only then would they be reimbursed.

From our perspective, these 15 patients who never did the therapy or who did it very briefly, present a problem in evaluating what our treatment can or cannot do, since the total population at this point is only 38. I have already discussed at length with Dr. Chabot, Dr. Antman and Dr. Jeff White our concern and regret that the study did not allow for a washout period of even a week, that would have eliminated from consideration most of these non-compliers.

Toward the letter's end, I made the point that due to the lack of available intravenous formulations of pancreatic enzymes, we necessarily relied on oral supplements exclusively. As a result, to comply with the therapy, patients must be able to swallow:

It is true that even under ideal situations, there are some obvious limitations to our treatment as we administer it today. Most importantly, pancreatic enzymes, the main anti-cancer element in our program, presently are legally available in the U.S. only as oral preparations. Consequently, to implement the program, patients must be able to get the pills down. Patients in an advanced terminal state, unable to swallow, will not be able to do the therapy. This obstacle, however, could be overcome. With industry or government support, injectable formulations of enzymes, akin to more conventional chemotherapy, could be developed easily and made available for use with very advanced patients who can't eat. In fact, in the 1960s, a Dayton, Ohio surgeon, Dr. Frank Shively, learned of Beard's work with enzymes from the early 1900s, and with the cooperation of a local drug company, created an injectable preparation that he used in 192 patients with advanced cancer, with some very unusual successes. However, in 1969 [sic, should be 1966] the FDA prohibited their use because government scientists at the time could not understand the need for an IM or IV form of digestive enzymes. No one since has had the interest, or in our case, the resources to study the efficacy of injectable enzymes as antineoplastic agents.

I then presented the significance of the staging disparity—and challenged Dr. Killen's contention that stage at the time of diagnosis had no influence over survival:

Now, I would like to discuss the actual survival data of the "control" chemotherapy arm presented during the December 13th meeting. The results at first glance go beyond anything previously reported for any chemotherapy regimen used in the treatment of the *usual* population of patients with inoperable pancreatic cancer. But on closer study, the documentation may show something quite different. As I reviewed the stratification in both arms by stage, an interesting phenomenon, which we discussed briefly December 13, emerged. In the nutritional arm, 35% of patients fall into stage II and III while 64.7% qualify as stage IV [note: by Dr. Chabot's chart, which differed from our numbers]. I could argue that Patient 1, listed as a stage II patient, might be more accurately classified as stage IV, not stage II, so if we include him as a stage IV the numbers change slightly, to 32% as stage II and III, and 68% as stage IV.

However, we find almost the reverse in the control arm. Here, 61.5% are listed as stage II and III and 38.5% as stage IV. Though the numbers are smaller in the chemotherapy group, I nonetheless found this to be a very unusual distribution of patients with inoperable disease. In my reading of the literature, the breakdown for newly diagnosed patients with unresectable (non stage I) pancreatic cancer usually follows what we see in the nutrition arm: at the time of initial diagnosis, 25–30% are generally classified as stage II and III and somewhere in the range of 70–75% as stage IV. In the Gemzar study from

1997, the authors describe a similar distribution, 28% falling into stage II and III, and 72% at stage IV.

In our pilot study, 8 of 11 patients presented at diagnosis as stage IV and 3 as inoperable or locally advanced stage II, again falling into a pattern consistent with the described literature.

When I made reference to this unusual difference in staging distribution between the two arms in the current trial, you were dismissive, and stated twice that it doesn't matter since stages II, III and IV patients show no difference in survival. I was perplexed both times you said this. I keep up with the literature as meticulously as possibly, particularly as regards issues of staging and survival. Over the years, I have always read that the stage at diagnosis has a significant effect on survival, and I have never read what you stated, that staging makes no difference. I would appreciate your providing me with the specific references to support your claim, for two reasons. First, it's important to correct my apparent ignorance and misconceptions, but it's also important to rectify the misstatements of Dr. James Abbruzzese of MD Anderson, recognized as one of the scholars of pancreatic cancer, and the author of the section on the disease in the DeVita text (6th edition). I think we will all accept this book as a most responsible effort. In his chapter Dr. Abbruzzese writes in three separate sections as follows:

> Patients with locally advanced, nonmetastatic disease have a median survival of 6 to 10 months. A survival advantage has been demonstrated for patients with locally advanced disease treated with 5-FU-based chemoradiation compared to no treatment or radiation therapy alone. Patients with metastatic disease have a short survival (3 to 6 months), the length of which depends on the extent of disease and performance status. pp 1130–1.

> Patients with unresectable pancreatic cancer due to locally advanced or metastatic disease have a median survival of 6 months; this duration of survival can be quite variable, ranging from 3 to 14 months depending on performance status and extent of disease. p 1143

> Patients with locally advanced, nonmetastatic pancreatic cancer have a median survival of 10 to 14 months (with current chemotherapy and chemoradiation regimens). p 1143

As we can see, Dr. Abbruzzese describes a very significant difference in survival between locally advanced, that is, stage II and III, and metastatic, stage IV disease. He provides the appropriate references, those with which I am familiar. If what Abbruzzese claims is true, the very odd stratification in the chemo arm, skewed as it is toward earlier stage disease, in contrast to the more typical distribution in the nutritional arm, helps explain, if not completely, the prolonged survival in the former group. After all, in the third quote above, he reports a 10–14 month **median** survival for locally advanced disease with pre GemTax regimens. The extraordinary survival of GemTax, while potentially still unusual, becomes less extraordinary. But if you believe Dr. Abbruzzese to be misguided, send the appropriate references, which I will then happily send on to him.

When I finally finished the letter, dated January 7, 2005, I sent it off to Dr. Killen and copied all the study supervisors including Dr. Chabot, Dr. Jeff White and Dr. Wendy Smith of the NCI, and Dr. Linda Engel of NCCAM. Three weeks passed with no word from anyone—not from Dr. Killen, not from the NCI team, and not from Dr. Chabot at Columbia. I began to wonder if anyone intended to respond at all. Then toward the end of January, via regular mail I received a copy of a letter typed on official NIH stationary and addressed not to me but to Dr. Chabot. Dated January 27, 2005 and written in response to my charges, the note was signed by Dr. Linda W. Engel, identified as the Special Assistant to the Director, NCCAM, and the Program Officer at NCCAM in charge of overseeing the project grant. This document would later prove invaluable in confirming our position that the study's data had little if any meaning.

Dr. Engel began with a vigorous and I thought unneeded, defense of Dr. Killen:

Dear Dr. Chabot:

As you know, Dr. Gonzalez sent a letter dated January 7, 2005, to Dr. Jack Killen at NCCAM. In it he outlined a number of concerns about questions asked by Dr. Killen at our meeting on December 13. As the Program Officer in NCCAM responsible for administering this grant, I am writing to you now in response to that letter, because it appears that Dr. Gonzalez seriously misinterpreted the motivation for and beliefs underlying Dr. Killen's questions to the group. . . . It is possible that Dr. Killen's style of questioning—which included both attempts to clarify points of uncertainty and also playing devil's advocate—may have led Dr. Gonzalez to conclude that he had ". . .a completely different agenda." . . . We thought it important to clarify for you, as Principal Investigator of the study, key points raised in the letter in order to ensure that they are clearly articulated for the entire team, and so that the record is appropriately corrected.

After reading the letter several times, I wasn't quite sure what record Dr. Engel sought to correct, since in the paragraphs that followed she disputed not a single one of my allegations about the conduct of the trial or its meaningless data. As the following excerpts indicate, she seemed to accept all my points as valid:

> There have been numerous and very difficult scientific, operational, and procedural challenges in carrying out this trial. These have been well documented and frequently discussed.

> The results of the trial, as contained in the most recent interim analysis, are both surprising (control arm) and disappointing (experimental arm), particularly in comparison with the historical data on which the protocol was based. . . .

> In spite of everyone's best efforts, it appears as if the current design and implementation of the study may have resulted in accrual into the two study arms of patient populations that are not comparable. As a consequence, it is very difficult (if not impossible) to ascertain treatment effect with certainty.

> Given all of the challenges, the surprising outcomes, and the uncertainties about balance between the two arms, it is highly likely (if not certain) that reviewers of the data from this study will raise substantive and legitimate concerns about the comparability of the two populations. As a consequence, it is virtually certain that the controversy surrounding the study will not be settled by the data from it.

Dr. Engel then questioned the value of continuing the study as it has been designed:

> The December 13 discussion with the team was very illuminating in that nothing materially altered this assessment. With respect to the specific matters raised in Dr. Gonzalez' letter, we will make only two brief comments.

> We discussed at considerable length his concerns about the probable accrual of patients unable to comply fully with the nutrition arm of the protocol. It

was our impression that everyone in the room basically agreed that, despite best efforts, there is in fact, reason to be concerned about this issue, and that it clouds interpretation of the data. Even if we assume, however, that this is the explanation for the disappointingly poor outcome of patients on the nutrition arm, accrual of 15 or 20 additional patients to the nutrition arm of <u>this comparative study, as it is designed and currently being implemented</u>, would only be appropriate if there is a chance that the interim results would change. . . .

In conclusion, let us say that we have tremendous respect and admiration for the team that has worked with extraordinary skill and care on this study. We are also disappointed that the current study has not yielded a clear answer to the question that it was designed to answer. . . .

Despite Dr. Engel's opening defense of Dr. Killen, she had, in a few thoughtful paragraphs, summed up the significant problems with the trial that had left us, after some six years, with a population of non-compliant nutrition patients, two groups that were not comparable, and meaningless data.

Subsequently, Dr. Killen himself responded to me, in a one-page letter dated February 2, 2005. The brief note, written in what appeared to be a spirit of reconciliation, represented I thought a complete turn-around from his brash attitude during the December 2004 meeting. Though he began by bluntly stating I had misunderstood his intent, he then lauded the pilot study as well as the efforts of those—including Dr. Isaacs and myself—involved with the current NCI-NCCAM trial.

Dear Dr. Gonzalez:

I am writing in response to your letter to me dated January 7, 2005. I was dismayed to discover that you apparently misunderstood my intentions at our meeting on December 13, and also that I did not have an opportunity to talk with you about these matters in real time. . . .

First, as a medical oncologist who trained at an institution that specialized in treatment of patients with GI cancer (Georgetown), I have always believed that the promising results of the pilot study merited investigation. Fully aware of the prognosis for, and limited options available to patients with advanced pancreatic cancer, I have watched this study with considerable interest (albeit from a distance) for years before joining NCCAM. Now, having learned about its implementation and progress, I also understand that the trial has presented many big challenges from many directions, and my respect and admiration for the team that has worked with such extraordinary diligence and care on the study has grown immensely.

Second, I assume that my direct, "devils' [sic] advocacy" style of questioning created confusion about my motives. On this point I assure you that my intention was (and is) to understand as best we can all of the information that we have to date about the treatments under investigation in the trial, and also about how well the trial is working to answer the specific questions that it was designed to address.

I laughed when I read Dr. Killen's opening comments that so closely resembled those of Dr. Engel. She claimed that I had "seriously misinterpreted" his motives, he wrote that I had "apparently misunderstood" the same. Both referred to his "devils' advocacy style of questioning" which had apparently "created confusion." But I had heard exactly what Dr. Killen said, that the clinical trial needed to be stopped with words to the effect that a "press release should be sent out as quickly as possible to counter the positive data of the pilot study." These were not difficult sentiments to interpret, understand—or remember.

Other than pointing out my intellectual shortcomings, nowhere did Dr. Killen counter a single *fact* presented in my 29-page single-spaced January 7, 2005 letter, nor did he deny making the remarks he actually did make during the December 13, 2004 group meeting—as witnessed by Dr. Isaacs and myself.

Dr. Chabot did not reply to my letter, so we wondered what he, as Principal Investigator, might have to say at the next group meeting scheduled for March 7, 2005 at his Columbia offices. We were also anxious to meet with Dr. Killen face to face, to hear his "real time" explanation for his behavior during the December 2004 meeting. However, to our disappointment and surprise, Dr. Killen did not attend.

Interestingly enough Dr. Chabot, in front of those present, disputed not a single one of my facts or charges, but instead affirmed for all to hear that I had essentially "outlined the problems with the study." My letter, he continued, provided the basis for the paper that would be written about the project and its many difficulties, at the same time expressing his wish that Dr. Isaacs and I remain fully engaged with the trial. With our continued involvement, he hoped that the study's many acknowledged shortcomings might be corrected, particularly that more appropriate, more compliant patients might be accrued in the future for treatment with us, to help insure we ended up with meaningful data. I wondered, as he spoke so congenially, if Dr. Chabot feared Dr. Isaacs and I might just walk out and quit the project.

We agreed to stay on board, but in subsequent weeks and months, despite Dr. Chabot's expressed good intentions the trial continued as before with none of the promised changes implemented. The study remained on hold for much of the first half of 2005 during which time Dr. Chabot entered only one patient into the nutrition arm, who, like so many of the others he had previously approved, could not stick with the regimen. When reimbursement delays continued, Dr. Isaacs and I announced we would not accept any new patients for treatment until those supervising the clinical trial found a way to resolve the payment problems. And though by June 2005 Dr. Chabot had approved four more patients for chemotherapy, the two arms still remained unequal in terms of total numbers and the staging distribution. As a result, the data had in our opinion become only more muddled.

With my various concerns mounting, I discussed the situation with my friend Beth Clay, a Washington-based consultant on alternative medicine issues, a former NIH employee, and at one time Senior Professional Staff specializing in health care for Congressman Burton. Ms. Clay, who had followed our project's course closely over the years and had seen my January 2005 letter to Dr. Killen, had kept the Congressman up-to-date with the situation. Based on recent events, she now suggested I write Congressman Burton directly, summarizing the trial's ongoing tribulations, and enclose a copy of my January 2005 Killen letter.

I followed Ms. Clay's suggestion, subsequently composing a six-page note to the Congressman dated June 9, 2005. I began with a summary of my background and the study's history to date, much of which I assumed he already knew. I then discussed in some detail selected problem areas, reporting also Dr. Killen's statement made during the December 13, 2004 meeting that the study should be stopped and the negative results publicized as quickly as possible.

I ended the letter expressing my enormous disappointment with the project's current course:

> Frankly, at this point, despite my hope six years ago, I see no new era of co-operation between alternative researchers and the NIH and NCI. I have come

to believe the study was set up to fail, it is failing, and there is the possibility the illegitimate results will be used to belittle my treatment, undermine my 20 years of hard work and research efforts.

In January, I wrote a 29 page letter to all involved with the study explaining, and documenting in great detail, my grave concerns about the issues discussed above, the entry of inappropriate patients, the biased and unfair entry of mostly early stage patients into the chemotherapy arm, the attempts by oncologists to undermine and deliberate sabotage patients in the study. Though at a subsequent meeting I was told orally that my criticisms were valued and taken seriously, I have not received one written statement indicating any of the problems would be addressed or corrected, and in fact they have not been corrected.

I need help, because we are just two doctors against a wall of indifference and the overt hostility of academic medicine. I am deeply concerned of course that this promising therapy, instead of receiving the legitimate research attention any promising treatment deserves, is falling prey to the business as usual institutional biases we have had to fight for 20 years. I also am concerned that NC-CAM has in my many year experience evolved into yet another bureaucracy promoting institutional bias, whose goals seem quite different from the intent originally outlined by the Congressmen such as yourself who worked so hard to set up that office. . . .

I hope you might have a suggestion how to proceed. At this point, I have no illusion that the study can be made to work; I am however concerned that the meaningless data from a poorly run study can now to be used to destroy my 20 years of research efforts. This I know was not the intention of any of us when we first worked together to get this clinical trial moving.

Thank you for all your help in the past, and any help you can give me now.

As I awaited the Congressman's response, Dr. Isaacs and I prepared for the approaching June 20, 2005 group meeting. With my frustration mounting, I decided to e-mail Dr. Chabot and the other supervisory personnel, documenting in writing my many concerns about the study's floundering direction. Below, I excerpt pertinent paragraphs:

After reviewing recent events, I felt a note to those involved with the current NCI-NCCAM clinical trial essential before the planned meeting for June 20.

The problems that have plagued this study virtually from the outset continue, in fact seem to be worsening, despite repeated recognition and discussions of such problems among all of us. I see no indication that the course of the trial will change, and that the problems will resolve so that our efforts might actually generate useful scientific information.

I will try, this time, to be brief:

1. **Payment difficulties.** From July of 2004 until May of 2005, as everyone knows, financial support for the study was withheld. This repeats the previous pattern in which for many months every fiscal year payments are withheld, for any number of reasons. I realize these repeated significant delays affect not just Dr. Isaacs, myself and the supplement company, but all of Dr. Chabot's staff at Columbia. We have been given many reasons for the delays over the years, many of which make little sense to me; if clinical trials were routinely run this way, no clinical trial could ever be completed effectively.

While such payment delays do affect many, they have created a particularly serious dilemma for Dr. Isaacs and myself. As everyone knows, all patients entered into the nutrition arm of the study have been told that the grant covers the cost of treatment. We felt this was a particularly humane aspect of the trial, since insurance virtually never pays for alternative treatments such as ours. . . .

Because of this financial underwriting promised, we think it inappropriate during such delays to announce to patients they need to begin themselves subsidizing the treatment regimen. Dr. Isaacs and I, working with the supplement company, have during all such delays paid for the treatment out of our own pockets. At times in the past, when there were a number of patients following the treatment, such expense has presented an ominous financial threat to us. Contrary to what our critics think, we are not floating in money, our expenses are enormous, the supplement company sells only to our patients and has a very small profit margin. And contrary to what our critics have claimed, Dr. Isaacs and I do not receive any money from the supplement company, even though we have designed most of the supplements we use in the treatment. . . .

Though the above may be repeating what Dr. Isaacs and I have said before, we believe at this point it is essential to document in writing these points. And I think it crucial to document, as I have said before, that I have never heard from any researcher, from Dr. Good, to Dr. Wynder to Dr. Guesry, who among them have run many hundreds of studies, of any government supervised clinical study where the investigator must, for long periods of time, subsidize the study. I have never heard of it. Here, I would be grateful, if I am wrong and this is a standard or common occurrence, if Dr. Smith and Dr. White, who represent the NCI, and Dr. Killen, out of the NIH, could please respond in writing with the name, or registration number of any federally supervised, federally funded clinical trial where this has happened. . . . I am beginning to suspect that this is indeed a first for the various institutions involved, but if I am wrong, please send the documentation to that effect.

2. **The long periods when the study is "on hold."** Over the past three years, the study has been in hiatus far more than it has been up and running and accruing patients. I estimate in the last year, the study has been active perhaps a total of three months. Again many reasons are given why this situation prevails, but I find the explanations perplexing. Unfortunately, the fact that the study is on hold more than it is active is far from secret; as I have said before, word spreads quickly in the alternative medicine world, and the word is out that this study is a problem. In recent months, we have been contacted by patients with appropriately diagnosed pancreatic cancer who seem to be ideal candidates in terms of psychology and determination, who want to become private patients and want no part of the study, even when they are told it is up and running. I have taken on a number of such patients who are complying perfectly, and even though suffering advanced disease, seem already to be responding. . . . At this point, the delays, for whatever reason they may have occurred, whether deliberate or not, have effectively corrupted the study.

As I have not heard of any NCI-NIH study in which the investigator routinely must for long periods of time subsidize the effort financially, I am also unaware of any clinical trial that has been beset with so many repeated stops and starts, and hold ups and delays. I've never heard of it. I know there are studies with problems, I know there are studies that take time to get started, to accrue patients, but I am simply unaware of a situation in which a clinical trial is on hold more than it is running, over a period of years. If there are such studies, and if I am simply ignorant or misinformed, I would appreciate being corrected, again in writing, by Dr. Smith or Dr. White at the NCI, or Dr. Killen at the NIH.

3. **Entrance of patients unable to comply with the treatment.** Of course, in my January letter I documented at great length the large numbers of non-compliant patients who had been entered into the nutrition arm. Since recently,

the study has been on hold far more than it has been actively accruing, in the past six months only one patient was entered for our treatment. . . . However, within ten days, she had to discontinue her treatment, and was hospitalized because she could not eat. . . .

Because our approach is not a chemotherapy drug administered in the clinic setting, where all the patient need do is show up, because this is a self-administered life style intervention requiring the patient be able to eat, be disciplined and motivated, we argued from day one the need for a lead-in period. I know I have brought this up to everyone over the years of the study.

But the lack of such a lead-in remains to me a big mistake with the design of the protocol, in view of the nature of our treatment, and in view of chemotherapy studies, such as the classic Gemzar efforts, that allowed a lead-in for pain control. Because our protocol lacks provision for this, we have seen emerge a largely untreated group of very advanced cancer patients, with very poor performance status who misrepresent their clinical status, who are now officially "Gonzalez treatment failures." Although I do not believe, based on my original conversations with Dr. Klausner, Dr. Rabson, Dr. Wittes, Dr. Wynder and Dr. Antman that anyone at that time hoped to pass off an untreated group as Gonzalez failures to discredit my work, the effect could be the same. . . .

To compound the problem, we were not permitted involvement in any way with the selection of patients, which was to be under the direct supervision of Dr. Chabot at Columbia. Our exclusion from the process never made any sense to us, because I have personally been researching this therapy for 24 years, since I was a medical student working under Dr. Good, and I would have thought our experience would have been helpful to avoid some obvious pitfalls with unsuitable patients. Our input could have helped weed out at least some of the patients who were compliance disasters. If everyone agreed that we needed to be distanced from patient selection, a reasonable lead-in period, even two weeks, would have eliminated from the study many of those who could not follow, or chose not to follow, the nutritional therapy.

Because of these ongoing issues that remain unresolved, we feel that unless there is some sincere interest in changing the direction of the study its continuance in its current form will have little benefit in terms of evaluating the treatment we are trying to evaluate. I still believe that some involved in the study see it as a nuisance, best completed as soon as possible regardless of the inherent severe problems. . . . If those involved really are tired of this study, have had enough, are not interested in changing it, or for whatever reason are really not interested in a truly fair and reasonable investigation, just say so. . . . After the experience of the past 12 months, with the ongoing financial hold ups, the long periods of non-accrual, and then finally the accrual of yet another patient unable to comply, we see little scientific justification for continuing the clinical trial as it now exists, if a fair exploration of our approach is the true intent. If indeed institutional indifference to what we do remains so pervasive, either passively or aggressively, that no clinical trial of our treatment can be done properly, I think this needs to be known, so that other researchers don't run into the same roadblocks we have faced.

Two days later, on June 15, 2005, Dr. Smith of the NCI responded via e–mail, without essentially answering any of my questions:

Dear Nick,

We appreciate your note and look forward to a more in depth discussion of these issues at our next meeting, this Monday, June 20. However, we would like to briefly comment on a couple issues [sic] regarding NIH in your email:

1. In your email, you have a statement that "financial support for the study was withheld from July 2004 until May of 2005".

To clarify, financial support for the study was not withheld by NIH. Due to internal processes at Columbia, the money was not able to be distributed until certain requirements were met. That is, the funds that were left in Columbia's account for this project were not available for use until IRB approval. . . . It is our understanding that Columbia processed your purchase order as quickly as possible.

2. You requested examples of other clinical trials with challenging administrative issues.

Trials where investigators face financial burden: Each clinical trial is unique and it is between the investigators of each trial to work out their roles and responsibilities (and payment arrangements for salary and supplies, etc.). As the nature of specific financial arrangements are not mandated by NIH, comparison with examples of other NIH funded trials would not provide additional understanding of this specific situation.

Trials in which accrual has been interrupted: Again, we believe a comparison with other trials wouldn't help to understand the challenges in this specific situation. What is important is whether the interruptions in accrual in this trial were for rational and appropriate reasons. If these were valid reasons and actions were based upon real events (and we believe this to be so), then the appropriate regulatory processes and monitoring occurred for this trial.

We look forward to discussing all the issues in your email in detail. We know this has been a frustrating experience at times, but we are fully committed to support the research team in their pursuit of scientifically meaningful data.

As the June 20, 2005 meeting approached, Dr. Isaacs and I prepared ourselves to walk out if we sensed yet another "business as usual" exchange, or more platitudes about correcting past problems. The day of the session, held as per usual at Dr. Chabot's Columbia offices, I asked to lead off by reviewing my most pressing concerns, including the interruptions in accrual, the entry of patients unable to comply with treatment, and the payment delays. I contrasted the trial patients with several we had accepted into our private practice during periods when the study was on hold who were not only following the regimen as prescribed but showed signs of a significant positive response.

After presenting my case, Dr. Chabot—who chaired the session—once again adopted a conciliatory pose, acknowledging as he had before the points I had raised, expressing his hope I would stay involved with the study. He assured me he intended to accrue more patients into the nutrition arm, at least 15 to be exact, to offset the compliance issues that had muddied the data. He also agreed to listen more closely if we challenged the admission of any subject whom we believed did not fulfill the explicit entry criteria of the written protocol. In a further olive-branch gesture, Dr. Chabot said he had spoken to the Director of the Columbia Cancer Center, who promised to underwrite all future costs whenever the powers that be, for whatever reason, withheld payments. At that point Dr. Chabot handed me a one-paragraph letter he had himself signed, stating:

Dear Nick:

Because I appreciate your concerns regarding timely reimbursement to you for pancreatic patient evaluations, supplements, and enzyme preparation material for study participants, I want to assure you that there will be no interruption in securing payments from Columbia University. This study is important to all involved and as the PI of this project I will do all that is possible to insure its conduct and completion [sic]

Sincerely,

John A. Chabot, M.D

It was at this meeting that Dr. Chabot first reported his new plan, already, he said, in operation, to counter any overt or subtle hostility to the trial on the part of those physicians entrusted with locally monitoring our nutritional patients. Either he or a staff member would contact the doctors of each newly entered subject, explain the details of the trial, and encourage their cooperation. As I remember, Dr. Chabot told us one of his staff had spoken with the oncologist who had agreed to follow the nutrition subject admitted in April 2005, the first since this new outreach program had been put in place. Though the physician promised unbiased assistance, the patient had long since quit the therapy by the time of the June meeting.

Everyone attending, especially Dr. Chabot, said, as they had before, all the right things about correcting past mistakes while proceeding toward a fair and honorable conclusion to the study. But with Dr. Chabot's new promise to ramp up accrual into the nutrition arm and allow us some say in the selection process, we agreed, despite our six years of bad experiences, not to resign from the project.

During the week that followed, Dr. Isaacs and I awaited the minutes of the June session with some unusual interest, hoping to see in writing official confirmation of Dr. Chabot's promises, particularly his intention to accrue another 15 nutrition patients. Though Dr. Smith at the NCI usually sent the first draft within days of the meeting, this time around the notes hadn't arrived after nearly a month, even though I e-mailed Dr. Smith requesting they be sent. And despite the assurances from him, Dr. Chabot admitted no new patients into the nutrition arm, so from our vantage point nothing had changed.

Chapter 5

The Problems Worsen

On August 11, 2005, I received a completely unexpected e-mail from Dr. Chabot informing me that the Columbia IRB had closed the study to accrual. His brief note made no reference to the conciliatory statements uttered during the June 2005 meeting, especially his plan to admit 15 additional nutrition patients:

> Wendy, Nick and Linda. The IRB has reviewed our 6 month renewal application. They have closed the study to new accrual until the 10th death on the chemo arm and the interim analysis are performed. The study remains approved for ongoing data collection and analysis. jc

That afternoon I called Dr. Chabot hoping for some clarification. He only repeated rather firmly what the e-mail implied, that—at least according to my understanding—the IRB, after reviewing the current data, felt the study had reached its conclusion demonstrating the superiority of chemotherapy and had shut down recruitment pending the tenth death in the chemotherapy arm. At that point the IRB, after analyzing the data, would make a final determination about stopping the trial for good.

When I asked Dr. Chabot pointedly if he had made clear to the IRB the many problems that plagued the study, confirmed in Dr. Engel's January 2005 letter, he said he had not. I responded by saying I didn't understand how the IRB could come to a reasonable decision about halting patient accrual or the trial itself if kept ignorant of the many issues undermining the data. I also asked him pointedly about the 15 additional patients he had promised to enter into the nutritional arm to compensate for the many that had not complied adequately. In turn he simply repeated what he already said, that the IRB had made its binding decision, period.

As I thought about Dr. Chabot's e-mail and our conversation, I did not understand why he had failed to inform the IRB of the trial's many flaws and the weaknesses of the data, and at first, I wasn't sure what to do. When I discussed the situation with Dr. Isaacs, we both saw 20-plus years of determined, hard research, along with a potentially useful therapy, disappearing into oblivion, the victim of a poorly conceived, poorly managed study.

With my concerns mounting, I once again contacted Beth Clay, my Washington contact and friend of Congressman Burton, describing to her the most recent turn of events. She listened intently, before explaining that the Congressman, who had read my June note carefully, was still pondering the best way to help me. Nonetheless, she suggested, based on the rapidly changing situation, that I should write him with an update.

Following Ms. Clay's advice, I composed a lengthy letter for the Congressman, dated August 16, 2005, which summarized the history of the trial and more recent events. Below I excerpt the most pertinent section:

> You may remember that my colleague Dr. Isaacs and I agreed enthusiastically to collaborate with the NCI and NCCAM to have our therapy evaluated because it seemed at the time in 1999, that the government agencies were entering a new era of cooperation and open-mindedness toward serious alternative approaches. Of course, had I believed otherwise, I never would have become involved with any clinical trial.
>
> Initially, the National Cancer Institute agreed both to supervise and fund the entire clinical investigation of our therapy. As the study developed, however, the administrators of NCCAM, or the Office of Alternative Medicine (OAM) as it was known at the time, felt understandably that their group should be involved. Since NCCAM seemed seriously determined to work toward a fair and honest study, I was happy for their support.
>
> I am sorry to say that my earlier optimism and enthusiasm were completely misplaced. After Dr. Stephen Straus assumed the Directorship of NCCAM some

years ago, I could sense from my first meeting with him an immediate change in attitude toward me specifically, and toward NCCAM's original mission, to evaluate fairly promising alternative treatments. The recent negative NCCAM study about echinacea published in the New England Journal, and the earlier negative study of St. John's Wort in the treatment of depression have helped confirm my fears. Both these studies were filled with flaws and could not but fail as designed, yet were disseminated widely in the press as legitimate objective investigations. I became more concerned when after the echinacea report appeared, newspapers around the country quoted Dr. Straus talking about the various negative studies his group has supervised. I suspect there are those now at NCCAM who feel that their career objectives are best served by promoting negative evaluations of alternative medicine approaches. . . .

In January, I wrote a 29 page letter to all those associated with the effort at NCCAM and the NCI, carefully documenting the many problems we've encountered. A copy and a summary of that letter were provided to your staff. In my June letter to you, I summed up these difficulties. More recently, I sent yet another letter reporting ongoing problems to the various government scientists involved. Repeatedly, I have been assured that all wanted a fair study, but despite such promises, this has not proven to be the case. I was told on August 11 that the study is over [as I thought], despite the previous promises that it would continue and new patients would be entered to help offset earlier problems with accrual of patients unable or unwilling to comply with the nutritional treatment. We are therefore left with very flawed and meaningless negative data, that I fear, as in the St. John's Wort and Echinacea study, will now be used to say my therapy "doesn't work." I am concerned as I have been before that 20 years of hard work is about to be destroyed, with no recourse on my part.

Not long after I sent off my note, I received a perplexing e-mail from Dr. Smith of the NCI announcing the next group meeting scheduled for the afternoon of Monday, September 12, 2005. If the study had closed to accrual, as Dr. Chabot seemed to be saying, I didn't understand the need for further group sessions. What would be the point? Since Dr. Chabot had left for vacation, after thinking about the situation, on August 17, 2005 I decided to e-mail Dr. Smith directly:

Wendy—

Before John went on vacation he called me and told me the IRB had decided "since there was no change in the data" the study was now over in terms of accrual—to my astonishment—period. After the 10th chemo death, then we are permitted to evaluate data etc. but as far as the IRB is concerned it's over. I asked John if he has discussed with the IRB all the problems with accrual [sic], with delays, with non compliance in the nutrition arm, with the disparity in staging distribution in the two arms, and he said he had not discussed any of those things at all, just given them the data. According to what John said the IRB believes there is no reason to continue the study at this point, the "question"—to use his word—has been answered, whatever that means. . . .

I expressed to John what I have said many times before, that there isn't any data about our treatment that can reasonably be evaluated without some more compliant patients and some attempt to equalize staging distribution. Needless to say, I wasn't pleased since this is not what we had agreed to in our last meeting. His e-mail seems ambiguous but when I guestioned [sic] him on the phone he specifically said the study was over as per the instructions of the IRB.

Consequently, I was surprised to read your e mail about next meetings, since if the IRB has decided the study is over, why are we meeting. I know John is away, but perhaps you can call the IRB and see what is going on.

On August 18, 2005, a week after my conversation with Dr. Chabot, and two days after I had sent my letter to Congressman Burton, at the suggestion of Beth Clay I wrote to the NCI Director, Dr. von Eschenbach. I described in detail the ongoing problems that had, in my estimation, wreaked havoc with the project:

Dear Dr. von Eschenbach:

I think you will remember me as a participant in the NCI supervised clinical trial of our nutritional approach to advanced pancreatic cancer. In April of 2003, I wrote you at the suggestion of Congressman Dan Burton's office, after ongoing severe difficulties with progress of the clinical trial. As I said in my letter at that time, I can only begin to imagine how busy you must be, so again I will try and be brief. I wouldn't be writing to you again unless I felt absolutely frustrated with the course and implementation of this clinical trial.

After I first contacted you two years ago, I subsequently received a letter from Wendy Smith assuring me everyone was trying hard to get the study to work. Though the thoughts were pleasant, in fact nothing changed, and the terrible problems with accrual, with entry of inappropriate patients, with unfair distribution of patients in the two arms (chemo and nutritional), with long term suspension of the study because of paperwork shuffling and with delays in reimbursement, continued without abatement. After further complaints, I was again repeatedly assured, most recently during a June meeting here in New York as well as by e-mail that all those involved, from Columbia, the NCI and NCCAM wanted the study to succeed, and that we move forward, and compensate for what I have identified as multiple egregious errors in protocol design and execution.

Therefore, I was quite astonished when on August 11th I learned from Dr. Chabot at Columbia that all accrual has stopped as the IRB at Columbia feels the study has already adequately made its point. I was dumbfounded, since the project in my opinion has been conducted so ineptly that no fair or meaningful data exists at this time.

After summarizing briefly the origins of the current effort, beginning with the pilot study and its results, in some detail I then described six major problems with the management of the trial: 1. Entry of unsuitable patients; 2. Disparity in stage between the nutrition and chemo arms; 3. Attempts by oncologists to sabotage the nutrition arm; 4. Effect of non-compliance in the nutrition arm; 5. Perpetual delays in the study; 6. Delays in reimbursement.

My letter continued:

I want to assure you that all I have written you has been, over the years of this study, repeatedly documented at length in one form or another. I have expressed my concerns in multiple e-mails to those involved with the study, and more recently in at least two lengthy letters, including one of 29 pages which I wrote in January of this year. This I sent in response to a December meeting in New York, at which time Dr. Jack Killen of NCCAM, whom I had not previously met, announced in front of everyone that NCCAM wanted to get the negative data out as quickly as possible "to counter the positive pilot study data." At that meeting, it became quite apparent to me that NCCAM's motivation and attitude toward me had changed considerably. In any event, I have enclosed a copy of my January letter, which goes into great detail about the issues I have summarized for you now. I have also enclosed a copy of a more recent and briefer follow-up.

During the meetings in New York since January, no one, including, interestingly enough, the NCCAM representatives, has questioned or countered any of my charges, concerns or complaints. In fact, at no time over the years in any document has the substance of any of these charges or complaints been denied. Unfortunately, though everyone seems to acknowledge the flaws described, in practice nothing has been done differently, and the study has always continued as before, with no problem resolved—not the problem of inappropriate accrual, of selection bias, of the delays in accrual and in payments for the treatment. Instead, I learn this week that as far as Columbia is concerned, we already have adequate data and the study is essentially over. . . .

We entered this study with good will, in good faith, and with a sincere desire to evaluate what we believe based on our extensive experience, is a useful treatment for poor prognosis cancer. . . .

Beth Clay has assured me that you really want fair evaluations of alternative treatments, and supported our study. But those under you responsible for this project have not met the challenge. I am at the point where I feel if, despite your good intentions, the NCI as an institution had no desire to pursue a true or fair investigation of my treatment, and if I perhaps misread what seemed to be Dr. Klausner's serious interest, those at the NCI responsible for the study should have just told me, and saved all this trouble. I would also suggest in a broader sense, that if the NCI has no motivation to investigate promising "alternative" treatments, again, the NCI should say so . . . then Dr. Isaacs and I could have avoided this six-year nightmare, and now the potential danger this adventure represents to our patients and the future of our research. . . .

Personally, I want nothing more than I wanted 20 years ago, the opportunity to share my results with colleagues, and to stimulate legitimate research for the benefit of patients with advanced cancer who have few options. Dr. Isaacs and I have no other motivation.

I know that when I wrote you before, and when earlier this year Beth Clay spoke to Dr. Rabson [note: Associate NCI Director] about the ongoing difficulties with the trial, the questions went back to Dr. Jeff White's office for consideration. From my perspective, I don't think it's going to be very helpful to expect solutions from those who for whatever reason are part of the problem.

I appreciate your time, and look forward to a response.

Before Dr. von Eschenbach had responded, on August 28, 2005 Dr. Chabot e-mailed me, stating, with some apparent annoyance, that I had misunderstood him during our last phone conversation. He wrote, to clarify:

Dear Nick, It seems very clear from your communication to Wendy Smith that you misunderstood me during our last telephone conversation. The IRB does not consider the study over and in fact the study is approved to continue but not approved to accrue further patients until the interim analysis is done. I find it difficult to understand how you would come to the conclusions you write about based on our conversation but I want to be sure you understand I did not intend to communicate your eventual understanding.

I do not know the internal deliberations of the IRB. I will try to be more precise in my communications with you in the future and I respectfully ask you to be very sure that we understand each other before you quote or paraphrase me. john

Not surprisingly, Dr. Smith had shared my e-mail sent to her with Dr. Chabot. Regardless, once again I was being accused, as had both Dr. Engel and Dr. Killen before, of "misunderstanding" what I thought I clearly "understood" and clearly "interpreted."

Technically the study would continue as of course I understood, to allow for data analysis and wrapping up loose ends, but I had hardly misinterpreted the main point, that the study had been closed to accrual until the 10th death in the chemotherapy arm, at which time the IRB would review the data. In our phone conversation Dr. Chabot had also reported that the IRB would most likely not allow us to enter additional patients, a statement he did not deny in his August 28 e-mail to me. And nowhere in his note did he deny his failure to inform the IRB of the trial's many managerial problems—problems, as reported in Dr. Engel's official January 27, 2005 letter, that left the two groups not comparable and the data meaningless. Indeed, I understood fully that the study was "approved to continue but not approved to accrue further patients until the interim analysis is done."

To make matters worse, despite the promises made in June, we still weren't certain the payment issue had been resolved and after nearly three months we hadn't received the official minutes of the June 20, 2005 group meeting. As the next session—set for the afternoon of September 12, 2005—approached, we debated with ourselves whether we should even bother attending. We felt uncomfortable sitting through another one of these lengthy talkathons when we still had no verification of what had been discussed in June. And, to complicate the situation further, the NCI personnel had already changed the date once, creating difficulties with our patient appointments.

I instructed my staff to leave the time open on September 12 so we could attend, but allowed them to schedule patients earlier in the day. Then on Friday, September 9, Dr. Smith informed us by e-mail the conference had been moved once again, this time from Monday afternoon to that morning. We were exasperated since all the study supervisors knew full well that our patients come from all over the world, often with plane reservations that cannot be changed so it is impossible for us to start juggling appointments at a moment's notice. I didn't know whether the NCI hoped the move would keep us from attending, but regardless of intent, the decision had in essence been made for us.

On Saturday, September 10, 2005, I e-mailed Dr. Smith:

> Thank you for your note. Since the meeting had been originally scheduled for the afternoon, I had scheduled patients Monday morning that can't be moved again. I had already moved patients since the time for the meeting had been changed before. At this point, even if I wanted, I could not attend.
>
> More importantly, for reasons that remain totally unclear to us, we still haven't gotten the minutes of the last meeting. Why is that? And, why have another meeting when the issues raised in the past meeting have not been documented.
>
> As per my previous e mail, Linda and I see no reason to attend.

When I checked my office e-mails the morning of Monday, September 12, 2005, I discovered that on the previous day, Sunday, September 11, 2005, Dr. Smith had forwarded the minutes of the June 20, 2005 meeting. She now could claim that the June 2005 record had been distributed before the September gathering, even if the day before, and on a Sunday no less.

I noted that after discussing some mundane procedural issues, in the minutes Dr. Smith described asking Dr. Chabot to clarify the number of patients entered into the trial—an issue we had been trying to resolve for many months. Beyond that point, to our surprise Dr. Smith's official summary of what was said did not reflect, for the most part, what Dr. Isaacs and I remembered. For example, she wrote:

> Interruptions in accrual—Dr. Gonzalez reported that interruptions in accrual have been experienced due to breaks in funding. There are 6–8 patients who meet the criteria to enter the trial but whom he turned away because he was not assured of prompt reimbursement.

Her statement here mischaracterized my comments regarding this particular issue. Contrary to her claim, we hadn't turned any suitable patients away; instead we had accepted them into our private practice during the lengthy periods when accrual was on hold. Neither they nor I expected reimbursement from the grant since they were not clinical trial patients. I could not understand how Dr. Smith could get such a simple point so wrong.

She then continued:

> Entrance of patients unable to comply with the treatment—Dr. Gonzalez repeated concerns regarding patient selection; specifically there are patients who are are [sic] entering the trial who can't do the treatment and how frustrating that has become. Dr. Chabot stated that he was not aware of any subject that was entered into the trial that didn't meet the entrance criteria; however he acknowledged that a subject could meet the criteria at the time of entrance and quickly thereafter experience conditions that would have made them ineligible for the trial or impair their ability to do the treatment.

I had no recollection of Dr. Chabot saying at any time during the June session that "he was not aware of any subject that was entered into the trial that didn't meet the entrance criteria." First of all, had he made such a statement Dr. Isaacs and I would have immediately reminded him of the many patients he had admitted we believed did not meet the written entry criteria, including the three for whom no evidence of signed consent seemed to exist, or those entered beyond eight weeks from diagnosis in obvious violation of the protocol requirements. We would have countered the case strongly, yet no mention of any such debate appeared in the minutes since the comment attributed to Dr. Chabot was not made and no argument from us ensued.

During the meeting Dr. Chabot did, on the other hand, acknowledge that many patients accepted into the nutrition arm had either never begun or adequately pursued the prescribed regimen. Of this statement, the minutes report nothing. Nor did Dr. Smith record anywhere in this official record that Dr. Chabot had promised to enter 15 additional patients for treatment with us to help offset the many who had complied poorly or not at all.

Dr. Smith also included an alleged summary of my conversation with Dr. Chabot regarding his plan to contact physicians who would be monitoring our newly admitted patients. To my surprise, her version differed drastically from my recollection of what Dr. Chabot actually said:

Dr. Chabot stated that he asks each patient to confirm that they have identified a physician who they describe as supportive. He also now telephones the
physicians to confirm that they are indeed supportive (he has made these calls
from early on). His question to patients is "do you have a local physician who
is supportive and will continue to take care of you once you are home?" Michelle Gabay, the research nurse on the trial has left Columbia and interviews
are currently taking place to find her replacement. Michelle was in contact
with the local physicians and Dr. Chabot now makes the calls. In her discussions with Dr. Chabot, she didn't indicate that any local physician had problems with the trial. Dr. Isaacs pointed out that there is a difference between
a physician agreeing to take care of immediate needs and being supportive of
using the Gonzalez regimen and mentioned other stories of negativity from
local physicians.

According to the notes, Dr. Chabot seemed to be claiming that either he or his
assistant Michelle Gabay had spoken with the physicians of most if not all patients admitted into the nutrition arm to assess their attitude toward the study,
if not from day one, from "early on," whatever that meant. But at the meeting
Dr. Chabot had said something quite different; first of all, he explained the plan
had only been recently conceived and set in motion in late 2004, and that only
one physician had been contacted. Never did he imply that the plan has been in
operation since "early on" or that multiple physicians had been called.

Further along in her notes, Dr. Smith mischaracterized our discussion regarding the promised financial support from the Columbia Cancer Center, should
reimbursement be delayed for any reason. She wrote:

> Payment difficulties—Dr. Gonzalez reported that he has experienced sub-
> stantial delays in receiving reimbursements for patient-related expenses. Dr.
> Chabot stated that the Columbia Cancer Center will now reimburse Dr. Gon-
> zalez for the expenses of this trial (the subcontract) regardless of any funding
> interruptions . . . Dr. Chabot gave Dr. Gonzalez a letter stating this from the
> Director of the Cancer Center, Dr. Riccardo Della-Favera. . . . Dr. Gonzalez
> stated that he appreciated this and thanked Drs. Chabot and Della-Favera.

In fact Dr. Chabot himself, not Dr. Della-Favera, had signed the brief letter,
which nowhere mentioned the Columbia Cancer Center.

When I discussed the e-mail with Dr. Isaacs we were troubled by the errors—
such as the reference to Dr. Della-Favera as the author of Dr. Chabot's letter.

And we were perplexed by the alleged exposition by Dr. Chabot as reported, in which he claimed all approved patients met the written entry criteria, since Dr. Isaacs and I remembered no such statement from him at the June meeting. We also wondered why Dr. Smith would ignore Dr. Chabot's clear promise to enter another 15 nutrition patients to balance the many admitted who had never adequately complied.

The following day, September 13, 2005, I sent a long e-mail to all those involved, expressing my concern over the errors in the official record:

Wendy:

Thank you for sending a copy of the minutes from the meeting of June 20, 2005. Since they were sent on Sunday, Sept 11, we were unable to review them before your meeting at Columbia of Sept 12. Our comments are below.

We would like to observe that it is unfortunate that these minutes were not prepared earlier, as we would expect that everyone's memories of the events of June 20 are quite unclear at this point.

There are a number of very serious errors in the minutes. Under point 2, you have a question about how many patients are in the enzyme arm. So do we. For quite some time now, we have been trying to get copies of the consent forms of two of the patients on the enzyme arm [#9 and #16], most recently in an e-mail to Dr. Chabot dated July 27, 2005. We still have not received these, and so we will now bring up the same question we brought up to him at that time. If the patients have consent forms, we want a copy, as the subcontract we were required to sign requires that we keep them. If the patients do not have consent forms, we would like to know if they are included in the clinical trial.

Under point 3, we would like to correct the entire paragraph. On May 27, 2005, we sent an e-mail stating that since it had taken 11 months to get the payment mechanism in place for the fiscal year 7/04–6/05, we did not want to start adding patients to the trial until the payment mechanism for the fiscal year 7/05–6/06 was in place. . . . The six to eight patients discussed were treated as private patients during the lengthy period earlier in the fiscal year when the trial was closed for various bureaucratic issues having nothing to do with our decision in May. . . .

Under point 4, we would like to state for the record that we do not recall Dr. Chabot saying that he was not aware of any subject that was entered in the trial that didn't meet the entrance criteria. I have no recollection of any such statement in this meeting or at any past meeting. Not only do we, Linda and I, not recall this statement, but we do not recall having the inevitable argument that would have ensued had he said it. Nor have I in fact received any statement challenging my description of the many patients who did not meet the entrance criteria as discussed in detail in my January letter.

In the second paragraph of this section, you state that Dr. Chabot telephones physicians to confirm that they are indeed supportive and has made these calls from early on. "From early on" is vague, and most readers would assume based on your report that these telephone calls were made to the physicians of the majority of patients. Our recollection is that this policy was only put into place in the last year, and that only after frequent discussions of the hostility of oncologists toward the study were such calls instituted. Frankly, even if calls were made, they had no effect. Patient —, for example, one of the later patients in the trial, reported constant negativity from his oncologist and private physician. If his physicians received a phone call, it certainly didn't make much difference in their attitudes.

Under point 6, you report some information about a letter about funding interruptions. A PDF copy of the actual letter we received is attached. As you can see, it is written by Dr. Chabot, not Dr. Dalla-Favera [sic], and nowhere in the body of the letter is the Columbia Cancer Center mentioned. Dr. Chabot may have said what you report about the Cancer Center reimbursing for patient expenses regardless of funding interruptions, but the letter does not state this.

That covers our comments on the meeting notes. We would appreciate receiving a copy of the finished document and a chance to comment on others' corrections if any.

Days passed with no response to my e-mail, and no corrected copy of the June 20, 2005 meeting minutes. However, on September 23, 2005, I received an e-mail from Dr. Chabot ignoring completely my earlier note, announcing that the Columbia IRB had suddenly re-opened the trial to accrual. This communication would set off yet another round of e-mail exchanges between us, ultimately culminating in his announcement that the IRB had closed the study to further patient recruitment.

His September 23, 2005 note read:

Nick, I've been trying to reach you this week by phone to give you the good news from the IRB. We have been approved to accrue patients to the study. I have tried to reach you to discuss whether you are willing to continue participating with additional patient accrual. Based on your last email, I am unclear on that issue. You know my position remains that we should accrue in both arms until our study design dictates that we stop and we then carefully evaluate all of the conditions that may have impacted the results. I hope to hear from you soon. jc.

Though Dr. Chabot referred to my September 13, 2005 e-mail in this brief note, he made no comment about the errors I had identified. Certainly, he denied nothing.

Despite his happy tone, we felt reluctant to resume accrual until the serious errors in the minutes of the June 20, 2005 meeting had been addressed in writing, to avoid further misunderstanding down the road. So on September 30, 2005, I replied to Dr. Chabot:

Dear John:

Thank you for your e-mail about the IRB allowing accrual to resume. . . .

One serious problem, which I discussed in a previous e-mail, is a lack of interest in the study in patients calling our office. The constant yearly delays and suspensions of accrual have had a significant negative effect—we hear it every day. The posponements [sic] have injured the study perhaps irreparably.

Regardless, we would prefer to delay further accrual until some issues have been sorted out. We believe that this is an ideal moment to do so. . . . After the letter from NCCAM in February [sic, it was January], which expressed concerns that the study as it is currently designed would not answer the questions it was meant to answer, we have done a lot of thinking about this issue, as you know from our e-mail before the June meeting. In the absence of a lead-in period, and with the difficulties in matching the two groups for stage and performance status, we are concerned that the study design and the ensuing data are irreparably flawed. . . . We discussed the matter at the June meeting, but we had questions about the minutes of that meeting which have still not been answered. We would therefore suggest the following before accrual begins again:

Please give us your feedback on our comments about the meeting minutes from June. . . .

Please give us your feedback on the letters we have sent and the comments we have made about the conduct of the trial so far. . . .

We look forward to your written response.

Nick Gonzalez

In an e-mail dated October 4, 2005, Dr. Chabot responded, ignoring my questions:

Thank You [sic] for responding. I am concluding from your message that you are not willing to participate with additional patients while awaiting answers to these questions. I expect the interim analysis will be finished and reviewed by the data safety and monitoring board prior to completing a written answer to your set of questions.

From what I had been previously told by Dr. Chabot, I understood that when the Data and Safety Monitoring Board (DSMB), another Columbia group responsible for supervising clinical trials along with the IRB, began its "interim analysis" accrual would be suspended. So if the DSMB had already begun their assessment, I wondered how the trial might be open to recruit new patients, as Dr. Chabot claimed it was in his September 23, 2005 e-mail to me. So seeking confirmation of what he meant, that same day I wrote Dr. Chabot:

Thank you for getting back to us so promptly.

We do not understand what you mean when you say that "I expect the interim analysis will be finished and reviewed by the data safety and monitoring board prior to completing a written answer to your set of questions."

That same afternoon, he responded:

I agree, that is a reasonable request. The interim analysis is underway and I expect to hear from the DSMB this week as to whether the study has reached its endpoint. If that is the case than further discussion about accrual is pointless.

As I had earlier thought, the trial for all practicalities had not reopened to new patient entries except for a brief period of several weeks, and the promised 15 additional patients seemed now an illusion.

On October 9, 2005, I e-mailed back, wishing to state my concerns in writing;

John:

I appreciate your latest e mail, and explanation. So apparently the data is up for review at Columbia, the study is indeed on hold again, and the study can be stopped for good presumably if the DSMB decides the point of the study has already been made.

However, in our prior phone conversation from several weeks ago, you stated that the IRB had not been informed about the problems with the data as it exists, such as the inequality of staging distribution, and most importantly, the large number of patients in the nutrition arm that did not comply for various reasons. I assume they are aware the study has been tainted by the long delays and suspensions of accrual since many of the delays seem to have been because of the IRB. However, am I then to assume that the DSMB is similiarly [sic] uninformned [sic] about the nature of the data, and instead will simply have raw numbers and will make their decision in ignorance of the study's flaws?

I do not see how either the IRB or the DSMB can make any decisions without being fully and appropriately informed about the study amd [sic] the problems with the data. And I do not understand, even after our phone conversation, why the IRB had not been so informed.

In our meetings and in any number of our conversations, you refer to the "data" as if there were evaluable data. There isn't. As I've said before, and as I feel I need to say yet again, basically a largely untreated control group of largely very advanced pancreatic cancer patients who will be labeled "Gonzalez treatment failures" are being compared to what appears to be a predominantly earlier stage group receiving not only aggressive chemotherapy, but based on Dr. Fine's publications, also very intensive supportive care—beyond anything I've ever seen reported for pancreatic cancer—in contrast to the virtual lack of support offered the nutrition patients. I don't know see [sic] how the DSMB or the IRB can make decisions about the study without this information.

I am troubled, that during the last meetings we attended, your emphasis was "getting the study done." I know this study has been a difficult one for everyone involved but getting it over with because it's been difficult is not to me an appropriate approach; I would hope we would all agree that the important goal of any clinical study, particularly one as controversial as this, is to get it done right. . . .

The data is worthless. And no one involved in the study from Columbia, the NCI or NCCAM has countered my arguments or my facts to make me feel otherwise. In fact, Dr. Engel's letter from earlier this year, in response to my long letter, only agreed with my perspective on the data.

So where do we go from here?

Regards

Nick

Three days later, on October 12, 2005, Dr. Chabot responded, again with some apparent annoyance. At that point, with his hurried admission of 11 chemotherapy patients over a four-month period, he had, at least according to his latest revamped data sheets which he sent me, resolved the staging disparity previously so apparent between the two groups. By removing two earlier stage chemotherapy patients and adding multiple stage IV patients to the group, he had actually managed to make the chemo patients appear now more advanced:

> You have seen the stage matched survival curves. I do not understand what more you can ask for with regard to stage matching. The trial is being evaluated now because we met the stopping rule that was determined prospectively. Changing the rules we wrote now, at the point of data analysis would be impossible to defend. The 10th death on the chemo arm occurred shortly after chemo started, however it is not likely to invalidate the statistical difference between the groups. We will need to follow the remaining patients on study before any final analysis but it is almost certain that accrual will cease. I will keep you informed of developments as they occur and I hope you will continue to be actively involved with the analysis. jc

Dr. Chabot did not address the additional issues I had raised in my previous note, issues that had rendered the data meaningless as confirmed in Dr. Engel's official NIH letter. He had also failed to give us an explanation for the two missing consent forms—after two years of our questioning his office about the problem. So I responded:

John:

We just wish to clarify one point from your e-mail below. You say that you hope that we "will continue to be actively involved with the analysis." We would just like to make it clear that we do not consider that we have been actively involved with the analysis up to this point. All we have done is come to the meetings and review the information we were given.

We have, of course, provided the data available for analysis for patients on the nutritional arm. We have sent copies of all records generated in this office as they were created. This information was then put in to whatever databases are maintained at Columbia. We have made repeated requests for an opportunity to proofread the data, since various errors have been presented at meetings in a way that, quite frankly, does not inspire confidence.

We are still waiting for an answer about the consent forms for [#16] and [#9]. Do they exist, or don't they? If they exist, we would like a copy as is required by the subcontract we signed. If they don't exist, we would like to know if the patients are included as data points in the study. We continue to request them because, although your office was entrusted with the job of getting consent forms, as a part of the subcontract we were required to sign, I am obligated to maintain copies of these consent forms. Linda started trying to get these consent forms in the summer of 2003. . . . We have repeatedly requested copies, or an indication of their status, since we were instructed to treat these patients as if they had met the criteria, including filling out consent forms.

Regards

Nick

Five days later, on October 24, 2005, after all the cross talk, Dr. Chabot sent a brief note:

Wendy and Nick, Please note that per the DSMB recommendation, the IRB has closed our study to further accrual. We remain open for followup and data analysis. jc

So 29 days after Dr. Chabot's September 23, 2005 e-mail announcing the study had reopened to recruit new patients, the Columbia IRB closed accrual for good with presumably no knowledge of the problems plaguing the study. According to what he himself had told me, Dr. Chabot had not informed either the IRB or the DSMB about the trial's managerial shortcomings or its flawed data.

Chapter 6

The Battle Moves to Washington

W hile Dr. Chabot and I continued our heated exchange, NCI Director Dr. von Eschenbach finally responded to my August 18, 2005 letter. In his note to me dated September 30, 2005, Dr. von Eschenbach, like Drs. Engel and Killen before him, disputed not one of my allegations or the problems I had earlier identified:

> I have reviewed the materials and asked the relevant NCI program staff to prepare this response to your issues. Although the challenges of conducting trials such as this are formidable, I have every confidence in the NCI's commitment to proper management of this supplemental award to the Herbert Irving Comprehensive Cancer Center at Columbia.

> It is important to note that the specific decisions and responsibility for the conduct of this trial rest with the Principal Investigator, Dr. John Chabot, and many of the issues you raise in your letter should be addressed to him. NCI staff have observed Dr. Chabot's dedication to the completion of this trial and to a fair evaluation of the results. I am informed that Columbia staff have repeatedly taken steps to address many of your concerns, such as the effort and recruitment of additional staff to increase accrual in the control arm, and the commitment from Columbia to cover your expenses from their own institu-

tion funds to avoid any delays in payments. . . . It is also my understanding that Dr. Chabot has acknowledged the methodological concerns you raise, has offered to discuss these in detail, and is committed to considering the inclusion of these issues in the manuscript that will result from the trial. . . .

This trial has been challenging both scientifically and administratively, and it is because of NCI's interest and commitment to seeking out scientific evaluation of non-mainstream approaches that our staff have been involved to this degree. We remain committed to finding new and innovative interventions that will move us to a time when no one suffers or dies from cancer.

Sincerely,

Andrew C. von Eschenbach. M.D.
Director
National Cancer Institute

I thought it important to note that in the second paragraph excerpted above, Dr. von Eschenbach documented for the written record that "Dr. Chabot has acknowledged the methodological concerns you raise . . . and is committed to considering the inclusion of these issues in the manuscript that will result from the trial." While Dr. Chabot may have disregarded these "concerns" in his e-mails to me, apparently he had "acknowledged" these same problems to someone at high levels within the NCI hierarchy. Unfortunately, the director offered no remedy, only the same reassurances about everybody's commitment I had heard for years.

As my frustration mounted, I had a long phone conversation with Berkley Bedell, former Congressman from Iowa, who had long argued for legitimate government-supported evaluations of promising alternative approaches. Many years earlier Congressman Bedell had, in fact, first suggested the federal government set up the Office of Alternative Medicine. I had known the Congressman for some time, and after explaining in detail the difficulties which I believed had compromised the trial, he suggested I contact his friend Senator Tom Harkin of Iowa, who had also been instrumental in creating OAM in 1991. I had previously met the Senator over breakfast in New York in 2001, after he had addressed the New York Academy of Medicine. At that time he had urged me to call his office should I have any problems with any government agency in the future.

So, at Congressman Bedell's request, I composed an eight-page letter to Senator Harkin, dated October 17, 2005. I began by reviewing the successfully completed pilot study before outlining the history of the current clinical trial and its problems, including the flaws in the study's design, the lack of a lead-in period, the hostility of the oncology community to the project, the epidemic non-compliance among nutrition patients, the constant delays and suspensions, and the tardy reimbursement of patient costs.

A week after I sent the letter, one of Mr. Harkin's staff contacted my office, informing me that the Senator had taken a particular interest in my treatment approach, our NCI-NCCAM clinical study, and its apparent troubled course. The aide further explained that the Senator wished to meet with me on October 26, 2005 in Washington, suggesting, if possible, I bring along one of my patients. I responded saying I was most grateful for this opportunity, and would do the best I could in terms of his request that a patient come along, given the short notice.

That same evening, I spoke to the person I thought ideally suited the Senator's request, a patient with advanced stage IV cancer who happened to live in the Washington, D.C. area. This individual, who had already long outlived by years the original dire prognosis given by the best at Sloan-Kettering and Harvard, enthusiastically agreed to accompany me to the session with Senator Harkin.

The following week my patient and I met with the Senator and two of his aides in a large office off the main Senate chambers. Senator Harkin, who remembered very well our meeting in New York some years earlier, seemed genuinely disturbed as I recounted the obstacles I had faced with the trial, as outlined in my letter to him. After listening intently, he told me that he personally had grown disenchanted with the current direction of NCCAM, which, we both agreed, seemed now more determined to discredit alternative medicine approaches than evaluate them fairly and objectively as he and Congress had originally intended.

He then turned his attention to my patient, whose story the Senator found quite remarkable. An hour later our meeting ended, with a promise from the Senator that he would write to NIH Director Dr. Elias Zerhouni to express his personal concern about the direction of my study in particular, and of NCCAM in general. As I departed for Union Station and the train back to New

York, I felt somewhat relieved. With a powerful Republican Congressman, Dan Burton, and a well-liked Democratic Senator, Tom Harkin, on my side, perhaps we could at least salvage our reputations if not the study itself.

In the days that followed, I kept in close contact with Monica Knab of Mr. Burton's staff, who informed me that the Congressman seemed exasperated by the recent turn of events, disturbed that the trial had veered so terribly off course. He was disappointed our study was not the breakthrough project he had hoped for, that might finally bring conventional and alternative researchers together for the benefit of science and of patients.

Subsequently Congressman Burton wrote a lengthy and thoughtful letter to NIH director Zerhouni, dated November 4, 2005, outlining the various problems with the study and vigorously stating his own concern over its management.

Mr. Burton began by confirming his support for appropriate evaluations of promising alternative treatments:

Dear Dr. Zerhouni:

As you may know, for years I have been a strong supporter for integrating alternative and complementary therapies into our traditional health care system. In fact, during my tenure as Chairman of the House Committee on Government Reform (1997–2002), I initiated a formal investigation into the appropriate role of complementary and alternative medicine in the US health care system. The impetuous [sic] of this investigation was the growing frustration of many cancer patients who wanted to explore complementary therapies in conjunction with conventional cancer approaches or, at times, to turn to alternative approaches entirely but were unable to because of an apparent bias against alternative cancer approaches within the medical community and the government research and regulatory agencies. These perceived bias [sic] created barriers to advancing understanding of when and how various nontraditional therapeutic approaches were beneficial, which in turn impeded the ability of many American cancer patients to make informed choices about therapeutic options. . . .

Congress created the Office of Alternative Medicine in the early 1990s, specifically to investigate and validate alternative therapies being used around the world so that patients—particularly cancer patients—could turn to the National Institutes of Health (NIH) for accurate and validated information.

In fact, when the OAM was created, more than 70% of the callers seeking information were calling regarding alternative cancer therapies. Regrettably, according to the reports I have received, it seems that OAM is paying too little attention to fully and fairly evaluating real world integrated cancer protocols—failing in one of the core missions Congress intended the agency to pursue.

I would draw your attention to one particular evaluation project that I am aware of involving Dr. Nicholas Gonzalez's pancreatic cancer treatment. I personally spoke with Dr. Richard Klausner, the previous Director of the National Cancer Institute (NCI) regarding the importance of a full, fair and appropriate evaluation of this therapy. I was assured that NCI was firmly committed to carrying out an evaluation of the Gonzalez protocol with an open mind, and a clinical trial comparing the Gonzalez protocol to the chemotherapy standard was organized, managed by Columbia University and funded by NIH.

Unfortunately, despite the assurances from NCI, it appears from reports I have received that a fair and appropriate evaluation of this important protocol has yet to take place. I understand that from its very inception there have been numerous irregularities and challenges with this clinical trial that employees at both the National Cancer Institute and the National Center for Complementary and Alternative Medicine (NCCAM) have either ignored or failed to address in a timely manner. For example, I am told that NCI chose not to notify oncologists of this important trial. In addition, it appears that many patients encountered so much physician bias against the Gonzalez protocol that some patients felt intimidated and withdrew from the study. . . . Finally, and perhaps most importantly, I understand that there was a demonstrable patient referral bias in favor of the chemotherapy protocol—possibly setting up the Gonzalez protocol for failure. . . . Additionally, he [Dr. Chabot] apparently also required Dr. Gonzalez to accept patients who did not fit the clearly established protocol. Because of these apparent irregularities, Dr. Gonzalez believes that none of the data gathered is worthy of publication, and he is greatly concerned that individuals could use this faulty data to justify statements indicating a negative outcome, when no such outcome has been determined through valid scientific investigation.

If these allegations of irregularities are true, it is deeply disturbing. The American people, particularly the pancreatic cancer community, deserve far better from the NIH than has apparently been provided to date on this issue. . . .

I believe—as do many other Members of Congress—that the NIH does have an institutional bias against complimentary [sic] and alternative medical therapies. . . . I have no doubt that Dr. Gonzalez has devoted his life and career to helping patients with cancer. I understand that he has reported excellent therapeutic results, particularly with pancreatic cancer in patients who fit the protocol and follow through with the treatment. Furthermore, I understand that Dr. Ernst Wynder, a leading and well-respected cancer researcher, reviewed the scientific basis of the Gonzalez protocol and in his later years became a champion of both the therapy and Dr. Gonzalez.

I respectfully ask you investigate the circumstances surrounding the Gonzalez evaluation and determine if the allegations reported to my office are accurate; namely that the NCI and NCCAM have failed—and perhaps deliberately failed—to manage this trial adequately and insure a full, fair and appropriate evaluation of this protocol. I have taken the liberty of providing as enclosures each of the letters and emails that have been provided to me regarding these concerns and which were apparently outlined in a letter provided to the Columbia researcher and to the NCI and NCCAM previously. I know that you have many demands upon your time, but I respectfully request a written response by December 15, 2005 addressing each of the issues presented in the enclosed documents as well as an explanation and timeline for the resolution of any issues you deem to be legitimate. Furthermore, if you determine that some type of scientific misconduct has taken place, I would appreciate an account of the disciplinary actions you intend to take in order to rectify the situation.

Then 12 days later, Senator Harkin wrote his own briefer letter to NIH chief Zerhouni:

Dear Dr. Zerhouni:

I am writing to share concerns that have recently been brought to my attention about the conduct of research into complementary and alternative therapies at the National Institutes of Health.

As you know, I led the effort in Congress first to create an Office of Alternative Medicine with NIH, and then to elevate the office to Center status with the creation of the National Center for Complementary and Alternative Medicine. The intent of Congress in creating NCCAM was to ensure that NIH had the authority and resources to improve and expand rigorous scientific review of alternative and complementary therapies for treating a range of illnesses. More than one-third of Americans turn to complementary or alternative therapies each year to treat both chronic and fatal conditions, or simply to promote good health. These consumers deserve unbiased, objective information about the potential benefits and potential drawbacks of these treatments.

Unfortunately, in recent months I have heard complaints from individuals in the alternative medicine field that NCCAM has strayed from its mission of promoting objective, unbiased research about alternative therapies. Instead, these researchers and advocates allege that NCCAM—at times in conjunction with other NIH centers, including the National Cancer Institute—has promoted flawed studies seemingly designed to call into question promising therapies without fully and fairly evaluating the benefits of the treatment.

Most recently, I met with Nicholas J. Gonzalez, M.D., who relayed his concerns about a clinical trial of his nutrition treatment regimen for cancer. The study is being conducted by NCI and is funded by NCCAM. Dr. Gonzalez outlined his belief that NCI and NCCAM have, from the early stages of the trial, sought to discredit his work rather than conduct a full and fair investigation of his treatments. These concerns are outlined in detail in a January 7, 2005 letter from Dr. Gonzalez to John Y. Killen, M.D., Jr., Director of the Office of International Health Research at NCCAM. I have attached that letter. . . . I would like your assurances that Dr. Gonzalez's allegations will receive a full and complete review. . . .

My office received similar concerns earlier this summer after NCCAM published a study on the use of Echinacea for the prevention and treatment of colds in adults. . . .

While I do not have the ability to independently evaluate these claims, they are very troubling to me. Congress did not create NCCAM with the intention that it would serve only to validate alternative medical treatments in every case, but there was the expectation that NCCAM would be an unbiased source of information. . . . Unfortunately, there is a growing sense in the alternative medicine community that this is no longer the case. And if practitioners of alternative medicine believe their treatments will not receive a fair and unbiased review from NCCAM, they will no longer agree to work with the Center, and consumers will lose what Congress believed would be the one independent source of information on promising alternative treatments.

Meanwhile, the study team planned its next meeting at Columbia, scheduled for December 12, 2005. Dr. Isaacs and I decided not to attend, since we still had received no response to our September 2005 e-mail asking that the many errors in the minutes of the June 2005 meeting be addressed. If the official record remained uncorrected, we intended to boycott all future meetings. By this point we had such little trust in the official minutes, Dr. Isaacs and I agreed all communication with any of the study personnel needed to be in writing.

To our surprise, shortly after the December 2005 session, we received via e-mail a copy of the minutes. This brief document, slightly more than a page, lacked even a reference to the errors we had identified in the June record. It was as if our September 2005 e-mail had never been sent.

Chapter 7

Dr. Zerhouni's Answer

Subsequently, in a four-page letter dated December 22, 2005, Dr. Zerhouni responded to Congressman Burton. In his reply, Dr. Zerhouni devoted the first 2½ pages to denying, vehemently, any mismanagement or wrongdoing by Dr. Chabot or anyone else associated with the study from the NCI or NCCAM. The trial, the director insisted without hesitation, had been impeccably run, implying, not too obliquely, that my complaints reflected only my disappointment that the data had not turned out to my satisfaction.

When I first read the document, I was surprised by the number of factual errors and mischaracterizations that easily could have been prevented had Dr. Zerhouni's staff investigated the situation appropriately:

Dear Representative Burton:

Thank you for your letter, dated November 4, 2005, in which you wrote to me out of concern for the National Institute of Health's (NIH) management and evaluation of complementary and alternative medicine projects, in particular the nutritional pancreatic supplement treatment protocol initiated by Dr. Nicholas Gonzalez. NIH appreciates your interest and commitment to advancing complementary and alternative medical research. I have consulted with the National Cancer Institute (NCI), which currently administers the grant for this project, and the National Center for Complementary and Alternative Medicine (NCCAM), which currently funds the grant, regarding the issues you raise and would like to take this opportunity to address all of your concerns.

The NIH is steadfastly committed to upholding its mission of providing accurate and validated health information to the American public, for both mainstream and non-mainstream treatments. Working under this mission, this study was based on very encouraging pilot data, submitted by Dr. Gonzalez, to NCI's Best Case Series Program. These data were so impressive that both the NCI and NCCAM's predecessor, the Office of Alternative Medicine, worked together with investigators at the Herbert Irving Comprehensive Cancer Center, Columbia-Presbyterian Medical Center, New York, to carry out a more definitive clinical trial of the regimen. Over the years, both NCI and NCCAM have provided funding and have maintained very active involvement on the study team. Dr. John Chabot of Columbia serves as the study's Principal Investigator and Dr. Gonzalez is a co-investigator.

Unfortunately, it was necessary to abandon the original randomized trial design in April, 2000 when it became apparent that patients and practitioners would not accept randomization. A matched cohort design was adopted. While less optimal because it will ultimately limit our ability to provide definitive conclusions regarding the comparison of efficacy, this was a necessary compromise in order to obtain information about the regimen that would be helpful to the many patients with pancreatic cancer and their care providers. Now that the results of the first prospective study of his regimen are nearing completion, Dr. Gonzalez has made allegations of irregularities concerning NCI's and NCCAM's management of his nutritional pancreatic supplement cancer treatment protocol. Based on our investigations, we have found no evidence supporting Dr. Gonzalez's allegations.

Dr. Gonzalez alleges that NCI failed to notify oncologists of his cancer treatment protocol, thereby limiting patient recruitment for the trial. NCI did in fact notify oncologists of this trial through its regular notification mechanism, listing the trial in the PDQ clinical trial database. This database of clinical trials is readily accessible to both health professionals and patients at www .cancer.gov and can be searched using a basic search form allowing selection of type of cancer, stage/subtype, type of trial, and trial location.

Dr. Gonzalez alleges that physician bias against his treatment has been so strong as to cause subjects to withdraw from the study. There is no objective evidence supporting this claim. Dr. Chabot, the Principal Investigator of the study, and his research staff at Columbia University's Herbert Irving Comprehensive Cancer Center have contacted the outside physicians to confirm their involvement in the management of the patients on the trial and have not received any direct reports of bias or intimidation. It is our understanding that, contrary to his allegation, very few subjects receiving Dr. Gonzalez's therapy withdrew from the study or elected to change their therapy.

Dr. Gonzalez alleges that NIH staff failed to ensure timely payments to the private clinic involved in the study's evaluation, causing Dr. Gonzalez and his partner, Dr. Linda Isaacs, to carry the NIH-funded study protocol with their own financial resources. As you may be aware, there are requirements that must be met before NIH releases funds for any trial. Perhaps Dr. Gonzalez is not familiar with this process, but these requirements were adhered to for this trial in the same way they are with all NIH-supported clinical trials. . . .

Dr. Gonzalez has raised very serious allegations against Dr. Chabot in terms of the conduct of the trial. Based on his interest and expertise in pancreatic cancer, Dr. Chabot agreed to direct the trial after the protocol was finalized. We have seen no evidence to support Dr. Gonzalez's assertion of scientific misconduct by Dr. Chabot or his staff. It is our understanding that rules of clinical trial management were strictly adhered to by the Columbia research staff at every point in this process. The protocol was prospectively set and followed in order to avoid any insertion of bias. Dr. Chabot remained steadfast to the predetermined trial design and discussed with Dr. Gonzalez the critical nature of maintaining a predetermined trial design and assuring its ethical oversight by an impartial data and safety monitoring board, which is charged with deciding whether the evolving safety and efficacy data in any clinical study warrants continued patient enrollment, treatment, and follow up.

Dr. Gonzalez alleges that there was a referral bias in favor of the chemotherapy protocol by Dr. Chabot. We have seen no evidence to support this claim. It is important to note that consideration of enrollment in either the Gonzalez treatment arm or chemotherapy arm of the study is based entirely on patient choice and not assignment by the PI. Therefore, patient referral bias based on the PI's actions is unlikely. In addition, Dr. Chabot, a surgeon, has explicitly stated that he has no bias towards either chemotherapy or alternative approaches. Secondly, it is NIH's understanding that a statistical analysis of all subjects entered to date reveals no meaningful difference in stage or functional status between the subjects who chose to be entered into the Gonzalez treatment arm and those who chose to be entered into the chemotherapy arm. Dr. Gonzalez's claim may be based on a preliminary look at the status of subjects in each arm when very few subjects had been recruited to the control arm. Now that all subjects have been enrolled, it appears that there are no statistical differences between the two groups on these measures.

Dr. Gonzalez alleges that Dr. Chabot required him to accept patients who did not fit the established protocol. We have seen no evidence to support this claim. Dr. Gonzalez wrote the majority of the eligibility criteria himself. Based on these criteria, Columbia staff screened subjects before sending them to Dr. Gonzalez's office. Due to the nature of pancreatic cancer, it is not unusual for patient status to change within days or weeks. Patients who meet the requirements at the time of enrollment may experience changes in their ability to meet the criteria over time. To date, there is no enrolled subject who failed to meet the entrance criteria at the time of enrollment. It is our understanding that Dr. Gonzalez contacted Dr. Chabot to discuss his reluctance to accept some subjects in the trial. It is our understanding that Dr. Gonzalez's reluctance to enroll some candidates into the study was based on his subjective assessment of whether the patient would be a good candidate for his therapy and not on the predetermined eligibility criteria. However, the Columbia team was bound by the predetermined entry criteria set by Dr. Gonzalez himself. Adhering to these criteria was necessary to avoid any insertion of bias from any source towards either arm.

From my consultation with NCI and NCCAM, I understand they have taken repeated steps to address Dr. Gonzalez's concerns. The concerns raised in your letter have been raised and thoroughly discussed at meetings of the study research team and have been recorded in meeting minutes, as well as in correspondence between Dr. Gonzalez and NIH staff. NCI and NCCAM staff involved in the management of the grant supplement used to support the study have addressed and managed each concern under their purview. Other concerns more appropriately handled by the Columbia staff have been forwarded to Dr. Chabot for response. . . .

About two months ago, Dr. Andrew von Eschenbach, Director of the NCI, reviewed correspondence and materials received from Dr. Gonzalez with these same allegations and provided a thorough response to his concerns. In his response to Dr. Gonzalez, Dr. von Eschenbach encouraged continued communication between Dr. Gonzalez and Dr. Chabot. I also strongly encourage continued dialogue between Dr. Gonzalez and Dr. Chabot. Dr. Chabot has repeatedly expressed willingness to discuss with Dr. Gonzalez all of these concerns and, moreover, is willing to consider inclusion of the raised issues in the manuscript that will result from the trial.

At this time the trial is still active. While enrollment has ended, survivors are still being followed. Trial data is still being collected and a final data analysis has yet to be conducted. NIH staff have closely monitored this trial and we believe that a fair evaluation is occurring. Dr. Chabot and the Columbia research staff have expressed their commitment to the trial's fair analysis. Once the data are complete and analyzed, the trial will be judged in the scientific community through its publication in a peer-reviewed journal. Through publication, the scientific community will have the opportunity to evaluate any methodological concerns of this independent trial.

Because we are committed to the fair evaluation of potentially therapeutic alternative therapies, NIH staff have diligently managed this trial and provided the necessary support to ensure that the investigators can bring this trial to a statistically meaningful conclusion. We hope that the information we have provided is useful to you. Please do not hesitate to contact me if you have additional questions or concerns.

Sincerely,

Elias A. Zerhouni, M.D.

The National Institutes of Health, the federal scientific overlord assigned the responsibility of conducting medical research in many fields, consists of 27 individual Institutes and Centers, such as the National Cancer Institute and NCCAM, each with its own director and budget. Dr. Zerhouni served during his tenure as the ultimate czar over the whole NIH oligarchy, with its overall annual budget in excess of $28 billion—and increasing yearly—and its staff of over 18,000, including 6,000 scientists at the main Bethesda campus alone. One might imagine that with these bountiful resources at Dr. Zerhouni's disposal, his staff could appropriately investigate questions of scientific interest and, as in this case, questions of scientific integrity. Therefore, it remains to this day inconceivable to me that with all the manpower and money available to him, Dr. Zerhouni would have put his signature to something that at best could be described as misguided.

As a start, when I first read a copy of the document which Congressman Burton's aide had e-mailed to me, I could not understand why the director of the NIH would send out an official letter dealing with such sensitive matters without having his office contact me, either by phone, e-mail, or old-fashioned snail mail. One would suspect that in his position, he would want to review any documentation in my possession that might support the serious allegations detailed in the Congressman's November 2005 letter. For whatever reason, Dr. Zerhouni and his staff felt no need to communicate with me in any way at any time.

Dr. Zerhouni himself—or whomever he assigned to the project—did, however, speak to unnamed individuals at both the NCI and NCCAM, whose every word he seems to have believed without doubt. Nonetheless, nowhere did he mention Dr. Engel's official letter of January 27, 2005, written in her capacity as "Program Officer at NCCAM responsible for overseeing the project grant." In this review of the study's data, Dr. Engel denied not a single allegation in my earlier 29-page letter from January 7, 2005, agreed with the most serious—and rather bluntly contradicted Dr. Zerhouni's rosy assessment of the study's management.

To quote again from her letter:

> There have been numerous and very difficult scientific, operational, and procedural challenges in carrying out this trial. These have been well documented and frequently discussed. . . .

> In spite of everyone's best efforts, it appears as if the current design and implementation of the study may have resulted in accrual into the two study arms of patient populations that are not comparable. As a consequence, it is very difficult (if not impossible) to ascertain treatment effect with certainty.

> Given all of the challenges, the surprising outcomes, and the uncertainties about balance between the two arms, it is highly likely (if not certain) that reviewers of the data from this study will raise substantive and legitimate concerns about the comparability of the two populations. As a consequence, it is virtually certain that the controversy surrounding the study will not be settled by the data from it. . . .

> We discussed at considerable length his concerns about the probable accrual of patients unable to comply fully with the nutrition arm of the protocol. It

was our impression that everyone in the room basically agreed that, despite best efforts, there is in fact, reason to be concerned about this issue, and that it clouds interpretation of the data. Even if we assume, however, that this is the explanation for the disappointingly poor outcome of patients on the nutrition arm, accrual of 15 or 20 additional patients to the nutrition arm of <u>this comparative study, as it is designed and currently being implemented</u>, would only be appropriate if there is a chance that the interim results would change.

Her statements in her capacity as NIH spokesperson made Dr. Zerhouni's letter seem to me incomprehensible. I suspected, as I reviewed his document, that the NCI and NCCAM staffers he trusted so much had not shared Dr. Engel's letter with him. Why else would he ignore an official NIH report that proved my point, that the study had fallen short on so many levels that the data lacked meaning?

Chapter 8

Dr. Zerhouni's Letter: Some Initial Remarks

I discussed Dr. Zerhouni's letter at length with Monica Knab, Congressman Burton's aide, who suggested strongly that I write a comprehensive rebuttal, answering each and every one of Dr. Zerhouni's points. My response to Dr. Zerhouni, written on weekends and during my odd free time when I wasn't consulting with patients, took nearly five months to complete and ran 352 pages with additional supporting documents provided in an appendix. Though initially I dreaded the task, in retrospect the undertaking turned out to be a blessing in disguise, for while composing my reply I came to realize as never before just how poorly this study had been managed. And it was during this time, as I pursued my analysis of the trial, that I first learned of Dr. Chabot's close relationship with Dr. Fine and the Columbia research team that had developed the GTX chemotherapy regimen used as the "control" counter to our regimen.

In the following sections and chapters, I dissect Dr. Zerhouni's letter in some detail, extracting from, and condensing, the information as it appeared in my monograph prepared for him. His first paragraph, in which he thanked Congressman Burton for his inquiry and identified the various institutions participating in this clinical trial, appeared innocent enough. But in the second paragraph, which purported to be a summary of the study's history, the errors began:

> The NIH is steadfastly committed to upholding its missions of providing accurate and validated health information to the American public, for both mainstream and non-mainstream treatments. Working under this mission, the study was based on very encouraging pilot study data, submitted by Dr. Gonzalez, to NCI's Best Case Series Program.

True, I did present a series of cases from my practice to the NCI in July of 1993 as part of their initial efforts to evaluate promising alternative treatments. As a result of that effort, subsequently, the NCI suggested I pursue the Nestlé-funded pancreatic cancer pilot study. In 1998 during the meeting with me in Congressman Burton's office, the then NCI Director Dr. Klausner, based on the preliminary pilot study results, promised financial support for a large-scale trial. However, I never presented my pilot study data to the Best Case Series Program at the NCI, about which I know little and which as far as I know didn't even exist back in 1993. Had Dr. Zerhouni's staff called me, I would happily have outlined the true sequence of events.

The third paragraph of the first page continued:

> Unfortunately, it was necessary to abandon the original randomized trial design in April, 2000 when it became apparent that patients and practitioners would not accept randomization.

I had no idea what Dr. Zerhouni meant when he said "patients and *practitioners* would not accept randomization." We predicted that the study would never succeed with a randomized format because *patients* seeking entry would most likely not agree to receive chemotherapy. Our predictions proved true, so that after a wasted year Dr. Antman and colleagues changed the format to matched cohort. But it was the patients who would not accept randomization, not the practitioners.

The next sentence read:

> Now that the results of the first prospective study of his regimen are nearing completion, Dr. Gonzalez has made allegations of irregularities concerning NCI's and NCCAM's management of his nutritional pancreatic supplement cancer treatment protocol. Based on our investigations, we have found no evidence supporting Dr. Gonzalez's allegation.

Here Dr. Zerhouni evoked what I believe to be the sour grapes defense, i.e., I complained only late in the game because the data didn't turn out in my favor, as if I had never voiced an objection previously. But as everyone involved with the trial well knew, Dr. Isaacs and I had been strongly voicing our concerns about the study's design and management from the very beginning in 1997–1998 when we correctly warned that the randomized design invited trouble. From the beginning—not at the end—we argued that a clinical trial assessing a lifestyle therapy such as ours should properly include a lead-in period to cull out patients who simply could not or would not follow the prescribed self-administered treatment plan.

As the trial progressed, we complained repeatedly about those patients Dr. Chabot qualified but whom we believed did not satisfy the written entry criteria. For example, as early as the fall of 2003—more than two years before Dr. Zerhouni's letter—we first expressed our concern about the two patients admitted without any evidence of the signed consent required by the written protocol, Columbia regulations, and federal law.

In my January 7, 2005 letter, written long before the study's termination, I described in detail and with ample documentation serious problems, including the staging disparity between the two arms as well as the rampant noncompliance among our patients that had left us with meaningless data. So Dr. Zerhouni's statement that I began complaining only when the data failed to meet my expectations couldn't be further from the truth.

Returning to Dr. Zerhouni's letter, it continued:

> Dr. Gonzalez alleges that NCI failed to notify oncologists of his cancer treatment protocol, thereby limiting patient recruitment for the trial. NCI did in fact notify oncologists of this trial through its regular notification mechanism, listing the trial in the PDQ clinical trial database. This database of clinical trials is readily accessible to both health professionals and patients at www.cancer.gov and can be searched using a basic search form allowing selection of type of cancer, stage/subtype, type of trial, and trial location.

Dr. Zerhouni appeared once again to be misinformed. The statement on the official NCI website—referred to above as the "PDQ" listing for "Physicians' Data Query"—went up *only* after constant prodding by Dr. Isaacs and myself, and only after the study had been up and running, as I remember, for about a year. We thought the delay perplexing, since the PDQ supposedly provided information on all NCI supervised and funded clinical trials in a timely fashion.

Regardless, we never doubted that the NCI had included our clinical study on its website (PDQ), since we ourselves had insisted on the posting. But the NCI-NCCAM staff Dr. Zerhouni contacted undoubtedly knew full well the real nature of my complaint, that they had failed to send out the promised letter to U.S. oncologists urging their cooperation with the study. The government supervisors also knew of our disappointment that the NCI had never taken out the proposed journal ads announcing the project, as it has done for other studies, to help accrual.

The beginning of the first full paragraph, second page read:

> Dr. Gonzalez alleges that physician bias against his treatment has been so strong as to cause subjects to withdraw from the study. There is no objective evidence supporting this claim. Dr. Chabot, the Principal Investigator of the study, and his research staff at Columbia University's Herbert Irving Comprehensive Cancer Center have contacted the outside physicians to confirm their involvement in the management of the patients on the trial and have not received any direct reports of bias or intimidation.

Each of the points raised by Dr. Zerhouni in the above paragraph warrants addressing. As a start, the director denied that any patient accepted into the nutrition arm dropped out because of physician bias against my therapy or against the NCI-NCCAM trial. Before I address this particular claim, I would like to make a general comment about the pervasive antagonism in the medical profession toward the project. Dr. Herbert's direct attempt to undermine the study by filing, in writing, an ethics complaint with the DHHS—I have a copy of his letter—or his widely disseminated verbal assaults carried in the media should be objective enough evidence for anyone that such bias existed.

We also knew physicians at times actively campaigned to discourage patients diagnosed with pancreatic cancer from considering our study as an option, as discussed in my January 7, 2005 letter. In that document I provided specific instances of such harassment, such as the notable episode at a major cancer center in which the consulting oncologist, according to a patient interested in exploring our trial, exclaimed in words to the effect that "there really was no Gonzalez clinical trial, that it was a total fraud meant to con patients." The physician then tried to talk him into entering a pet clinical study.

I don't have a tape recording of the session, but the patient's very believable wife confirmed the story. In this case, despite the verbal harangue this young man did apply for entry and was admitted—though unfortunately, like so many others he was too ill to stick with the therapy beyond several days. Nonetheless, from him we learned, in vivid detail, just how pernicious physician hostility toward us and the study could be. We wondered in how many similar situations potentially suitable trial candidates, faced with an oncologist hostile toward us, simply chose not to investigate the trial or contact us.

Of course, Dr. Zerhouni, in the above quote, specifically denied that any patient *withdrew* from the study because of physician bias. In response to this point, in my January 7, 2005 letter to Killen I discussed five participants who dropped out for precisely this reason. This antagonism took several forms, including overt ranting as well as more subtle prodding to forgo the nutritional regimen and change over to a more conventional treatment. Here I excerpt the relevant section:

> Patient 23, with a long history of depression, was on high doses of two antidepressants when first seen in our office. Though the protocol for the study precludes entry of patients with psychiatric illness, she was nonetheless admitted to the nutrition arm. From the day she started our treatment, her local oncologist badgered her to quit the protocol and instead begin chemotherapy. She followed his advice, and died. . . .

> Patient 27, who is now out more than 14 months, did the program well for the first six months after entry, but began feeling so well he unfortunately slacked off the supplements. On a reduced program, his situation quickly deteriorated. His local oncologist, who had been negative about our therapy even when the patient was doing well, repeatedly emphasized that "it (our treatment) isn't working." Patient 27 never resumed our therapy fully, eventually quitting completely before trying Gemzar. However, he became so ill on chemotherapy he refused to continue after only a few sessions and currently is doing no treatment.

> In the case of Patient 29, her local physicians effectively convinced her the situation was hopeless, and that she would be "dead any day." After a brief effort, she quit the program so she could eat whatever she wanted for whatever time remained. She felt there was no reason to try, and died less than two months later.

> Two patients—Patient 30 and Patient 31—quit the program after relentless pressure by their oncologists to do chemotherapy, or in the case of Patient 30,

vaccine treatment. Patient 30 did follow the program fairly well for at least a year, before quitting. I say fairly well, because she was only at best partially compliant with the diet. She liked to eat what she wanted, and tended easily to fall off the prescribed diet.

In my Killen letter I did discuss the one and only patient whose doctors, at least most of the time, supported his choice of an alternative treatment:

The only patient in our current study that I can say has for the most part enjoyed the support of his local physicians has been our star Patient 1, who was career military, and whose primary oncologists and gastroenterologists are all salaried officers in the Air Force. Frankly, they have no financial incentive to get the patient off the trial and onto chemotherapy, and seem to have no emotional incentive either. To the contrary, from the beginning his doctors have for the most part encouraged him, have done everything needed to help him, and generally have done nothing medically without discussing it with me. Their help has been invaluable since Patient 1 lives in —, and initially, with his advanced disease and unstable diabetes, had a very rocky course. Their astute and appropriate interventions, usually with the goal to keep him on this clinical trial, have helped him stay alive now three years since diagnosis. But even in this case, the going has not always been so smooth. Several months ago, Patient 1's previous oncologist, who had been quite supportive, was transferred to another base. The new oncologist Patient 1 now sees regularly has been cooperative, but has expressed, according to the patient, no interest in the treatment, in his prolonged survival, or in the clinical trial. But nonetheless, Patient 1 should teach us that cooperative doctors can make a difference, in fact a significant difference in patient compliance, and patient survival.

The above examples illustrate that bias against us existed, that it probably dissuaded suitable patients from considering the trial as an option, and that five subjects entered into the nutrition arm—#23, 27, 29, 30, and 31 by our identifiers—withdrew directly as a result of it. It's important to remember that none of the supervisors of the project, including Dr. Chabot, ever challenged or questioned my assessment of these patients as described in my January 7, 2005 letter to Killen.

Reading the above quotation from Zerhouni's letter, one might believe that Dr. Chabot or his staff had been contacting the local physicians of our patients since the study began. In fact we first suggested Dr. Chabot intervene for this purpose years into the study, when physician bias remained such a persistent problem. Based on his own statements, Dr. Chabot did not put the plan into action until late 2004, after 38 patients had already been admitted into the nutrition group. And, he intended to call only those physicians of newly qualified subjects, not those already dead or actively being treated. As far as I know—though the story seemed to change—his office contacted only one such physician, who denied any bias. Regardless, in this case the patient could not follow through with the therapy.

Chapter 9

Withdrawal of Patients from the Clinical Trial

D r. Zerhouni's letter continued:

It is our understanding that, contrary to his allegation, very few subjects receiving Dr. Gonzalez's therapy withdrew from the study or elected to change their therapy.

His statement requires two responses, the first to address the total number of patients who dropped out for whatever reason, and the second, to document the number who quit specifically to change treatment. The numbers on both counts are hardly "few."

In the following section, I evaluate all those who withdrew from the study. For my Zerhouni monograph I divided these patients into two groups, the first consisting of those who never started the prescribed nutritional regimen or who stopped it within a month, and the second, those who followed the regimen for more than four weeks before discontinuing treatment.

Patients who never began the therapy or quit within a month: In my January 7, 2005 letter I described 13 patients who never began the therapy after being approved for entry or who initially pursued treatment but then discontinued it within a month:

One of these, Patient 2, developed projectile vomiting before taking a single supplement because of a gastric outlet obstruction. Despite duodenal stenting, he could never subsequently follow the protocol.

Another seven who could hardly eat at the time of entry had already, from our perspective, deteriorated into the terminal spiral of the disease, when appetite precipitously declines. For example, Patient #3, after only three days on the supplements, required hospitalization for management of severe pain and vomiting, then quickly began radiation and chemotherapy. She never resumed her nutritional protocol.

Patient 4, who at the time of entry had been diagnosed with pleural effusions, followed the therapy only intermittently after the first eight days because of poor appetite and repeated hospitalizations necessitated by pulmonary distress.

Patient 5 reported very poor appetite within 13 days of entry into the trial, was hospitalized and discharged on hospice. He never continued the treatment.

Patient 6, who had difficulty eating from day one on the regimen, developed a biliary obstruction within six weeks and never thereafter pursued the therapy.

During the first appointment with Dr. Isaacs, Patient 7 reported severe nausea that never relented, and precluded any significant compliance with the supplement program. After being diagnosed with a gastric outlet obstruction, she underwent bypass surgery, but afterwards did not pursue the therapy.

Patient 8 arrived in our office already on Megace because of very poor oral intake. Once home, he never could follow the diet, instead relying on Ensure for nourishment. I estimate he never got more than half the pills down, and deteriorated very quickly.

Patient 9 had lost more than twenty pounds because of poor appetite over a several-week period before acceptance into the study. During my initial consultation with him, I never thought he would be able to do the treatment because of his severe anorexia and general weakness. He went home, began Megace, and quit the therapy within four weeks.

Patient 10, with extensive carcinomatosis, tried hard to do the program, but had so much difficulty eating I doubt he did the therapy for more than two weeks. He ended up doing his "own version" of the treatment, to use his wife's words, before pursuing the GemTax chemotherapy regimen at Columbia. He died very quickly, far faster than any patients described in the GemTax arm of our study. Nonetheless he will be considered a Gonzalez failure.

Two patients could eat somewhat normally but never could follow the treatment because of significant concurrent medical problems related to their pancreatic cancer. At the time of entry, Patient 11 had a history of pulmonary emboli, and was so debilitated he arrived in our office for his first appointment in a wheelchair, with a resting pulse of 120. He appeared to us to be in the terminal phase of his illness, and did his therapy fully for less than a month. In our private practice we don't accept pancreatic patients this fragile, because we know they are too weak to do it.

Patient 12 also seemed to be in an end stage condition when first seen by Dr. Isaacs. Visibly cachectic, with a BMI of 19, he was so weak during the initial interview he could barely hold up his head. When asked about his appetite, his wife prompted him, "You're eating three meals a day, right, honey?" Within six days of his initial visit he was hospitalized for treatment of dehydration, and after discharge was promptly re-admitted because of coffee-ground emesis and biliary stent blockage. Then, while undergoing evaluation for PEG tube placement less than a month later, he was found to be completely obstructed. He never could follow the therapy.

In the case of two patients, Patients 15 and 16, we attribute their disastrous non-compliance within the first month to psychosocial issues. Patient 15 misrepresented her family situation, had in fact no family support whatsoever, and quit after trying for two weeks.

Patient 16, a problem from day one, appeared attracted to the study primarily because it offered, as he said, "free benefits." During the first session with me, he asked repeatedly for me to explain what expenses would be covered. I think he had hoped the grant would subsidize his rent! Though he never took a single supplement, he will be considered a Gonzalez failure.

Patient 16 would never have come to us as a private patient, if he had to pay for it. I also believe a patient like this would not have been interested in joining the pilot study, which required the patient pay out themselves for the treatment during the first two months, until we were sure they were going to do it, and only then would they be reimbursed.

Dr. Chabot admitted the final nutrition patient, #39, in April of 2005, four months after my January 7, 2005 Killen letter had been written and sent, so she was not included in the above discussion. Regardless, within ten days of beginning treatment, this unfortunate woman quit the trial because of an esophageal stricture associated with severe, painful inflammation. Unable to resume her nutritional regimen, she chose to pursue aggressive chemotherapy before dying three months after her formal entry.

So in total, 14 patients never started the nutritional therapy or quit within the first month. Of these, 12—patients # 2, 3, 4, 5, 6, 7, 8, 9, 10, 11, 12 and 39—dropped out for largely if not entirely physical reasons, that is, they were too sick to follow the regimen for any length of time. Another two—patients #15 and 16—did not begin or quit due a social situation or psychological problems that helped undermine compliance with the therapy plan. Two of these 14—patients #2 and 16—never took a single supplement.

Patients who followed the regimen for more than four weeks before quitting: For my Zerhouni manuscript, I also included a section from my January 7, 2005 letter describing nine patients who complied with the prescribed regimen for at least four weeks, but subsequently withdrew from the study:

> Patient 18, who at the time of diagnosis had some 15 tumors in her liver, after beginning her treatment developed severe, unrelenting pain that persisted despite high dose morphine. Her [local] doctors seemed unable to get the problem under control, and eventually, because of nausea and loss of appetite, she quit the program. Despite these difficulties and her terrible disease at the time of presentation she survived seven plus months from diagnosis.

> Two patients, 23 and 24, quit the program within two months after each developed pulmonary emboli. Patient 23, with a long history of depression, was on high doses of two antidepressants when first seen in our office. Though the protocol for the study precludes entry of patients with psychiatric illness, she was nonetheless admitted to the nutrition arm. From the day she started our treatment, her local oncologist badgered her to quit the protocol and instead begin chemotherapy. She followed his advice, and died.

> Patient 26 lacked the internal resources to follow the program, though we have not included her in the initially non-compliant group. She never seemed to understand even the simplest aspects of the program . . . .

Patient 27, who is now out more than 14 months, did the program well for the first six months after entry, but began feeling so well he unfortunately slacked off the supplements. On a reduced program, his situation quickly deteriorated. His local oncologist, who had been negative about our therapy even when the patient was doing well, repeatedly emphasized that "it (our treatment) isn't working." Patient 27 never resumed our therapy fully, eventually quitting completely before trying Gemzar. However, he became so ill on chemotherapy he refused to continue after only a few sessions and currently is doing no treatment.

Patient 28, who is now more than two years out from her diagnosis, complied well for the first four months on trial, until she developed a gastric outlet obstruction. After surgery, she then resumed the program but then lapsed into a depression brought on by family problems. She had no support as far as we can tell for her treatment choice and eventually quit before proceeding with a course of Gemzar. She is not doing great, but is still alive.

In the case of Patient 29, her local physicians effectively convinced her the situation was hopeless, and that she would be "dead any day." After a brief effort, she quit the program so she could eat whatever she wanted for whatever time remained. She felt there was no reason to try, and died less than two months later.

Two patients—Patient 30 and Patient 31—quit the program after relentless pressure by their oncologists to do chemotherapy, or in the case of Patient 30, vaccine treatment. Patient 30 did follow the program fairly well for at least a year, before quitting. I say fairly well, because she was only at best partially compliant with the diet. She liked to eat what she wanted, and tended easily to fall off the prescribed diet.

Overall, at best eight patients—32, 33, 34, 35, 36, 37, 38, and Patient 1—might be considered to have stuck with the program as prescribed fairly well, though even among this group, compliance often deteriorated. Patient 32 for example was in and out of her local hospital because of recurrent stent infections, and when hospitalized she could not pursue her treatment. Patient 36 initially did well, with regression of most of his liver metastases, but then decided to tour the U.S. in an RV, despite our arguments against such an expedition. While traveling, he developed a gastric outlet obstruction, so that he could not continue the treatment.

Of the nine patients described above who quit the study more than a month after entering, two—Patients #18 and 24—stopped treatment with us because they were too sick to continue. Another two—patients #26 and 28—discontinued our therapy because of psychosocial reasons, and five—#23, 27, 29, 30, and 31—due to relentless physician opposition to our alternative approach.

In summary, of the 39 total patients entered into the nutrition arm, 14 never started or quit within a month, while another 9 dropped out after four weeks. Overall, 23 patients of a total of 39, or 59%, discontinued the nutritional therapy. Of these, seven patients—#3, 10, 23, 27, 28, 31 and 39—quit to begin chemotherapy, and one, #30, withdrew to pursue an experimental vaccine treatment. These numbers hardly supported Dr. Zerhouni's claim that "very few subjects receiving Dr. Gonzalez's therapy withdrew from the study or elected to change their therapy."

Since all but one of the above case reports appeared in my January 7, 2005 letter, if Dr. Chabot or the government scientists supervising the study doubted any of my facts, it would have been their responsibility to challenge me in writing, and in a timely fashion. Yet in the year after I sent that letter, not one of the institutional managers—not Dr. Chabot from Columbia, not Dr. Smith nor Dr. White from the NCI, not Dr. Engel nor Dr. Killen from NCCAM—expressed a single reservation or objection to the data I had presented, either verbally or in writing.

Chapter 10

Payment Delays

In the second paragraph, second page, Dr. Zerhouni attributed my complaint over the payment delays—which he apparently considered inconsequential—to my ignorance of standard clinical trial procedures:

> Dr. Gonzalez alleges that NIH staff failed to ensure timely payments to the private clinic involved in the study's evaluation, causing Dr. Gonzalez and his partner, Dr. Linda Isaacs, to carry the NIH-funded study protocol with their own financial resources. As you may be aware, there are requirements that must be met before NIH releases funds for any trial. Perhaps Dr. Gonzalez is not familiar with this process, but these requirements were adhered to for this trial in the same way they are with all NIH–supported clinical trials.

I certainly hope, for the sake of Dr. Zerhouni, the NCI, the NIH, and medical science, that the reimbursement delays we perpetually faced in our clinical trial represented a unique, rather than a typical, situation. Regardless, nowhere in any document at any time, or in any conversation, did I ever allege "NIH staff failed to ensure timely payments." In my conversation with Dr. Straus about the issue, the NCCAM Director blamed the NCI directly for the problem. In her June 15, 2005 e-mail to me, Dr. Smith of the NCI essentially held Columbia responsible. But never did I myself single out any particular individual or institute over this issue because I had no idea why bills remained unpaid, often for many months at a time. I only knew that they were unpaid.

True, I admit I have never personally been responsible for filing the complicated paperwork that inflicts all NIH funded clinical studies, nor am I an expert in the stringent requirements that govern the release of allocated monies. But over the years, I have witnessed first hand—and participated directly with—many clinical and laboratory studies, both government and industry supported. During my five-year tutorship, including my research fellowship training, under Dr. Good—with 2000 papers to his credit—I witnessed many laboratory and clinical efforts come into being, most federally funded. During the decade of my close friendship with Dr. Wynder—with his 700-plus publications—I again observed many research projects take shape from inception to completion, including multi-million dollar, multi-institutional NCI and NIH supported epidemiological trials.

My good friend and supporter Dr. Pierre Guesry, former Medical Director of the Pasteur Institute, retired Vice President for Research at Nestlé, supervised during his distinguished career hundreds of investigations of all types, from basic science lab work to human clinical trials. It was because of Dr. Guesry's enthusiasm for my work that Nestlé agreed to fund the pilot study, including treatment costs for all entered patients. Though Nestlé is not the NCI or the NIH, the company never withheld or delayed any payment for any reason, from the beginning to the end of the project. At the Eppley Cancer Center at the University of Nebraska Medical Center, Nestlé later subsidized the animal studies evaluating the anti-cancer effect of my enzymes. For this series of experiments, all requiring institutional approval and oversight, Nestlé provided the promised funding as needed and, as far as I know, always on time.

For a three-year period beginning in 1995, The Procter & Gamble Company allocated many millions of dollars in support for our efforts, under the direct supervision of Dr. J.P. Jones, at the time Vice President for Research in Health Care at P&G, and responsible during his much lauded career for supervising many scores, if not hundreds, of projects. In the 1980s Dr. Jones arranged for P&G to underwrite Dr. Barry Marshall's pioneering work linking the bacterium *Helicobacter pylori* to most ulcers—a concept derided as quackery at the time. Without the help of Dr. Jones and P&G, Dr. Marshall's innovative research might have been relegated to the medical junk pile, instead of garnering him the Nobel Prize in Medicine in 2005. During our own tenure together, P&G funded basic laboratory studies of our enzymes, requiring close working relationships with scientists both at the company and at contract institutions.

P&G always paid the bills as promised and when promised, with never a single delay. Dr. Jones, now retired, still a close personal friend and advisor, seems as perplexed as I by the troubled reimbursement history of this project.

So though I may not know how to file the paperwork, I have observed, up close, research studies of a variety of types financially supported in a variety of ways for some 30 years. During this time I have never heard of any NCI-NIH or industry financed trial plagued by repeated funding suspensions lasting for months, during which time the investigator must underwrite the cost of the research. I will say that in my opinion, Dr. Zerhouni's attitude, as expressed in his letter, reflected that of the lower level government bureaucrats assigned to oversee our study. Whenever Dr. Isaacs and I broached the reimbursement problem, all seemed remarkably indifferent, though patients' lives were involved, and offered only a "this is the way we work, too bad" response. Should these delays be typical for NIH studies, as Dr. Zerhouni assured us they are in his letter to Congressman Burton, I question how any clinical trial could ever reach a meaningful conclusion or why any scientist would agree to cooperate with that government institution. I also wonder if Dr. Zerhouni's own personal staff would have continued working for him if each had to pay for the privilege of coming to the office every day, to the tune of tens of thousands of dollars a year—with the carrot stick of payment held out but only at some vague undefined time in the future. I suspect the director would have been forced to do a lot of his own typing.

Chapter 11

Supposed Allegations Against Dr. Chabot and Denials of the Referral Bias

T he third paragraph, page 2 of Dr. Zerhouni's letter, read:

Dr. Gonzalez has raised very serious allegations against Dr. Chabot in terms of the conduct of the trial. Based on his interest and expertise in pancreatic cancer, Dr. Chabot agreed to direct the trial after the protocol was finalized. We have seen no evidence to support Dr. Gonzalez's assertions of scientific misconduct by Dr. Chabot or his staff. It is our understanding that rules of clinical trial management were strictly adhered to by the Columbia research staff at every point in the process. The protocol was prospectively set and followed in order to avoid any insertion of bias. Dr. Chabot remained steadfast to the predetermined trial design and discussed with Dr. Gonzalez the critical nature of maintaining a predetermined trial design and assuring its ethical oversight by an impartial data and safety monitoring board, which is charged with deciding whether the evolving safety and efficacy data in any clinical study warrants continued patient enrollment, treatment and follow up.

In response, up to the time of Dr. Zerhouni's letter I had made no "assertions of scientific misconduct by Dr. Chabot or his staff." In all the scores of e-mails and letters I had written over the years to document the problems with the trial prior to December 2005, I can find no evidence that I ever once used the word "misconduct." The term did appear in Congressman Burton's letter to the director, but only in a general sense, not as a specific accusation aimed at Dr. Chabot. Specifically, Congressman Burton had written:

> Furthermore, if you determine that some type of scientific misconduct has taken place, I would appreciate an account of the disciplinary actions you intend to take in order to rectify the situation.

Of course, Congressman Burton's words reflected the documentation I provided his office, but even in this context he made no allegation, only requesting that if the Director uncovered "misconduct," appropriate disciplinary action would be taken.

Though I myself had never used the word "misconduct" anywhere up to that time, I did not believe, contrary to Dr. Zerhouni's assertion, "that rules of clinical trial management were strictly adhered to by the Columbia research staff at every point in this process." Perhaps one might dispute whether a particular patient could eat "normally" at the time of entry or not, but by the time of the director's letter no one could deny that Dr. Chabot had mishandled informed consent with at least three patients. I didn't know who in Dr. Zerhouni's staff crafted his response to Congressman Burton, but the consent form violations already evident and documented by December 2005 made the director's defense of Dr. Chabot incomprehensible.

Dr. Zerhouni's letter continued:

> Dr. Gonzalez alleges that there was a referral bias in favor of the chemotherapy protocol by Dr. Chabot. We have seen no evidence to support this claim. It is important to note that consideration of enrollment in either the Gonzalez treatment arm or chemotherapy arm of the study is based entirely on patient choice and not assignment by the PI. Therefore, patient referral bias based on the PI's actions is unlikely. In addition, Dr. Chabot, a surgeon, has explicitly stated that he has no bias towards either chemotherapy or alternative approaches. Secondly, it is NIH's understanding that a statistical analysis of all subjects entered to date reveals no meaningful difference in stage or functional status between the subjects who chose to be entered into the Gonzalez treatment arm and those who chose to be entered into the chemotherapy arm. Dr. Gonzalez's claim may be based on a preliminary look at the status of subjects

in each arm when very few subjects had been recruited to the control arm. Now that all subjects have been enrolled, it appears that there are no statistical differences between the two groups on these measures.

It is still inconceivable to me that Dr. Zerhouni's staff would have allowed him to write something so off target. Here, the director referred specifically to the significant staging disparity between the chemotherapy and nutrition groups which first became evident during the December 13, 2004 meeting and which I documented at length in my January 7, 2005 letter to Dr. Killen. Congressman Burton had sent Dr. Zerhouni a copy of my letter providing the relevant information about the staging issue, so the director had the documentation in his hands.

During the December 2004 meeting and later in my January 2005 letter, I pointed out that this serious imbalance made any comparison between the two arms impossible. True, on paper Dr. Chabot did subsequently "correct" the problem, first by eliminating without explanation two early-stage chemo patients, then in a four month period, during which time he would enter no one into the nutrition arm, approving nine stage IV subjects for chemotherapy. Concurrently he also disqualified two stage IV nutrition patients, again without discussion, and downstaged another five—with no reason given. With such adjustments, the disparity not only disappeared, but the chemo patients as a group seemed more advanced than ours.

While Dr. Chabot, a "surgeon" as Dr. Zerhouni pointed out, may have claimed impartiality to either treatment, by that point he had co-authored multiple articles in the scientific literature with Dr. Fine's research group, the originators of the very GTX protocol serving as the "control" in our clinical study. This obvious conflict of interest not only warned of potential bias but should have in our opinion required Dr. Chabot to step down as PI.

I can only describe as perplexing Dr. Zerhouni's statement that "Dr. Gonzalez's claim [about the staging disparity] may be based on a preliminary look at the status of subjects in each arm when very few subjects had been recruited to the control arm." The staging imbalance surfaced in December 2004, when the study had been up and running a full five years and 38 nutrition patients had been entered, 97.5% of the 39 who would be ultimately be qualified. At that point, the chemotherapy group consisted of 14 patients, or 60% of the 23 that would finally be admitted. These numbers hardly conformed to a "preliminary look."

Even if we were to assume Dr. Chabot legitimately resolved the staging issue, the two groups were still not comparable for another serious reason Zerhouni completely ignored, the many "nutrition" patients who could not or would not comply with the prescribed treatment. This problem had been extensively discussed in my January 2005 letter to Killen, then confirmed by Dr. Engel, the official NIH spokesperson on the study, in her January 27, 2005 response addressed to Dr. Chabot:

> We discussed at considerable length his concerns about the probable accrual of patients unable to comply fully with the nutrition arm of the protocol. It was our impression that everyone in the room basically agreed that, despite best efforts, there is in fact, reason to be concerned about this issue, and that it clouds interpretation of the data. Even if we assume, however, that this is the explanation for the disappointingly poor outcome of patients on the nutrition arm, accrual of 15 or 20 additional patients to the nutrition arm of this comparative study, as it is designed and currently being implemented, would only be appropriate if there is a chance that the interim results would change.

No correction in the staging disparity, however implemented, could ever undo the compliance issue.

Chapter 12

Admission of Patients Who Did Not Fulfill One or More Entry Criteria

In the second paragraph of the third page of his letter, Dr. Zerhouni once again lauded Dr. Chabot and the government team, the stalwarts of scientific honor and integrity, while attributing my claims of mismanagement to my fundamental lack of character. He wrote:

> Dr. Gonzalez alleges that Dr. Chabot required him to accept patients who did not fit the established protocol. We have seen no evidence to support this claim. Dr. Gonzalez wrote the majority of the eligibility criteria himself. Based on these criteria, Columbia staff screened subjects before sending them to Dr. Gonzalez's office. Due to the nature of pancreatic cancer, it is not unusual for patient status to change within days or weeks. Patients who meet the requirements at the time of enrollment may experience changes in their ability to meet the criteria over time. To date, there is no enrolled subject who failed to meet the entrance criteria at the time of enrollment. It is our understanding that Dr. Gonzalez contacted Dr. Chabot to discuss his reluctance to accept some subjects in the trial. It is our understanding that Dr. Gonzalez's reluctance to enroll some candidates into the study was based on his subjective assessment of whether the patient would be a good candidate for his therapy and not on

the predetermined eligibility criteria. However, the Columbia team was bound by the predetermined entry criteria set by Dr. Gonzalez himself. Adhering to these criteria was necessary to avoid any insertion of bias from any source towards either arm.

For a number of reasons Dr. Zerhouni's response seemed to me simply ludicrous. First of all, the main point in the paragraph, "To date, there is no enrolled subject who failed to meet the entrance criteria at the time of enrollment" was factually incorrect and could easily be countered. By this point in the study, Dr. Chabot had already acknowledged admitting three patients with no evidence of the required signed consent form, as discussed at length in Chapter 3. All involved with the study knew of this serious oversight, and the mishandling of informed consent in these cases should have been evidence enough to disprove Dr. Zerhouni's statements as written above.

To help assess the number of nutrition patients approved in violation of the entry rules, all we need do is refer to the written protocol, the ultimate rule book for the trial. In its various incarnations from first draft to last, written between 1997 and 2000, this document provided a clear description of the eligibility requirements which remained fairly constant through the study's duration. For example, the April 2, 1998 protocol edition defined these criteria in section 3.0, beginning on page 5. I include not all, but only the most pertinent points:

3.1 . . . No prior treatment, except surgery with noncurative intent (such as biopsy or palliative bypass).
Diagnosis within 8 weeks of beginning therapy. . . .

3.3 Since the Enzyme-Nutritional Therapy will be administered by the patients at home, they and their families must be willing to undertake the required work. . . .

3.5 Non pregnant, non lactating
Able to eat solid food, three meals per day . . .
Supportive live-in spouse or other family member . . .

3.8. Informed Consent: Each patient must be completely aware of the nature of his/her disease process and must willingly give consent after being informed of the procedure to be followed, the experimental nature of the therapy, alternatives, potential benefits, side-effects, risks, and discomforts.

3.9 No serious medical or psychiatric illness preventing informed consent or intensive treatment (e.g., serious infection).

The category entitled "Patient Entry" provided additional relevant instructions:

4.2. All prospective patients must undergo extensive interviewing to determine their willingness to follow, and their suitability for Enzyme-Nutritional Therapy, a complex dietary program that involves major changes in lifestyle and it is not suitable for all patients.

4.4. Registration: To register the patient, fax or deliver the completed Eligibility Criteria Form and signed Informed Consent to the Cancer Center Protocol Office. . . .

4.5 Required forms:
Eligibility Criteria Form
Informed Consent

By late 2005, Dr. Isaacs and I estimated that *conservatively* 16 of the 39 patients approved by Dr. Chabot for our nutritional therapy did not fulfill the written entry criteria *when approved*—and not days or weeks later as Dr. Zerhouni claimed in his letter. These 16 could be divided into five distinct categories, based on the nature of the protocol violation: patients entered more than eight weeks after biopsy confirmation of disease; patients who could not eat adequately at the time of entry as required by the protocol; patients with psychiatric illness; a patient lacking family or social support; and finally, patients with no evidence of signed informed consent. In the following section, I provide brief summaries of these cases to make the point, with several more notable illustrations discussed at greater length.

Patients entered more than eight weeks after biopsy confirmation of diagnosis: Since those diagnosed with pancreatic cancer deteriorate so quickly—as Zerhouni himself pointed out in his letter—at the time we wrote the first protocol draft we all agreed trial candidates needed to be accepted for treatment soon after diagnosis. We ultimately chose eight weeks from biopsy as the upper limit for eligibility, though I personally thought a two month time frame still too generous with a disease as rapidly progressive as this particular malignancy. Regardless, by the time of Zerhouni's letter I had identified three patients Dr.

Chabot entered into the nutrition arm in violation of this rule, Patients #14, #16 and #34.

In the two cases of Patients #14 and #34, the lapses in judgment were straightforward. Dr. Chabot admitted patient #14 on January 23, 2003, *nearly 11 weeks* from the biopsy of November 8, 2002. He interviewed and approved patient #34 on September 6, 2001, ten weeks after the biopsy dated June 28, 2001. At the time Dr. Chabot admitted each of these two I pointed out that the lag between diagnosis and entry of greater than eight weeks disqualified them. Nonetheless he instructed us to begin the treatment process without offering a reasonable explanation for his decision.

The situation in the case of Patient #16 was somewhat more complex. This gentleman underwent exploratory surgery and biopsy proving pancreatic cancer on December 20, 2002. I did not consult with him for my initial office visit until February 6, 2003, nearly seven weeks later, but still within the allowed time frame. However, at that point his eligibility had not been determined, since Dr. Chabot had scheduled his own intake interview several days after my first session with the patient. At times, because of his scheduling problems, Dr. Chabot would send a patient to us to start the treatment process though he had not yet completed his evaluation. We thought this arrangement peculiar, but since Dr. Chabot was in charge, we abided by his rules.

After meeting Patient #16, Dr. Chabot postponed his final decision in this case until the Columbia pathologists reviewed the biopsy slides. By March 5, 2003, nearly a month later, Dr. Chabot still had not come to a conclusion about the status of Patient #16—who unfortunately, I learned, hadn't begun his treatment. By that point nearly 11 weeks had elapsed since the biopsy, so the patient no longer qualified. Even though we were instructed to begin the treatment process as if he had been approved, Dr. Chabot would later claim *this patient had never been admitted.*

I want to emphasize that by this time in 2001, the NCI had already given Dr. Chabot complete arbitrary authority over the selection of trial patients. Once he determined the eligibility of a particular candidate, we had no choice but to defer to his judgment, with no appeal possible. In essence, we believed we had only two choices, treat these patients on trial, or quit. At that time Dr. Isaacs and I were still grateful after years of hard work for the chance to have our therapy evaluated in a formal academic setting. So, we were once again willing to give Dr. Chabot the benefit of the doubt, hoping his decision-making process would improve with time.

Patients who could not eat adequately at the time of entry as required for the protocol: Since our therapy consists in large part of a prescribed diet and ingestion of some 150 capsules or more throughout the day, patients must be able to eat fairly normally to follow the regimen. Those who cannot do so will be unable to comply with the treatment plan.

According to the entry criteria, trial candidates, to be admitted, needed to be consuming three meals daily. As written, this provision appeared somewhat vague, but in our many discussions with Dr. Antman and Dr. Wynder as we wrote the initial protocol drafts, we all intended that patients must be able to eat *normally* to qualify. Furthermore, the final version of the official consent form dating from 2000, at which time the trial design had changed from randomized to matched cohort, more clearly defined the requirement in this way.

The relevant section from the consent document appeared on the first page, under "Study Purpose":

> Seventy to ninety patients will participate in this study. You were selected as a possible participant because you have been diagnosed with adenocarcinoma of the pancreas and have not previously received chemotherapy or radiation. Furthermore, you are able to eat normally and care for yourself, both requirements for entrance into the study.

The phrasing could not have been clearer.

By the time of Dr. Zerhouni's December 2005 letter, we had already identified ten patients whom Dr. Isaacs and I believed should have been disqualified because of extremely poor appetite at the time of their initial evaluation with Dr. Chabot. Below, I discuss in some detail two of the more obvious examples, Patient #8 and Patient #9, approved, we believe, in violation of the explicit entry criteria. I also include descriptions of eight additional cases as appearing in my January 7, 2005 letter to Dr. Killen.

Patient #8: In our opinion, Dr. Chabot's approval of Patient #8 for treatment with us represented perhaps the most significant violation of the provision requiring a normal appetite.

I first met with Patient #8 on January 16, 2002, before he had been seen by Dr. Chabot or formally approved for the study. During this session it became clear to me that Patient #8, because of his extremely inadequate food intake, should be excluded. When I discussed this issue pointedly with him and his wife, she cried upon learning that he might not be eligible. Out of a sense of fairness, I did agree to treat him for free if he didn't ultimately qualify, as Dr. Isaacs and I had done with other study candidates we believed to be unsuited for the trial.

In my note from that day I documented the patient's situation:

> The patient reports that his surgeon, Dr. M— also told him that chemotherapy would not be particularly helpful and actually suggested he think of alternatives. One of the biggest problems is that the patient's appetite has been "terrible." A week ago one of his doctors (and he's not sure which one) started him on Megace 2-tsp [teaspoon] day. With this his appetite has improved although it's still down. He reports a 20–25 lb. weight loss.

The drug mentioned above, Megace, is a synthetic progesterone originally developed as a treatment option for estrogen-responsive breast cancer. Oncologists soon learned that for some women in the terminal stages of their disease, Megace seemed to increase appetite, even if only temporarily. Eventually, physicians began recommending the drug for both women and men with all types of cancers, even for those with advanced HIV, to offset the poor food intake and the devastating weight loss of progressing malignancy or chronic infection. In this day and age, a patient with pancreatic cancer would be prescribed Megace for only one reason: a grossly reduced capacity to eat.

I immediately called Dr. Chabot after my session with Patient #8, arguing that he should be disqualified, a conversation I documented in the "Assessment" section at the end of my note from that day:

> The patient was tentatively approved for the clinical trial but he doesn't meet the criteria at this point. . . . He has no appetite and he's on Megace for appetite. An inability to eat precludes his entrance into the trial. I discussed this with Dr. Chabot.

In the "Plan" section I wrote:

> I am willing to start the patient on a program but I'm going to have to discuss with the various investigators whether he's appropriate for the clinical trial.

Before Patient #8 had been seen or approved by Dr. Chabot, in three separate places in the chart I wrote of his "terrible" appetite, and in two places my belief that he did not meet the entry criteria. I also specifically reported that after meeting with the patient, in a phone conversation with Dr. Chabot I expressed my opinion that he should not be admitted into the study. All this transpired before Dr. Chabot had concluded his intake evaluation, making incomprehensible Dr. Zerhouni's claim that patients deteriorated only after they had been appropriately approved.

After our phone discussion I also e-mailed Dr. Chabot, documenting in writing my opinion that this trial candidate should be excluded based on the written entry criteria:

> Since then he's lost 25 pounds, admitted he wasn't eating, couldn't eat and had no appetite until his Local MD put him on Megace a week ago. He is eating some now, but we have never had any success with a patient staying on the program who had to be put on Megace because of appetite. . . . I know from my experience he's already missed his window and I doubt he will stay on the program ten days.

The following day, Patient #8 planned to meet with Dr. Chabot for his formal intake interview, before returning to my office for the second session to review the prescribed treatment. Dr. Chabot did call me after his consultation with Patient #8, informing me he would order some blood tests before making a final determination about his eligibility. The written protocol required that certain blood parameters fall within a specific range, so Dr. Chabot wanted to make sure the patient's blood counts and chemistries met the predetermined criteria. I thought Dr. Chabot's decision perplexing, since the patient's poor appetite should have disqualified him at once, whatever the lab tests revealed.

Nonetheless, Dr. Chabot instructed me to proceed with my second session as if Patient #8 had been admitted. My note from that day documented my willingness to treat him regardless of his status on the study:

> [Patient #8] came in with his family. We spent 2 hours reviewing his protocol. I spoke with John Chabot as well regarding his eligibility for the protocol.

> Dr. Chabot agrees that we need to check his blood work and have more recent blood work. I explained this to Mr. [Patient #8]. He wants to do the program regardless. I won't charge him, if he's not eligible.

On January 22, 2002, five days after our second meeting, the blood tests all came back within the acceptable range. At that point I thought Dr. Chabot would most likely approve the patient despite his poor appetite.

I recorded these events in the patient's file:

> [Patient #8]'s blood work came in. It actually looks within the parameters of the clinical trial.

> I called Mrs. [Patient #8] and told her that we don't have a final decision. I'm waiting on Dr. Chabot . . . he is eating.

In my comment about his eating I did not mean to imply a reasonable food intake, only that he was getting some food down. I did not say he was "eating normally," only that he was "eating."

Two days later, on January 24, 2002, I documented that Dr. Chabot still had not notified the patient or me about his status:

> His wife called wondering whether he had been formally approved for the clinical trial. I have not heard from Dr. Chabot although I faxed the blood work and have called 3–4 times. I told her I would let her know as soon as possible.

Eventually, as I expected but to my disappointment Dr. Chabot accepted the patient for entry. Unfortunately, he never could fully comply with the treatment, and my own records described his subsequent downward spiral before he succumbed on April 23, 2002.

In a note dated April 15, 2002, dictated shortly before patient #8 died, I expressed my concern that Dr. Chabot had admitted yet another patient who did not follow the prescribed regimen:

> [Patient #8] is not doing well. He had to be hospitalized over the weekend. . . .

> The problem is he hasn't been able to eat since he started the program and he just wasn't really a suitable candidate for the protocol. That's the problem; he never was able to do it.

That same day I e-mailed Dr. Chabot, recounting the situation:

> Not unexpectedly, [Patient #8], though well meaning, has not been able to follow the diet virtually from day 1, and has been living on milk shakes. I am

amazed he has lasted nearly four months since diagnosis with his stage IV disease and doing half the protocol. You may remember that he was on Megace when seen in your office because he couldn't eat, and hasn't been able to eat. . . .

We are concerned that another two patients haven't been able to do it. . . . Maybe we should have a meeting to discuss all this?

Dr. Chabot never responded.

Patient #9: As per Dr. Chabot's instructions, I first met with this patient for his initial visit on February 5, 2003, before he had been seen at Columbia for his formal evaluation. On page 2 of my note from that day I described someone who, far too ill to proceed with the therapy, should be excluded:

> Currently, he does not seem to be doing well. Frankly, I think he is too sick to enter into the clinical trial. He has developed chronic, dull lower back pain that is resolved with Darvocet. His appetite is down. He lost about 20 pounds in the last six weeks. . . . His appetite is very poor and it sounds like he is starting to deteriorate.

In the "Assessment" section, the summary of my findings, I repeated my concern:

> Widely metastatic pancreatic cancer. He [sic] last blood work is already a month old. I suspect it is much worse than it was. Liver function tests were elevated at the time. In the last week, there has been significant deterioration in his clinical status. I do not believe he is going to be strong enough to do the program. I think it is too late. I think he is probably not going to last very long. I will e-mail Dr. Chabot at Columbia and let him know about my feelings on this patient.

That same day I e-mailed Dr. Chabot, expressing my reservations about this patient's eligibility:

> I saw Mr. [Patient #9] today for his first session, you will be seeing him Friday. . . . However, he looked like a patient who is about to crash very soon. From my experience, I know he isn't going to make it. Over the past week, he and his wife both said there has been a significant deterioration, he is having trouble eating, he is getting pale, he gets short of breath going up stairs (his lungs sounded clear on exam so I suspect it's anemia). His window of opportunity has passed.

149

Though Dr. Chabot had not yet conducted his intake interview, he instructed me to proceed as if Patient #9 had been approved. So the following day, February 6, 2003, I met with Patient #9 a second time to review the prescribed regimen. In my record from the session, I documented my strong belief that the patient did not qualify, though as in similar situations I offered to treat him off protocol and for free if Dr. Chabot rejected him from the study:

> My feeling is that he is too sick and I suspect his liver functions tests will have worsened since they were done a month ago. He is going to discuss these issues with Dr. Chabot. He wants to do the program regardless of whether he is on the clinical trial or not and I agreed of course to do that.

Nonetheless, I later learned in a phone conversation with Dr. Chabot that despite my objections he had approved this patient for treatment with us. He defended his position by telling me Patient #9 had been able to "walk up and down the hallway without any problem," an accomplishment I thought irrelevant to the issue at hand, his inability to eat.

Though Patient #9 to his credit tried to comply with the regimen, he simply was too ill and his appetite too poor. A comment in my files dated February 18, 2003, dictated just 12 days after the patient's second visit with me, described a phone conversation in which he admitted he could not eat:

> [Patient #9] complains he cannot eat. I thought he was far too sick to do the program. He is trying to get the pills down but it is difficult.

Two days later, on February 20, 2003, I e-mailed Dr. Chabot expressing my belief he had admitted another patient unable to follow through with the therapy. Once again, I gave Dr. Chabot the benefit of the doubt, suggesting that perhaps during the initial interview with him patients might be misstating their true clinical status in order to gain entry into the study:

> I am concerned about Mr. [Patient #9]. He called after five days on the supplements to tell me he has no appetite and "can't eat." This was my concern when I first worked him up. I think patients like this are so desperate to get on the clinical trial they mislead you about their eating. We've had three patients recently who couldn't do it. . . .

In a chart note dated March 10, 2003, I described another phone conversation with Patient #9, and repeated my belief that he should never have been qualified:

> I called [Patient #9] to see how he is doing. He is not doing well. I do not think he should have ever been entered into this clinical trial. He cannot eat. His local doctor put him on Megace because he cannot eat. His pain is poorly controlled with morphine and Darvocet.

On April 29, 2003, I e-mailed Dr. Chabot, once again questioning his approval of this patient:

> I had started to get suspicious about [Patient #9] from —. I hadn't heard from him for weeks. I called several times leaving messages, but no call back. Today his wife called saying he had died two weeks ago, not doing his program.

> As it turns out, for the record, within days of returning to — after his meetings with us his oncologist locally started him on Megace because he "couldn't eat." This was my concern about entering him into the study because he had lost some 20–25 pounds in the weeks before coming to New York and he and his wife said to us he couldn't eat well.

Dr. Chabot never replied, nor did he ever counter my charge that the patient, by the rules of the study, was unsuited. In this particular case I don't think the record could more strongly illustrate that Patient #9, because of his debilitated condition and very poor appetite, should not have been approved, and that I strongly argued against his admission directly with Dr. Chabot to no avail. Unfortunately, despite the significant non-compliance, as per the intent-to-treat provision of the trial, Dr. Chabot considered this patient as properly vetted, fully treated, and a "Gonzalez failure."

In my January 7, 2005 letter to Dr. Killen, I referenced a total of ten patients, including Patient #8 and Patient #9, with inadequate food intake at the time of entry. Though previously excerpted (in another context), below I include these case reports to illustrate this specific point, that Dr. Chabot admitted many patients who could not eat:

> One of these, Patient 2, developed projectile vomiting before taking a single supplement because of a gastric outlet obstruction. Despite duodenal stenting, he could never subsequently follow the protocol.

> For example, Patient 3, after only three days on the supplements, required hospitalization for management of severe pain and vomiting, then quickly began radiation and chemotherapy. She never resumed her nutritional protocol.

Patient 4, who at the time of entry had been diagnosed with pleural effusions, followed the therapy only intermittently after the first eight days because of poor appetite and repeated hospitalizations necessitated by pulmonary distress.

Patient 5 reported very poor appetite within 13 days of entry into the trial, was hospitalized and discharged on hospice. He never continued the treatment.

Patient 6, who had difficulty eating from day one on the regimen, developed a biliary obstruction within six weeks and never thereafter pursued the therapy.

During the first appointment with Dr. Isaacs, Patient 7 reported severe nausea that never relented, and precluded any significant compliance with the supplement program. After being diagnosed with a gastric outlet obstruction, she underwent bypass surgery, but afterwards did not pursue the therapy.

Patient 8 arrived in our office already on Megace because of very poor oral intake. Once home, he never could follow the diet, instead relying on Ensure for nourishment. I estimate he never got more than half the pills down, and deteriorated very quickly.

Patient 9 had lost more than twenty pounds because of poor appetite over a several-week period before acceptance into the study. During my initial consultation with him, I never thought he would be able to do the treatment because of his severe anorexia and general weakness. He went home, began Megace, and quit the therapy within four weeks.

Patient 10, with extensive carcinomatosis, tried hard to do the program, but had so much difficulty eating I doubt he did the therapy for more than two weeks. He ended up doing his "own version" of the treatment, to use his wife's words, before pursuing the GemTax chemotherapy regimen at Columbia. He died very quickly, far faster than any patients described in the GemTax arm of our study. Nonetheless he will be considered a Gonzalez failure.

Patient 12 also seemed to be in an end stage condition when first seen by Dr. Isaacs. Visibly cachectic, with a BMI of 19, he was so weak during the initial interview he could barely hold up his head. When asked about his appetite, his wife prompted him, "You're eating three meals a day, right, honey?" Within six days of his initial visit he was hospitalized for treatment of dehydration, and after discharge was promptly re-admitted because of coffee-ground emesis and biliary stent blockage. Then, while undergoing evaluation for PEG tube placement less than a month later, he was found to be completely obstructed. He never could follow the therapy.

I want to emphasize that all of these ten patients reported significant problems with appetite during the initial sessions with Dr. Isaacs or myself, not days or weeks later.

Patients entered with psychiatric illness: The rule in section 3.9 of the protocol, requiring exclusion of any candidate with a history of "psychiatric illness preventing informed consent or intensive treatment," was hardly harsh or unusual. Many studies over the years have confirmed that any form of mental disease, including depression, significantly and negatively affects compliance with lifestyle treatments. In all major dietary modification clinical trials we have reviewed, including the famed Women's Health Initiative, depression counted as a reason to disqualify a candidate.[36]

In *Compliance in Healthcare and Research,* Burke and Ockene describe a history of a psychiatric disorder as predictive of poor adherence with any treatment regimen:

> there is no "stereotypical" nonadherer. This has obvious implications for detecting nonadherence. . . . There are two exceptions to this generalism: first, difficult social circumstances such as marital discord, social isolation, and unemployment, adversely affect adherence. Second, patients with mental disorders, particularly those with paranoid or depressive features, tend to be less adherent.[24(p5)]

I want to emphasize that Dr. Isaacs and I insisted that mentally ill patients be excluded from our trial for their benefit and their protection. We know from our experience that those battling psychological disability cannot stick with the therapy, that their non-compliance always creates enormous stress for them, and for their own good they need to find a more suitable approach.

In any event, we believe three patients Dr. Chabot admitted to the nutrition arm, Patients #14, #16 and #23, should never have been approved because of an evident psychiatric disorder. Below I include descriptions of these three from my January 7, 2005 letter, beginning on page 6:

> Patient 14's course was uniquely peculiar. Because of a long history of severe depression and suicidal ideation, Dr. Chabot did not immediately approve her

for the trial, but instead requested she be seen by a psychiatrist for further evaluation since active mental illness is grounds for exclusion. Nonetheless, Dr. Isaacs did agree to see her and begin the treatment process before a final decision about eligibility had been made, so the patient could get started with the program. Unfortunately, the psychiatric work-up dragged on for a month, and though seen by us 12/20/02, she was not officially accepted into the trial until 1/24/03, **a full five weeks later**. During this period, the patient did not begin any aspect of the therapy because, as she told us, she didn't want to follow the regimen if she wasn't going to be a part of the study, and therefore had to pay for the supplements herself. Her husband also inquired if the supplements would stimulate her rapidly deteriorating appetite (they don't). Though quite debilitated, she thereafter struggled to follow the treatment plan and did survive 40.6 weeks from the time of her initial biopsy. In this case, her lack of urgency about the situation caused a critical loss of valuable time.

Dr. Chabot ultimately approved this patient based on a single, one-hour evaluation by a psychiatrist. To this day I don't know how Dr. Chabot could believe, whatever a psychiatrist said after such a brief examination, that this patient, with a long history of severe depression and suicidal ideation, was a suitable candidate for our clinical trial. The written protocol specifically precluded entry of any candidate diagnosed with a "medical or psychiatric illness preventing informed consent or intensive treatment." The patient's own behavior during the five week period after her first visits with Dr. Isaacs and Dr. Chabot, during which time she did none of the prescribed regimen, already confirmed her inability to comply. By the time she decided to begin treatment, her appetite had deteriorated to the point she could not possibly follow through sufficiently. Though these issues were brought to the attention of Dr. Chabot, he still insisted she be admitted and that we treat her. We believed then and believe today that this individual would have been better served had she been disqualified after the first visit with Dr. Chabot, so she could begin chemotherapy, a treatment that would not have required her active participation.

Continuing on page 7 of my January 7, 2005 letter:

> Patient 16, a problem from day one, appeared attracted to the study primarily because it offered, as he said, "free benefits." During the first session with me, he asked repeatedly for me to explain what expenses would be covered. . . .

Though he never took a single supplement, he will be considered a Gonzalez failure. Patient 16 would never have come to us as a private patient, if he had to pay for it. I also believe a patient like this would not have been interested in joining the pilot study, which required the patient pay out themselves for the treatment during the first two months, until we were sure they were going to do it, and only then would they be reimbursed.

Patient #16 also reported he lived alone with no social support, another reason, as defined in section 3.5, for exclusion. After I had seen this patient, Dr. Chabot's own assistant called me and expressed her dismay that Dr. Chabot would even consider admitting him since she felt he most likely would not comply with our rigorous nutritional regimen. As it turned out he never took a supplement, yet as far as we knew at the time of Zerhouni's letter, Dr. Chabot considered him to be a treatment failure.

I described the third patient in this category, #23 on page 12 of my January 7, 2005 letter:

Patient 23, with a long history of depression, was on high doses of two anti-depressants when first seen in our office. Though the protocol for the study precludes entry of patients with psychiatric illness, she was nonetheless admitted to the nutrition arm. From the day she started our treatment, her local oncologist badgered her to quit the protocol and instead begin chemotherapy. She followed his advice, and died.

To this day, I do not understand the rationale of admitting a patient on high doses of two powerful antidepressants into the clinical trial.

A patient lacking family or social support: Dr. Chabot approved Patient #15 for entry into the nutritional arm of the study despite no evidence of family support, live-in or otherwise, as required by the *written* eligibility criteria 3.3 and 3.5 listed above.

These provisions, like the others, were neither odd nor unkind. First of all, Dr. Isaacs and I had learned long ago that a lack of proactive live-in family contributes to poor compliance with our rigorous nutritional regimen, and ultimately treatment failure. Beyond our personal experience, by the time of our trial considerable evidence in the scientific literature had already confirmed the value of caretakers within the home environment to help patients stick to a prescribed medical therapy, particularly those requiring lifestyle modifications. During the early days of our own project, a relevant article discussing just this issue appeared in the *Journal of Advances in Nursing*. In this report, the authors provided evidence that the immediate family and social environment greatly influenced adherence to a complex regimen administered to diabetic patients, as nicely summed up in the abstract of the article:

> Patient non-adherence is a well-recognized although poorly understood phenomenon that affects patients in all areas of health care. Failure to comply with health regimens is extremely costly both in economic terms and the health status of individuals. This study assesses factors which correlate with the expected success of health regimen adherence in 146 insulin-dependent diabetes mellitus (IDDM) subjects. The results indicate that success in complying with a health regimen is associated with good family support and rapport with health professionals, an absence of chronic stress and the capacity to take up the challenges posed by the disease. *Health professionals have a role in engendering optimism, in maintaining enthusiasm, and facilitating and encouraging maintenance in health behaviours.*[37] [Italics mine]

The writer here also stated quite convincingly that the physician's attitude toward a "health" regimen can greatly affect patient behavior. Such findings, which should hardly surprise, suggested that in terms of our study, a family missing in action at a critical time and/or a physician hostile toward the therapy could easily sabotage compliance and in turn lead to a poor outcome.

I discussed Patient #15 on page six of my January 7, 2005 letter:

> Patient 15 misrepresented her family situation, had in fact no family support whatsoever, and quit after trying for two weeks.

We believed this patient, who never should have been approved for our study, would have been far better off pursuing a more conventional option.

Patients with no evidence of signed informed consent: The two patients, #9 and #16, for whom no evidence existed for the required signed consent form (and who did not pursue the nutritional treatment) should never have been sent to us for treatment, nor counted as valid "data points." Similarly, the third patent lacking a signed consent form, whom Dr. Chabot did ultimately disqualify after she died, also should not have been admitted.

In closing, the multiple patients Dr. Chabot approved for the nutrition arm who did not initially meet the eligibility requirements should readily disprove Dr. Zerhouni's claim: "To date, there is no enrolled subject who failed to meet the entrance criteria at the time of enrollment."

Chapter 13

Authorship of Entry Criteria

T he long paragraph excerpted from Dr. Zerhouni's letter in Chapter 12 stated that: "Dr. Gonzalez wrote the majority of the eligibility criteria himself." This claim requires some clarification. Speaking literally, I did write most of the entry rules in the *original version of the protocol,* but only in consultation with Dr. Antman. However, it is important to note that the protocol went through multiple revisions after the fall of 1997, all written with no input from either Dr. Isaacs or myself.

For the initial draft completed in September 1997, Dr. Antman suggested that I work directly from the lengthy computerized template used at Columbia for their chemotherapy studies, so the format is hardly my creation and many of the admission requirements I thought appropriate for our project had already been clearly defined. For example, most if not all chemotherapy clinical trials require that certain laboratory blood values, such as kidney and liver function tests, fall within a certain range. Dr. Isaacs and I did argue successfully for changes in some of the numbers, though for others we simply used what was already in place.

The Columbia document included two sections on informed consent which I found quite adequate, and here I changed not a word. Ironically, the admission of the three patients with no evidence of signed consent violated the requirements of the standard Columbia clinical trial form, as excerpted here:

3.8. Informed Consent: Each patient must be completely aware of the nature of his/her disease process and must willingly give consent after being informed of the procedure to be followed, the experimental nature of the therapy, alternatives, potential benefits, side-effects, risks, and discomforts. . . .

4.4 Registration: To register the patient, fax or deliver the completed Eligibility Criteria Form and signed Informed Consent to the Cancer Center Protocol Office. . . .

4.5 Required forms:
Eligibility Criteria Form
Informed Consent

I did write, with Dr. Antman's approval, the criteria that patients be entered within eight weeks of biopsy, that they be able to eat normally, be free of mental disability, have a live-in family member willing and able to help with the treatment, and be fully committed to following the required lifestyle changes. I include the relevant sections below.

Time requirement for entry:

3.1. . . . No prior treatment allowed, except surgery with noncurative intent (such as biopsy or palliative bypass procedures).

Must be diagnosed within 8 weeks of beginning therapy.

Rule for adequate appetite:

3.6 Clinical Parameters

Able to eat solid food, three meals per day

Dr. Antman suggested I keep this section brief, with the understanding among us that "three meals per day" meant three typical, normal meals.

Criterion prohibiting entry of patients with mental disability:

3.9 No serious medical or psychiatric illness preventing informed consent or intensive treatment (e.g., serious infection).

Requirement for supportive live-in family member(s):

3.10 Since the Enzyme-Nutritional Therapy will be administered by the patients to themselves at home, patients assigned to this arm and their families must express a willingness to undertake required work.

Need for commitment to our treatment:

4.2 Evaluation by Dr. Gonzalez **or staff trained by him:** All prospective patients must undergo extensive interviewing to determine their willingness to follow, and their suitability for, the Enzyme-Nutritional Therapy. This treatment is a complex dietary program that involves major changes in lifestyle and it is not suitable for all patients.

This first draft of the protocol did not specify the minimum number of patients we would need to enroll in order to determine a statistically valid treatment effect, since such considerations were beyond my expertise. Subsequently, Dr. Wynder and his staff, working with Columbia scientists, agreed that, for the trial to achieve mathematical significance, we must enter at least 72 total subjects, counting both arms together—considerably more than the 62 admitted before the project closed to accrual.

This number first appeared in section 13.2 of the March 20, 1998 edition of the protocol:

Our primary objective is to compare survival rates in the two arms. Randomized clinical trials suggest that the median survival on gemcitabine is roughly 6 months, and data from an uncontrolled pilot study suggest that the median survival on enzyme-nutritional therapy is roughly 18 months. . . . We will enroll between 72 and 90 patients over a period of up to 36 months. If enrollment is low, we will enroll as few as 72 patients. . . . If enrollment is high, we will enroll 90 patients. . . .

Dr. Wynder and I, working closely together, did write a lengthy section on compliance monitoring that we included in the March 20, 1998 protocol draft:

5.3   **Evaluation of compliance:**

There are two elements that require compliance monitoring. One addresses activities such as taking the various pills and the other prescriptive activities, such as coffee enemas and liver flushes. We will assess the degree of compliance to this part of the intervention through a detailed questionnaire administered by an individual trained to conduct this process. As part of this questionnaire we will also determine the extent to which the patient has spousal or other support in the conduct of this regimen.

Nutrient intake will also be monitored. Since nutrition is an important component of the Pancreatic Enzyme Protocol, we will conduct bi-monthly assessments of nutrient intake. This will be accomplished through the collection of three unannounced 24-hour telephone recalls at baseline and every other month during the trial. Each dietary recall period includes one weekend day and one weekday. Patients will be instructed on how to provide the recall data. The Pennsylvania State University's Dietary Assessment Center is an expert in this area and will conduct the calls. In addition to calculating the various components of the diet, the [sic] will also collect information relative to the specific dietary recommendations of the protocol (i.e., organic foods, and eating 10 almonds twice a day).

Through studying the participant's adherence to the prescribed protocol, we will be able to assess whether a positive outcome can be related to the degree of compliance. The compliance part of the protocol is a vital component in evaluating the affect [sic] of pancreatic enzyme therapy in pancreatic cancer.

Though written into the protocol Dr. Zerhouni referenced in his letter, I am unaware of any effort by Dr. Chabot or his staff to monitor compliance to the degree required above, nor have we seen any evidence that Columbia ever approached the Penn State group.

Finally, though Dr. Antman did give me considerable latitude as I wrote this first version, she did deny the request of both Dr. Wynder and myself for a lead-in period. This omission proved to be, in my estimation, a disastrous mistake.

Chapter 14

Screening of Prospective Patients

Before moving on with Dr. Zerhouni's letter, I would like to analyze several additional points made in the section quoted in Chapter 12:

> Based on these criteria, Columbia staff screened subjects before sending them to Dr. Gonzalez's office. Due to the nature of pancreatic cancer, it is not unusual for patient status to change within days or weeks. Patients who meet the requirements at the time of enrollment may experience changes in their ability to meet the criteria over time. To date, there is no enrolled subject who failed to meet the entrance criteria at the time of enrollment.

It is precisely because the status of patients with pancreatic cancer can "change within days or weeks" that the team supervising the Gemzar study allowed for a one week lead-in period, to eliminate those subjects who could not be stabilized in terms of pain, or who might decline so rapidly after entry that a fair evaluation of the treatment might be difficult if not impossible. Regardless, Dr. Zerhouni's claim that "To date, there is no enrolled subject who failed to meet the criteria at the time of enrollment" was, as we have seen, simply wrong. The director ignored the many patients who, based on the written entry criteria, should never have been admitted in the first place. These include the three patients we identified whom Dr. Chabot approved more than eight weeks after their biopsy diagnosis, the 11 who could barely eat when first seen at Columbia, the three diagnosed with, or exhibiting signs of, mental disability, the one patient lacking social or family support, and the three for whom no evidence existed of the required signed consent form.

The director then continued:

> It is our understanding that Dr. Gonzalez contacted Dr. Chabot to discuss his reluctance to accept some subjects in the trial. It is our understanding that Dr. Gonzalez's reluctance to enroll some candidates into the study was based on his subjective assessment of whether the patient would be a good candidate for his therapy and not on the predetermined eligibility criteria.

This statement is preposterous. As the official trial documents show, and as I have previously documented at length, on multiple occasions throughout the trial I communicated with Dr. Chabot by phone, by e-mail, and even verbally during the group meetings my concerns about the many patients he admitted who failed to meet the explicit entry requirements. Our objections were hardly "subjective" but based only on the protocol rules Dr. Zerhouni referenced.

Dr. Zerhouni then stated:

> However, the Columbia team was bound by the predetermined entry criteria set by Dr. Gonzalez himself. Adhering to these criteria was necessary to avoid any insertion of bias from any source towards either arm.

Now having denied any patient had been inappropriately admitted, Dr. Zerhouni implied that I had repeatedly requested Dr. Chabot bend the regulations which I myself had imposed on the project. In truth, though I did contact Dr. Chabot on multiple occasions to discuss patients I believe had been improperly admitted, never once did I call or write or e-mail, as Dr. Zerhouni's letter stated, to suggest he evade or ignore the entry requirements for my own self-serving ends. I wished only that he abide by the clearly written protocol.

Despite his unfortunate statements, Dr. Zerhouni inadvertently made an important point, by warning that failure to abide by the "predetermined entry criteria" would allow for the "insertion of bias"—precisely what I warned about for years. In their failure to follow the rules, these "predetermined entry criteria" Zerhouni referenced, the "Columbia team"—along with the NCI and NCCAM supervisors—I believe permitted the "insertion of bias," the whole point of my January 7, 2005 letter. Interestingly enough, not until Zerhouni contacted the NCI and NIH after receiving the letters of Congressman Burton and Senator Harkin in late 2005 did any of the study staff deny the easily verifiable fact that multiple patients had been admitted improperly.

Chapter 15

Dr. Zerhouni Believes "Concerns" Addressed and Managed

D r. Zerhouni then wrote:

From my consultation with NCI and NCCAM, I understand they have taken repeated steps to address Dr. Gonzalez's concerns. The concerns raised in your letter have been raised and thoroughly discussed at meetings of the study research team and have been recorded in meeting minutes, as well as in correspondence between Dr. Gonzalez and NIH staff. NCI and NCCAM staff involved in the management of the grant supplement used to support the study have addressed and managed each concern under their purview. Other concerns more appropriately handled by the Columbia staff have been forwarded to Dr. Chabot for response or referred back to Dr. Gonzalez for discussion with Dr. Chabot.

I found the first sentence above quite revealing, for a number of reasons. In the many paragraphs in the prior 2½ pages, Dr. Zerhouni had systematically denied every single one of my "concerns" and "allegations." His letter to this point was in fact a litany of categorical rebuttal. The phrase "We have seen no evidence to support this claim" appeared in one form or another four times. Dr. Zerhouni not only rejected outright every one of my assertions, but went so far as to imply that I sought to have Dr. Chabot bend the rules in my favor. Yet here he seems to be inexplicably changing tack, suggesting—in total contradiction to his previous statements—that the various supervisors essentially accepted my allegations about the study's difficulties and missteps as legitimate, legitimate enough to require management. He does not write that those in charge challenged, denied, dismissed, or rejected my claims but instead that they "had taken repeated steps to address Dr. Gonzalez's concerns." Webster's, among its interpretations of the word "address," defines its meaning as "to deal with." Presumably the various NCI-NCCAM personnel referred to above must have taken my "concerns" seriously, or why else would these complaints have to be addressed, that is, dealt with, and repeatedly?

In his second sentence above, Dr. Zerhouni referred to Congressman Burton's letter:

> The concerns raised in your letter have been raised and thoroughly discussed at meetings of the study research team and have been recorded in meeting minutes, as well as in correspondence between Dr. Gonzalez and NIH staff.

Indeed, over the years of the trial's history Dr. Isaacs and I had "raised" our "concerns" at many of the group meetings, though not all the details of all such discussions made their way into the official minutes. As early as 1998, we challenged Dr. Antman's insistence that the study be randomized, suspecting this format would be unworkable as it turned out to be, and lead to biases worse than those it intended to prevent. From the beginning we argued the case for a lead-in period, akin to that used in the Gemzar clinical trials, to help prevent the admission of patients who might prove unwilling or unable to comply with our self-administered lifestyle therapy. Early on we both warned that the hostility of the oncology establishment toward me and my therapy could influence patient accrual as well as the compliance of those who chose to proceed with our nutrition treatment—as ultimately it did on both counts. When we first realized Dr. Chabot frequently accepted patients into the nutrition arm whom we believed did not meet the written entry criteria and who in many cases could not possibly follow the prescribed treatment program, we objected, strenuously.

As the study then proceeded along its oft-delayed path, we advised that the persistent suspensions of accrual had undermined interest among patients beyond repair. We objected politely and at times less politely to the annual and lengthy reimbursement delays which we thought an unfair burden for any researcher associated with an NCI-NIH study.

As recruitment dropped to near zero levels throughout 2004, as the shortfall in total patients became an obvious and serious threat to the trial's legitimacy, I warned and warned again at the group meetings that we were heading toward a statistically nonsensical conclusion. Then during the December 13, 2004 session, five years into the trial, I first learned of the significant numbers and staging inequality between the two arms of which we had not previously been aware. I made my concerns about these issues known verbally at that meeting, in my lengthy January 7, 2005 letter, subsequently during the March and June 2005 meetings, and in multiple correspondences throughout 2005 with Dr. Chabot, the respective government personnel involved, Dr. von Eschenbach, Congressman Burton, and Senator Harkin. Yes indeed, the "concerns raised" in Congressman Burton's letter "have been raised and thoroughly discussed at the meetings of the study research team" because Dr. Isaacs and I insisted they be.

The next sentence read:

> NCI and NCCAM staff involved in the management of the grant supplement used to support the study have addressed and managed each concern under their purview.

Here, Dr. Zerhouni once again assured Congressman Burton that these issues I had "raised," to use his term—and which prior to this paragraph he had discounted as valid—were taken very seriously by the study supervisors, so seriously they were not only repeatedly discussed at the formal group meetings, but also *"managed."* The verb "manage" is an important word for the director to have chosen, implying as it does intervention to correct an evident shortcoming, lapse, or error in the conduct or supervision of the trial. While I do appreciate Dr. Zerhouni's reversal in position, acknowledging there were serious problems that required addressing, I do thoroughly disagree that any of these "concerns" had been "managed" effectively, or in a timely manner.

Despite my vehement objection to the randomized format from the first time I heard the term in connection with this trial, only when the study failed dismally did the powers that be agree we needed to change to matched cohort (or case-control). By then, a precious year had been wasted, with the study's reputation tarnished.

No one listened when Dr. Isaacs and I insisted that for a study evaluating a lifestyle treatment such as ours, a lead-in period would allow us to disqualify non-compliant patients and in turn help insure we would end up with meaningful data.

Though for years I warned that the obvious hostility of the oncology profession toward us and our treatment approach was influencing and would continue to influence not only accrual of new subjects but compliance of those patients admitted to the nutrition arm, the supervisory personnel did little. For example, the NCI never did distribute the letter urging oncologists to cooperate with the study (nor did it take out the proposed ads in medical journals).

Repeatedly, sometimes gently, sometimes more aggressively, Dr. Isaacs and I questioned the approval of those nutrition patients who did not meet the written entry criteria—such as those accepted beyond eight weeks from biopsy diagnosis, or those who could not eat. For years I warned, again sometimes gently, sometimes more aggressively, that the admission of so many patients into the nutrition arm who could not or would not follow the prescribed regimen made reasonable evaluation of my therapy impossible. Nonetheless Dr. Chabot continued to send patients to Dr. Isaacs and myself for treatment who lacked the physical capability, the psychological stability, or the social resources to pursue or stay with the therapy.

For years I warned that the ongoing and lengthy suspensions in accrual had helped destroy interest in the project among potential candidates, but the suspensions continued. For years Dr. Isaacs and I tried to find some way to fix the endless and dreaded reimbursement delays, yet after 5½ years the funding problems persisted. Only in mid-June 2005, after the last nutrition patient had been admitted and died, did Dr. Chabot finally assure us in writing that Columbia would subsidize any future patient costs. But the offer had no real meaning, since four months later the study closed for good.

True, in the waning six months of the study Dr. Chabot tried to correct, or to use Dr. Zerhouni's term, sought to "manage" the shortfall in total patients entered into the trial, the imbalance in numbers between the two groups, and the glaring disparity in staging distribution. These efforts to compensate for five years' worth of mistakes came only after my January 7, 2005 letter, only after Dr. Engel's response confirming the two arms could not be reasonably compared, and only after the letters of Congressman Burton and Senator Harkin reached NIH director Zerhouni.

Chapter 16

Reference to Dr. von Eschenbach in Dr. Zerhouni's Letter

D r. Zerhouni's letter continued:

About two months ago, Dr. Andrew von Eschenbach, Director of the NCI, reviewed correspondence and materials received from Dr. Gonzalez with these same allegations and provided a thorough response to his concerns.

I too found Dr. von Eschenbach's letter very relevant to the issues at hand, though I was surprised Dr. Zerhouni would refer to it. After all, in his communication with me the NCI director, unlike Zerhouni, denied not a single "concern" or "allegation" of mine but instead validated my assertions about the troubled study. Though he may have referenced Dr. von Eschenbach's letter, Dr. Zerhouni seems not to have read it.

In his note to me dated September 30, 2005, Dr. von Eschenbach wrote:

I am informed that Columbia staff have repeatedly taken steps to address many of your concerns, such as the effort and recruitment of additional staff to increase accrual in the control arm, and the commitment from Columbia to cover your expenses from their own institution funds to avoid any delays in payments due to issues regarding your subcontract with Columbia.

So Dr. von Eschenbach agreed with me that "many" of my "concerns" had warranted addressing, an indication of just how seriously he, and the "Columbia staff," must have considered my complaints. In terms of specifics, he acknowledged that the disparity between the two groups in the trial represented a serious problem, so serious that Columbia planned, he claimed, to add personnel to help recruit additional patients. I do not remember much about the promised extra staff, but Dr. Chabot did manage to find the 11 new patients for the chemotherapy arm during the narrow window when the study was open to accrual for a total of four or so months. Regardless, his efforts didn't resolve the epidemic non-compliance among the nutrition patients which still made any comparison between the two groups meaningless.

Dr. von Eschenbach also did not deny the payment problems, but reported that the Columbia Cancer Center agreed, in June 2005, to cover any future patient costs to offset delays in reimbursement. Though I appreciated his tacit acknowledgement of this serious issue, the NCI director misstated the facts somewhat; as we have seen the letter given to me by Dr. Chabot promising Columbia's financial backing had been signed only by him, not by the interim director of the Cancer Center. We doubted the letter had any legal clout, but since Dr. Chabot admitted no additional patients into the nutrition arm after April 2005, the issue became moot.

Dr. von Eschenbach thus confirmed my allegations about the numbers and staging inequality between the two arms as well as the reimbursement delays, and the need for correction in each case. Then in the next sentence of his letter, Dr. von Eschenbach added his coup de grâce:

> It is also my understanding that Dr. Chabot has acknowledged the method-ological concerns you raise, has offered to discuss these in detail, and is com-mitted to considering the inclusion of these issues in the manuscript that will result from the trial.

This is an important point, certainly one of the most important points of this entire story, for here Dr. von Eschenbach, in his official capacity as director of the National Cancer Institute, stated clearly and unequivocally for the record that Dr. Chabot himself, the Principal Investigator of the study, far from disparaging or rejecting my allegations "has acknowledged the methodological concerns" I had raised. This statement in an official government document could not be clearer.

Consequently, I find it interesting, perhaps ironic, that NIH director Zerhouni would have referenced Dr. von Eschenbach. In his letter to Congressman Burton, Zerhouni had spent the first 2½ pages strongly denying my every claim about the trial's poor management, while vigorously defending Dr. Chabot. He then admitted that there were problems with the trial requiring both addressing *and* managing. But here he effectively undermined his earlier arguments completely by acknowledging Dr. von Eschenbach's response to me, which not only accepted as legitimate many allegations I had raised, but stated Dr. Chabot agreed with me about the study's "methodological" flaws. To sum up, the NIH director used, in his defense, a document written by the NCI director which actually supported *my* position and not his—or I should more accurately say, not Zerhouni's position as presented in the first 2½ pages of his letter, when he insisted that the study was in all ways well-supervised by Dr. Chabot.

As Dr. Zerhouni continued, he adopted a remarkably conciliatory tone, echoing Dr. von Eschenbach's comments:

> Dr. Chabot has repeatedly expressed willingness to discuss with Dr. Gonzalez all of these concerns and, moreover, is willing to consider inclusion of the raised issues in the manuscript that will result from the trial.

Here Dr. Zerhouni stated, for the record, that Dr. Chabot "is willing to consider inclusion of the raised issues in the manuscript that will result from the trial." If my many allegations and protestations were nonsensical, as the director had *earlier* in his note implied, why would they ever need be mentioned in a scientific paper? Of course, Dr. Chabot would have agreed to discuss these points in writing for official public consumption only if he understood that my charges were, at least in part, valid. I can come to no other reasonable conclusion.

When I came to this point, and tried to sort out the internal contradictions within the Zerhouni letter—are my concerns legitimate or are they not, do they need management or not, does Dr. Chabot agree with them or not—I thought of something the late Linus Pauling told me decades ago. Though I would hardly claim that the eminent scientist was a close personal friend, we did talk occasionally over a period of many years. He was a source of great encouragement and inspiration to me, directly influencing my decision to pursue medicine as a career. Though controversial, he won not one but two Nobel Prizes, two more than most of us humble drones would ever think of earning. During one of our conversations, he said something that has been with me for 25 years: "The difference between a man of intelligence and, well, someone lesser, is internal consistency."

Chapter 17

The Usefulness of Peer Reviewed Publication

A s his letter neared its end, Dr. Zerhouni assured Congressman Burton that the NIH remained determined to bring this trial to a fair conclusion:

> At this time the trial is still active. While enrollment has ended, survivors are still being followed. Trial data is still being collected and a final data analysis has yet to be conducted. NIH staff have closely monitored this trial and we believe that a fair evaluation is occurring. Dr. Chabot and the Columbia research staff have expressed their commitment to the trial's fair analysis. Once the data are complete and analyzed, the trial will be judged in the scientific community through its publication in a peer-reviewed journal. Through publication, the scientific community will have the opportunity to evaluate any methodological concerns of this independent trial.

Dr. Zerhouni seemed certain that through presentation of the data in a medical journal everything would work out for the best, though I didn't understand why he assumed any paper from this project would be handled with more care than informed consent. I suspected Dr. Engel to have been far more on target in her January 27, 2005 letter to Dr. Chabot in which she dismissed any notion

177

that an article about the study, in view of how it had been designed and managed, would serve any useful purpose:

> Given all of the challenges, the surprising outcomes, and the uncertainties about balance between the two arms, it is highly likely (if not certain) that reviewers of the data from this study will raise substantive and legitimate concerns about the comparability of the two populations. As a consequence, it is virtually certain that the controversy surrounding the study will not be settled by the data from it.

I could not agree more with Dr. Engel and thought, as I pondered Dr. Zerhouni's letter, that with a study so flawed in design and implementation as this one, any publication of its data would only lead to confusion, conflict, and recrimination.

Undeterred, his optimism only more resolute, Dr. Zerhouni then proceeded:

> Because we are committed to the fair evaluation of potentially therapeutic alternative therapies, NIH staff have diligently managed this trial and provided the necessary support to ensure that the investigators can bring this trial to a statistically meaningful conclusion.

Once again, Dr. Engel did not share Dr. Zerhouni's enthusiasm that the study was managed "diligently," as she stated in her letter to Dr. Chabot:

> In spite of everyone's best efforts, it appears as if the current design and implementation of the study may have resulted in accrual into the two study arms of patient populations that are not comparable. As a consequence, it is very difficult (if not impossible) to ascertain treatment effect with certainty.

The Webster's definition of "implement" comes pretty close to that of Zerhouni's favored word "manage"—they mean the same. So though the NIH director deferred to the NIH-NCCAM staff repeatedly in his letter, he seemed unaware of that most important evaluation of the trial written by one of them, Dr. Engel's January 2005 letter. If Dr. Engel as a spokesperson for the NIH believed the data to have been essentially meaningless, why did Dr. Zerhouni think otherwise?

Chapter 18

The Battle Heats Up

T hroughout the early months of 2006, I continued work on my rebuttal to Zerhouni. At one point we received notice announcing the next group conference, scheduled for March 20, 2006, as if we were still part of the research team and as if nothing had changed. We had no intention of attending: though we had not resigned, the error-filled minutes from the June 2005 session still remained uncorrected and we were only more convinced that all communications between the group members and us needed to be in writing.

By that point, Dr. Isaacs and I began to suspect that Dr. Chabot and his colleagues might try to place an article about the study in a medical journal, even without our cooperation, and as if the many documented protocol violations had never occurred. Subsequently, the official record of that March 20 meeting—which Dr. Smith dutifully sent to us—confirmed our suspicions that the group intended to move ahead toward publication. Though relatively long compared to earlier versions, the minutes made no mention of the study's management lapses which I had repeatedly raised, Congressman Burton's November 4, 2005 letter, or Dr. Zerhouni's lengthy reply.

The author of the notes, presumably Dr. Smith, divided the document into five categories, headed with Roman numerals. In section II, "Status of control subjects," Dr. Smith wrote:

> When asked about a stopping rule for the length of time control subjects needed to be followed, the investigators stated that the data is robust enough at this time so no stopping rule is now necessary.

I found this sentence a warning sign, since it ignored Dr. Engel's letter of January 7, 2005 which made clear the data was hardly "robust."

In section III, titled "Analyses," Dr. Smith continued:

> The investigators have moved forward on analyses that can be conducted on all accrued subjects: i.e. Demographics, etc. A table has been constructed that illustrates that there are no statistical differences between groups on any of the demographic variables with 2 exceptions (these two blood tests were both in the normal range so the statistical difference between the mean levels of each group are not meaningful or relevant—both groups have levels within the normal range for these tests). In response to Dr. Gonzalez' concerns about potential differences in severity of illness between the enzyme arm and the control arm, Dr. Smith raised this specific issue with the research team. The table includes the p values which indicate no significant differences between groups for stage of illness or for functional status.

As a footnote to the above, even if we accept as true the statement that there was "no significant differences between groups for stage of illness or for functional status," the two arms remained incomparable because of the epidemic non-compliance among the nutrition patients, as clearly defined in Dr. Engel's January 2005 letter.

Four paragraphs later, within the same section, the note read:

> Dr. Chabot has not heard anything from Dr. Gonzalez but again welcomes his participation and continues to consider Dr. Gonzalez a part of the research team. Unless he hears differently from him, Dr. Chabot plans to continue to invite him and Dr. Isaacs to future meetings and to welcome Dr. Gonzalez' participation in the development of the manuscript as originally planned.

Dr. Chabot had heard nothing from me since after six months, we had heard nothing from any of them regarding the errors we had identified in the June 2005 minutes. But he correctly considered us part of the research team, since we had not quit the study.

In section IV, titled "Administrative and other issues," the team finally addressed the missing consent forms, as well as the errors we had identified in the June 2005 minutes:

1. <u>Number of subjects in the enzyme arm and missing consent forms:</u>

The Columbia staff investigated this issue. Two consent forms from subjects entered in the enzyme arm are missing. Their follow up into this issue revealed that there are notes in both subjects' medical charts indicating that they were consented and in at least one of these cases, it is recalled that the patient requested to take the form with them and planned to return it. It appears that both these patients 'walked off' with their forms. The IRB was informed of this and as both charts note that subjects were consented, the IRB left it up to the investigators to decide about inclusion of this data. The investigators conducted the statistical analyses both with and without these two subjects and there is no effect on the statistical conclusions.

I have addressed the history of the consent forms in detail earlier. In this particular version of his story, Dr. Chabot admitted the documents were missing, but claimed that both patients "walked off" with the forms—an odd occurrence, to say the least.

Under point #2 in section IV, Dr. Smith acknowledged the errors in the June 2005 minutes regarding the payment delays. Then under point #3, she wrote:

3. <u>Entering subjects on trial-issues of entrance criteria:</u>

It was Dr. Smith's notes from the meeting on June 20th that stated that Dr. Chabot stated that he was not aware of any subject that was entered in the trial that did not meet the entrance criteria. Dr. Gonzalez writes in his email that he does not recall that statement at that meeting or any other. Dr. Chabot isn't sure whether he made that statement or not at the June 20th meeting, but states that it is accurate and that regardless of whether he stated it then, he restated it at this time.

Dr. Gonzalez also states that he has not received any statement that challenges his description of patients who he states did not meet the entrance criteria as detailed in his January letter. Dr. Chabot said he would review each of the cases in that letter and respond in writing.

For the official record Dr. Chabot had denied approving any patients who did not meet the entry criteria a mere two paragraphs *after* he had acknowledged in two cases no evidence existed of signed informed consent—in itself an admission of a serious protocol violation. I am truly surprised that no one present pointed out the irony in this contradiction.

Under point 4, Dr. Smith wrote:

4. <u>The PI phone calls to physicians and hostility to the trial:</u>

Dr. Gonzalez responded to the June 20th minutes in which the notes state that Dr. Chabot calls the outside physicians to confirm that they are supportive of their patients' participation in the trial from "early on". Dr. Gonzalez states in his email that he thinks "most readers would assume based upon your (*Dr. Chabot's—added by ws*) report that these telephone calls were made to the physicians of the majority of patients." Dr. Chabot does not recall what percentage of the subjects' physicians were called but confirmed that if patients reassured him that they had a supportive physician and that Columbia had the documentation, he would not have typically called that physician. If there was any concern about the supportiveness, that is if the patient mentioned anything to him or if it didn't appear that there was a cooperative physician, he would give them a call to assess whether they were interested in having their patient on this trial, whether they have a problem, and whether they are willing to care for the patient on the trial. In some situations, Dr. Chabot found that the patient had a physician supportive of their patients' participation in the enzyme arm but upon recognition of increased disease, the physician then acted to facilitate the patient moving to other therapy.

As previously discussed, Dr. Chabot's statement made no sense to us for a number of reasons. We had first suggested Dr. Chabot begin contacting physicians of newly approved trial subjects in mid-2004. At that time we all had agreed that such calls were to be made *at the time of entry* to assure future cooperation, not afterwards as the patients pursued our treatment. The statement as reported above that "Dr. Chabot found that the patient had a physician supportive of their patients' participation in the enzyme arm but upon recognition of increased disease, the physician then acted to facilitate the patient moving to other therapy" implied he was communicating with multiple physicians when patients already admitted into the trial began to deteriorate under our care.

However, we are unaware of any call made by Dr. Chabot or anyone in his office to any physician of a patient already proceeding with our therapy.

Furthermore, by the time this process had been put in place, 38 patients had been already accepted into the nutrition arm. Only one more patient would be subsequently qualified for treatment with us, in April 2005, before Columbia closed down accrual for good, so few calls would have been made. Regardless, at the earlier June 2005 meeting, as reported in the minutes of that session, Dr. Chabot stated that his assistant, Michelle Gabay, and not he, had called physicians until she quit sometime in the spring of 2005. After she moved on, he claimed he called the physicians. Here, during the March 2006 meeting he said for the record that he made all the calls from the beginning. We suspected only one physician might actually have been contacted by his office, and believe Ms. Gabay actually made the call.

Even if we allow for the sake of argument that Dr. Chabot did call physicians of patients already undergoing treatment with us, in his attempted explanation he admitted to yet another management lapse. As discussed in Chapter 2, the written rules of the study allowed Dr. Isaacs and me, with the patient's permission, to adjust the therapy, specifically the dose of enzymes and/or their timing, should the disease progress. Consequently, any physician who "acted to facilitate the patient moving to other therapy" without consulting us had allowed for a protocol violation, apparently with Dr. Chabot's direct approval.

Under point #5, Dr. Smith addressed her error in the June 2005 notes, in which she claimed that the Director of the Columbia Cancer Center had assured us in writing we would be promptly reimbursed out of his funds:

5. Columbia letter about funding interruptions:

Dr. Gonzalez's email states that the letter was written by Dr. Chabot and that the Columbia Cancer Center is not mentioned. The letter is signed by Dr. Chabot and states "Because I appreciate your concerns regarding timely reimbursement to you for pancreatic patient evaluations, supplements, and enzyme preparation material for study participants, I want to assure you that there will be no interruption in securing payments from Columbia University." Dr. Chabot noted that there were no additional interruptions in payment and that to his knowledge, Dr. Gonzalez has been paid in full according to his subcontract.

There were no further interruptions, since no additional patients had been entered for nutritional treatment with us—though Dr. Chabot did correctly report that by that point, all past bills, after years of battling, finally had been paid. Nonetheless, the March 20, 2006 meeting minutes illustrated how errors continued to make their way into the official records of this study.

Chapter 19

Dr. Chabot's
April 22, 2006 Letter

L ittle more than a month after the March 20, 2006 group meeting, via regular mail I received a short letter written by Dr. Chabot and dated April 22, 2006. Along with this, Dr. Chabot had also sent the final data chart for the study that listed all patients entered into both arms, along with the stage and length of survival of each.

I thought the note seemed carefully crafted as yet another defense of his management of the study. After all, by this point he must have known Congressman Burton and Senator Harkin had written to Dr. Zerhouni, and of the director's subsequent response to Mr. Burton.

Dr. Chabot's letter read in part:

> It is my understanding that you are waiting for a written response to several issues that you have been concerned about over the past year. I hope the following satisfies those concerns.

> Enclosed with this letter, is a table that identifies patients by study ID number, which arm of the study they are included in, and their start date. The stage, characterized in column four, refers to metastatic disease versus those patients with locally extensive disease that precludes surgical resection. . . .

Other concerns that have been raised by you at investigative meetings include three particular patients that you imply should have been excluded from entry into the study. I have carefully reviewed the three charts that I believe you are referring to, and upon review, I believe our inclusion criteria were met. Two of the patients had well documented depressive disorders that were effectively treated. You imply that a psychiatric disease is an exclusion criteria. If you revisit the study protocol documents, please note the exclusion criteria refers to patients who have psychiatric conditions that preclude the ability to obtain informed consent. Upon reviewing each of the two charts in question, I believe that both individuals were appropriate to the study, given the extent of their psychiatric conditions. An additional patient was being treated with Megace as an appetite stimulant. There is nothing in the protocol that specifically would exclude a patient who is being treated with Megace. Both you and I saw the patient on several occasions and note that his appetite was improving steadily over the initial phases of our contact with him. Your office notes suggest significant improvement in his appetite and ability to eat. Based on my review of his chart, I believe that we made the appropriate decision, both prospectively and upon retrospective review of his performance, based primarily on follow-up notes in your records.

In my January 7, 2005 letter, I had described at least ten patients who could not eat at the time of entry, along with three who in my opinion should not have been admitted because of a strong history of psychiatric illness. So I had no idea why Dr. Chabot would say I questioned his approval of only three patients in total, when I had earlier referenced many more who failed to meet various eligibility criteria.

As I considered his comments, I thought Dr. Chabot, not I, needed to revisit the written protocol. He stated the study rules required exclusion of those "patients who have psychiatric conditions that preclude the ability to obtain informed consent," but as written, they prohibited entry of any patient with any psychiatric condition severe enough to prevent appropriate informed consent *or intensive treatment*. The relevant paragraph from the final protocol version read:

No serious medical or psychiatric illness preventing informed consent or intensive treatment (e.g., serious infection).

Dr. Chabot left out the second half of the sentence.

The two patients he referenced diagnosed with psychiatric illness were Patients #14 and #23, discussed previously. In terms of the third patient Dr. Chabot described, he was technically correct when he wrote: "There is nothing in the protocol that specifically would exclude a patient who is being treated with Megace." Though neither the written entry criteria nor the informed consent form mentioned Megace specifically, both required for admission a "normal" appetite. A patient diagnosed with pancreatic cancer would be prescribed Megace only because of severely inadequate food intake.

Furthermore, I had absolutely no idea what Dr. Chabot meant when he wrote: "Both you and I saw the patient on several occasions and note that his appetite was improving steadily over the initial phases of our contact with him." Patient #8, as described previously at length, the only patient documented to be taking Megace at the time of entry, died some three months after his admission into the study. He lived more than a thousand miles away, so after his intake interview with Dr. Chabot and his initial two visits with us, he never returned to New York. There were no further visits, no "several occasions," as the records clearly prove.

It isn't too hard to sort out the truth of this man's poor appetite, which I described in my initial and lengthy consultation note:

> The patient reports that his surgeon, Dr. M., also told him that chemotherapy would not be particularly helpful and actually suggested he think of alternatives. One of the biggest problems is that the patient's appetite has been "terrible." A week ago one of his doctors (and he's not sure which one) started him on Megace, 2-tsp. day. With this his appetite has improved although it's still down. He reports a 20–25 lb. weight loss. [note: in a period of about six weeks]

At the end of the note, I summarized my thoughts about this patient very succinctly:

ASSESSMENT:

1. History of metastatic pancreatic cancer. The patient was tentatively approved for the clinical trial but he doesn't meet the criteria at this point. He hasn't had liver function tests in 7 weeks and this has to be done. He has no appetite and he's on Megace for appetite. An inability to eat precludes his entrance into the trial. I discussed this with Dr. Chabot.

Between January 17, 2002, when I completed my in-office session with Patient #8, and April 23, 2002, the day he died, I documented in writing 12 individual phone conversations with either the patient or his wife. In a number of our early contacts, I answered simple questions about the mechanics of the program, but thereafter the record is one of a terminal cancer patient in rather rapid decline. For example, my note from January 24, 2002 indicated that he called because of severe diarrhea. On January 31, 2002, he called with a simple question about water filters, but eight days later, on February 7, 2002, his wife informed me that her husband had been admitted to the hospital with dehydration, but had been discharged. My note reported "He is eating," and "To me, it sounds like he's doing better," but this must be seen in the context of a patient so debilitated he had to go to the local emergency room for dehydration, which implied poor intake of not only water, but food as well. After his discharge from the hospital his oral intake improved, but only minimally. To claim my notes implied a normal or significantly improving appetite would be preposterous.

On February 28, 2003, when his wife and I again talked she reported that Patient #8 had resumed the Duragesic patch, a very powerful synthetic morphine derivative usually reserved for terminal cancer patients suffering intense pain. My note stated:

> The last couple of days she said he's struggling. He's having trouble getting all the pills down.

In a note from March 20, 2002, three weeks later, I wrote:

> He's doing much better. I spoke with his wife. She said over the last few days, he really seems to have turned a corner.

Here I transcribed his wife's assessment, not that of the patient, who was too weak to come to the phone to speak for himself. So this note, as the others, must be seen in context. Yes, his wife thought he was doing somewhat better, but better relative to nearly dying.

Less than three weeks later, on April 7, 2002, his wife indicated he was deteriorating quickly:

> I called Mrs. [Patient #8]. I wanted to follow up on him.

> His local doctor is taking care of the low potassium. He hasn't been doing well. He's been off his program for 10 days. He has ascites. They think he has an intestinal infection. They took him to the emergency room 2 nights ago.

They let me [sic] out today. So he hasn't been on his program at all and he's not feeling well. He just wasn't suitable for the protocol. He couldn't eat when he started.

The following day, I spoke to Patient #8's wife again:

I had a long talk with Mrs. [Patient #8]. His family had sent me a note. They're very concerned that the pain isn't being managed properly locally. The pain doctor that they had been seeing was away for 2 weeks. He's back tomorrow. He's not eating. His gut seems to have shut down. The workup of stool specimens was all negative. . . .

They're very concerned about him.

Thereafter, he quickly declined and on April 15, 2002, Patient #8 had to be hospitalized once more, this time with a life-threatening deep venous thrombosis. My note stated:

They thought he might die this weekend but they got him home. He's actually home and he's back on his enzymes, so he's certainly trying.

The problem is he hasn't been able to eat since he started the program and he just wasn't really a suitable candidate for the protocol. That's the problem he never was able to do it.

Two days later, on April 17, I reported:

[Patient #8]'s not doing well. He's almost comatose. He has a visiting nurse every day so he's comfortable.

The family was very grateful. His wife said it just took them too long to diagnose him and he was too sick and I agree.

Six days later, on April 23, Patient #8's wife called to let me know he had died at home.

I spoke with Mrs. [Patient #8].

[Patient #8] passed away on April 19. He died at home. The family was extremely grateful. He had been off his program for a number of weeks at the time he died.

It is true that at times his wife reported he was doing better after being hospitalized, but nowhere in my notes did I imply his appetite "was improving steadily over the initial phases of our contact with him," as Dr. Chabot claimed in his letter. Nowhere did my "office notes suggest significant improvement in his appetite and ability to eat." My statement describing an improved appetite referred to some increased food intake after being hospitalized due to his inability to eat or drink at all. My notes would seem to demonstrate the exact opposite of what Dr. Chabot claimed.

In his letter Dr. Chabot implied I had only complained about a single patient I believed couldn't eat adequately, Patient #8. Here I review the other nine I described in my January 7, 2005 letter to Killen presenting with very poor appetites at the time Dr. Chabot approved each for entry. Though previously excerpted, below I include this information to illustrate what Dr. Chabot ignored in his April 2006 letter to me:

> One of these, Patient 2, developed projectile vomiting before taking a single supplement because of a gastric outlet obstruction. Despite duodenal stenting, he could never subsequently follow the protocol.

> For example, Patient 3, after only three days on the supplements, required hospitalization for management of severe pain and vomiting, then quickly began radiation and chemotherapy. She never resumed her nutritional protocol.

> Patient 4, who at the time of entry had been diagnosed with pleural effusions, followed the therapy only intermittently after the first eight days because of poor appetite and repeated hospitalizations necessitated by pulmonary distress.

> Patient 5 reported very poor appetite within 13 days of entry into the trial, was hospitalized and discharged on hospice. He never continued the treatment.

> Patient 6, who had difficulty eating from day one on the regimen, developed a biliary obstruction within six weeks and never thereafter pursued the therapy.

> During the first appointment with Dr. Isaacs, Patient 7 reported severe nausea that never relented, and precluded any significant compliance with the supplement program. After being diagnosed with a gastric outlet obstruction, she underwent bypass surgery, but afterwards did not pursue the therapy.

> Patient 8 arrived in our office already on Megace because of very poor oral intake. Once home, he never could follow the diet, instead relying on Ensure for nourishment. I estimate he never got more than half the pills down, and deteriorated very quickly.

Patient 9 had lost more than twenty pounds because of poor appetite over a several-week period before acceptance into the study. During my initial consultation with him, I never thought he would be able to do the treatment because of his severe anorexia and general weakness. He went home, began Megace, and quit the therapy within four weeks.

Patient 10, with extensive carcinomatosis, tried hard to do the program, but had so much difficulty eating I doubt he did the therapy for more than two weeks. He ended up doing his "own version" of the treatment, to use his wife's words, before pursuing the GemTax chemotherapy regimen at Columbia. He died very quickly, far faster than any patients described in the GemTax arm of our study. Nonetheless he will be considered a Gonzalez failure.

Patient 12 also seemed to be in an end stage condition when first seen by Dr. Isaacs. Visibly cachectic, with a BMI of 19, he was so weak during the initial interview he could barely hold up his head. When asked about his appetite, his wife prompted him, "You're eating three meals a day, right, honey?" Within six days of his initial visit he was hospitalized for treatment of dehydration, and after discharge was promptly re-admitted because of coffee-ground emesis and biliary stent blockage. Then, while undergoing evaluation for PEG tube placement less than a month later, he was found to be completely obstructed. He never could follow the therapy.

I want to emphasize that the majority of these ten patients either reported or exhibited evidence of significant problems with food intake during the initial sessions with Dr. Isaacs and myself, not days or weeks later. And keep in mind that neither Dr. Chabot nor the other supervisors of the study ever disputed any these case descriptions included in my January 2005 letter. To this day, we believe all of these patients should have been excluded.

Chapter 20

Dr. Chabot's April 2006 Data Sheet

D r. Chabot's two-page chart accompanying his April 22, 2006 letter listed every single subject supposedly entered into the chemotherapy and nutrition groups, the date of their admission, and their stage. Since by this point the study had long since closed to accrual, this document represented the final official description of all patients approved for each arm of the study.

With this information before me, I could sort out the details of just when Dr. Chabot managed to enter the last 11 chemotherapy patients in 2005 when the trial was often closed. In comparison, between December 17, 2003, and March 8, 2005—a period of some 15 months—Dr. Chabot admitted exactly one patient for chemotherapy, on May 12, 2004. He then accepted four between March 9, 2005 and April 8, 2005, a period of four weeks. From June 13, 2005 until July 6, 2005, a total of some 23 days, he approved another five patients for chemotherapy, including one each on June 13, 15, and 16, and two on July 6. This collection of nine qualified between March 9, 2005 and July 6, 2005 approximated the total number Dr. Chabot had accepted for chemotherapy during the first three years of the study in its matched cohort design.

193

Two more subjects were admitted on September 22 and September 23, bringing the total for the chemotherapy arm to 23, the number reported at the December 12, 2005 group meeting. As I looked at the data, I was amazed that Dr. Chabot could find these 11 patients so quickly over a six month period, when so few had been entered in the previous five years.

Since Dr. Chabot classified nine of these 11 subjects as stage IV, on paper the staging of the chemotherapy group now conformed to the usual pattern for inoperable pancreatic cancer, with 34.7% at stage II and III, 65.2% at stage IV.

As I reviewed the chart, his data for the nutrition patients left me somewhat perplexed. First of all, Dr. Chabot provided information for only 37 nutrition subjects, not the 39 we had been counting since the last entry into the group a year earlier in April 2005. Once again, he had changed the numbers without an explanation, apparently discounting two stage IV patients who had been included as of the March 2006 meeting. Of the 37 Dr. Chabot now listed as properly admitted, 22 subjects (59%) he identified as advanced stage IV, and 15 (40.5%) at earlier stages. This distribution seemed consistent with what he had claimed on earlier charts, but differed considerably from our calculations which confirmed that 76% of the nutrition group should be classified at stage IV, 24% at stages II and III.

Since Dr. Chabot had, on this new document, separately identified each patient and their stage, I could finally pinpoint the discrepancy between his numbers and ours. First of all, the stage IV subjects Dr. Chabot had excluded, patients #9 and #16, were the two for whom no evidence existed of signed consent. Each had been sent to us for treatment in clear violation of the stringent criteria of the written protocol. Nonetheless Dr. Chabot continued (or at least it seemed to us he continued) to count both as valid "Gonzalez patients" throughout most of the study, though neither followed the prescribed regimen and both died quickly. Certainly, their exclusion late in the game made the staging disparity less significant.

Dr. Isaacs and I have identified another five of our patients on the chart Dr. Chabot still counted as valid entries, but at a lesser stage than what we had reported and what appeared to be correct. I have no idea when Dr. Chabot would have designated any of this group as non-stage IV, whether he did so at the point of entry or some time later. After all, I had not seen his assessment of any individual patient's stage prior to the April 2006 chart, sent to us long after the study had closed. Nonetheless, Dr. Isaacs and I had categorized each of these five particular subjects—all approved by October 2003—as stage IV at the time of entry on every one of our own data sheets, copies of which we had provided to all personnel during each group meeting. Not once did Dr. Chabot or any of the other study supervisors question our staging assignments for any patient, including these five.

One, Patient #26, whose diagnosis was based on a biopsy of a pancreatic tumor, also showed obvious evidence of liver metastases on CT studies at the time of diagnosis. Though the liver tumors were not themselves biopsied, they appeared, based on the official radiology report, to be so consistent with metastatic cancer that this patient can only be legitimately classified as stage IV. In oncology, a clinical diagnosis of stage IV disease does not require a tissue diagnosis of distant tumors in the context of reasonable radiographic evidence.

Two others arrived with biopsy evidence of metastases. For Patient #3, a sample taken from the peritoneal lining of the abdomen confirmed the diagnosis of stage IV disease. In the second case, Patient #27, a biopsy from a lesion on the omentum—the fatty blanket of tissue that covers and protects the intestinal tract—documented metastatic cancer. By the accepted standards of clinical oncology, this finding also required a stage IV classification.

In the fourth case, Patient #14, we had biopsy evidence of metastasis in a peripancreatic lymph node, that is, a lymph node adjacent to the pancreas, in and of itself suggesting stage III cancer, but a CT scan showed multiple enlarged nodes far removed from this region as well as encasement by tumor of major abdominal blood arteries. Evidence of spread to distant nodes, as opposed to purely local involvement, as well as invasion of large blood vessels, both justify stage IV status.

For the fifth, Patient #33, a pancreatic biopsy had confirmed cancer, but CT scans performed at a local hospital at the time of the original diagnosis showed no evidence of metastatic disease. Thereafter, Patient #33 traveled to MD Anderson Cancer Center in Houston, Texas, for a consultation with Dr. James Abbruzzese, the renowned expert in pancreatic malignancy. There, a new set of CT scans apparently demonstrated clear-cut evidence of metastases into the liver; I say apparently because we do not have the official radiology report of this specific study, only the patient's—and his wife's—description given to us of their visit to Houston. Unfortunately, Dr. Chabot, whose office was solely responsible for gathering medical records of trial patients, failed to provide us with this document. Consequently, we do not have in our possession a copy of the radiology report indicating liver metastases.

After the patient died and I began working on my response to Dr. Zerhouni, we tried unsuccessfully to contact surviving family ourselves hoping for their help in retrieving the MD Anderson records, so to date, the document remains missing.

Overall, of these five "Gonzalez patients" Dr. Chabot identified at a lower stage, four were clearly at stage IV. The fifth in question seemed most likely to have been stage IV at the time of admission to our study, but for now must remain "indeterminate" due to the absent radiology report from MD Anderson.

So in summary, not only did Dr. Chabot find 11 chemotherapy patients—nine at stage IV—as the study came to its end, but by eliminating two stage IV nutrition subjects and downstaging another five he made our group appear less advanced than those entered for GTX. I want to add that neither Dr. Isaacs nor I have ever reviewed the actual charts of any patient entered into the chemotherapy arm to confirm Dr. Chabot's staging assignments for this group, so we have only his April 2006 data sheet as a guide.

Chapter 21

The Battle Continues

In early May 2006, after some six months of hard work, I finally finished my response to Dr. Zerhouni. Totaling some 352 typed pages, the manuscript began with a discussion of the enzyme treatment going back to Dr. Beard, a history of the pilot study and an analysis of its data, and a summary of the problems undermining the NCI-NCCAM clinical trial. I then proceeded with a detailed, point-by-point, line-by-line rebuttal of Dr. Zerhouni's various claims. With the task completed, we had 25 copies of the manuscript bound up, along with supporting documentation.

I sent one to Beth Clay as well as to Congressman Burton whom, I learned from his aide Monica Knab, intended to contact the NIH director yet again after reviewing the monograph. Ms. Knab also suggested I send a copy directly to Dr. Zerhouni, along with an explanatory cover letter.

Below I include excerpts from my lengthy May 16, 2006 note to Dr. Zerhouni accompanying the book:

> I have now reviewed your response to Congressman Burton's November 4, 2005 letter, in which you dispute the concerns he raises regarding the handling of the NCI-NCCAM clinical study of my nutritional therapy. It was suggested I answer your letter point by point in detail. I have done so, in the accompanying document.

With all the resources available to you, including the standard telephone, the extraordinary number of factual inaccuracies in your letter profoundly surprise me. The errors, which serve no benefit to anyone including yourself, could easily have been avoided had your staff contacted me either in writing, by e-mail or by phone, and asked to review my documentation which I would happily have provided. I would of course have been willing to go to Washington to meet with any representative of your office, just as I was quite willing to meet in person with Senator Harkin. Whomever you assigned to the task felt no need to fact check. This unfortunate tack ignores the "due diligence" required in such a situation, solves nothing, and only serves to worsen an already volatile situation.

I would strongly suggest that you read this document yourself, as daunting as it might seem. Frankly, if I were you I wouldn't put a lot of faith in your staff to give you a reasoned and reasonable assessment. However, I thought that a preview might perhaps pique your interest—and convince you that you need to put more thought into any future letters that carry your signature.

In your letter to Congressman Burton, in the second paragraph, page 3 you write with great certainly [sic] "To date, there is no enrolled subject who failed to meet the entrance criteria at the time of enrollment." Let me advise you that in Chapter 20 of my manuscript, entitled, "Alleged Allegations Against Dr. Chabot," I report the fact that Dr. Chabot, the Principal Investigator, repeatedly admitted patients into the nutrition arm who did not sign the informed consent document for the study, as *required* by the written protocol you repeatedly reference, Columbia IRB regulations, NCI rules and Federal law. Not only did he accept patients without properly signed consent, he failed to inform Dr. Isaacs and myself of this serious oversight, leaving us with the false impression all informed consent had been properly obtained. Dr. Isaacs and I spent two and a half years trying to find out what happened to the forms.

As it turns out, though we were told specifically that Dr. Chabot was to conduct all intake interviews, at one point in time he assigned a fill-in nurse to the chore who seems to have been the source of the negligence. For this breach of trust alone, which put all of us in legal jeopardy, Dr. Chabot needs to be removed from his role as Principal Investigator, and reprimanded. Furthermore, the NCI personnel supervising this study, who seemed totally unconcerned by Dr. Chabot's violation of protocol, need a lecture on proper clinical trial management. . . .

Since you have in your letter denied any wrongdoing by Dr. Chabot in any way at any time, you have in essence signed off in writing on a violation of the written protocol and Federal law. Such disregard of the basic rules of your own Institute doesn't inspire confidence.

To make matters worse, as my document clearly reports, Dr. Chabot turns out hardly to have been a disinterested, objective third party referee, as is required for anyone assuming the position of Principal Investigator. As you know, in this clinical effort one group of patients received my nutritional treatment, the other the aggressive chemotherapy regimen, GTX, developed at Columbia by a colleague of Dr. Chabot, Dr. Robert Fine. According to what I have read in the medical literature (see for example *ONCOLOGY NEWS INTERNATIONAL* March 2004, page 44) Dr. Fine credits Dr. Chabot as being an integral part of the research team at Columbia who helped create and test GTX. His significant ties to GTX helps explain Dr. Chabot's inappropriate enthusiasm for the data on the chemotherapy patients. This obvious conflict of interest should have disqualified Dr. Chabot long ago as Principal Investigator. Though his failure to obtain informed consent in several patients—and his refusal to explain in a timely fashion the oversight—alone should warrant his removal from any supervisory function, his role as a co-researcher of one of the two therapies being studied requires he be dismissed, at once.

Finally, I recently received a letter from Dr. Chabot, dated April 22, 2006, that had as an attachment a chart listing the most recent data on survival and staging for both the chemotherapy and nutritional patients. Though he denies once again any wrongdoing, I was dumbfounded to see that he has now left off his list two stage IV patients . . . and describes four patients as stages II or III though the medical records indicate metastatic stage IV cancer. . . . the nutrition group as a whole now appears to be less advanced in terms of staging distribution than the chemotherapy arm. . . .

Consider my letter a formal complaint for unprofessional conduct, scientific misconduct, against Dr. Chabot, Dr. Wendy Smith and Dr. Jeff White of the NCI along with any other NCI personnel responsible for misleading your office. Please include in my complaint the individual or individuals on your staff who put together your letter. . . .

You had within your power the opportunity to help resolve a difficult situation but instead have chosen, for whatever reason, a contrary approach by denying what the facts clearly prove.

I look forward to your prompt response.

Several weeks later, Congressman Burton's office also sent a copy of my monograph to Zerhouni, along with a lengthy letter dated June 13, 2006:

Dear Dr. Zerhouni:

Thank you for your letter, dated December 22, 2005, responding to my concerns regarding the National Institutes of Health's (NIH) handling of Dr. Nickolas [sic] Gonzalez's nutritional pancreatic supplement treatment protocol.

I took the liberty of sharing your response with Dr. Gonzales [sic] and several other experts, and based upon their review, I am deeply concerned that your response appears to contain some errors of fact. I understand that Dr. Gonzales [sic] has completed an extensive response (enclosed) pointing out his perceived problems with the handling of the study. These problems, according to Dr. Gonzalez, include but are not limited to, questions about:

1) Changes in the protocol.
2) Failure by the principal investigator to inform of a conflict of interest in heading this trial.
3) Failure of the principal investigator to obtain signed informed consent documents.
4) Failure of the principal investigator to fairly assign a balanced number and staging of patients to both arms of the study.
5) Failure to ensure all patients met the enrollment criteria.

I also understand that Dr. Gonzalez contends that the principal investigator exerted an undue influence over the study by apparently requiring that Dr. Gonzales [sic] count patients who never truly participated in the study as nutrion [sic] arm failures (skewing the data set); and may have recently acted to change some of the original staging data in an apparent attempt to cover-up the obvious imbalance.

Clearly these are very serious accusations that warrant investigation. However, I understand that Dr. Gonzales [sic] contends that these apparent ethical problems may not be confined simply to the principal investigator, but may also involve NIH staff, both at the National Cancer Institute (NCI) and the National Center of Complimentary [sic] and Alternative Medicine (NCCAM). It is my understanding that Dr. Gonzales [sic] routinely informed NCI and NCCAM staff of his concerns about the principal investigator's actions but staff apparently failed to address these serious allegations of scientific fraud and unethical handling of patients with a life-threatening disease.

Given the importance of conducting safe, fair and statistically significant evaluations of all potentially beneficial medical protocols, and the seriousness of the allegations of scientific misconduct and improper management by both NIH employees and principal investigators, I would respectfully ask you to investigate the circumstances and NIH staff decisions surrounding Dr. Gonzales' [sic] study in much greater detail than to date; and, if appropriate, refer the matter to the NIH Inspector General for further action. I would also greatly appreciate if you would keep Monica Knab with my staff regularly informed of the status of your investigation, as well as, whether or not you ultimately decide to refer the matter to your Inspector General.

Finally, I would respectfully ask you to give serious consideration to not publishing or making any public pronouncements or endorsements about any alleged outcomes of the Gonzales [sic] study until all of the questions regarding this study have been fully explored and resolved. To do otherwise would, in my opinion, run the risk of perpetuating a grave injustice by misleading the public in general and the cancer community specifically.

Your diligent investigation and detailed response will be greatly appreciated.

I appreciated the Congressman's letter for many reasons, most particularly because he warned against publication of meaningless data.

Chapter 22

The Feds Step In

B y mid-June 2006, we had moved ahead on a number of fronts. Both Congressman Burton and I had sent copies of my exhaustively documented manuscript to Dr. Zerhouni for his perusal. But after the director's defensive response to the Congressman's November 2005 letter and his categorical denials of any wrongdoing on the part of the study supervisors, Dr. Isaacs and I hardly believed his office had the motivation to proceed as aggressively as the situation demanded. After all, Zerhouni's insistence in writing that the protocol rules had been steadfastly upheld when in fact Dr. Chabot had admitted multiple patients without evidence of the required signed consent—an easily verifiable fact—hardly inspired our confidence in the NIH bureaucracy.

As we waited for Zerhouni's reply, Dr. Isaacs discussed our study and its many problems with her sister, a physician and former head of the Institutional Review Board at a large Midwestern medical school. When Dr. Isaacs told her the story of the missing consent forms and that the IRB at Columbia, at least according to Dr. Chabot, had given him a pass on the issue, she was aghast. Unsigned or absent consent forms, she reported, represented a serious violation which no IRB can dismiss or ignore arbitrarily after the fact. As a remedy, she suggested we contact two Washington oversight agencies, the Office for Human Research Protections (OHRP) and the Office of Research Integrity (ORI), both within the Department of Health and Human Services, the umbrella organization above NCCAM, the NCI, and the NIH. These two groups, she explained to Dr. Isaacs, had been given the authority to investigate allegations of mismanagement and/or misconduct occurring in federally funded, federally supervised research activities.

After Dr. Isaacs shared this information with me, I checked out the OHRP website and its mission statement summarizing the office's purpose and jurisdiction:

> The Office for Human Research Protections (OHRP) supports, strengthens and provides leadership to the nation's system for protecting volunteers in research that is conducted or supported by the U.S. Department of Health and Human Services (HHS).[38]

The ORI website provided an equivalent mission statement:

> The Office of Research Integrity (ORI) promotes integrity in biomedical and behavioral research supported by the U.S. Public Health Service (PHS) at about 4,000 institutions worldwide. ORI monitors institutional investigations of research misconduct and facilitates the responsible conduct of research (RCR) through educational, preventive, and regulatory activities.[39]

On June 19, 2006—six days after Congressman Burton sent his letter to Dr. Zerhouni—I called the OHRP offices and spoke to Dr. Kristina Borror, Director, Division of Compliance Oversight, about our study and its possible mismanagement. She seemed receptive to my complaints, explaining that her office would consider evidence of protocol violations, whereas the ORI specifically investigated alleged instances of misconduct. She was particularly interested in the three patients admitted without evidence of the required signed informed consent—an oversight, she explained, that represented a violation of strict federal regulations. After I discussed some other areas of possible mismanagement, such as the entry of patients beyond the eight-week cutoff from biopsy diagnosis, Dr. Borror recommended I compose a letter to her detailing my concerns. Since misconduct might be involved, she also suggested I contact Dr. John Dahlberg, Director of the ORI's Division of Investigative Oversight. As per our phone conversation, I subsequently spoke by phone with one of Dr. Dahlberg's associates, who assured me she would be in touch with Dr. Borror so they could coordinate their efforts.

The day of my first contact with Dr. Borror I composed a seven-page letter to her, reading in part:

I am writing in response to our phone conversation earlier today, in the hope for much-needed intervention in a federally funded, National Cancer Institute clinical trial run out of Columbia University in New York. The clinical trial numbers are above. My colleague Dr. Linda Isaacs and I have been directly involved in this study and witness to repeated instances of protocol violations including failure to obtain required signed informed consent, and what we believe to be violation of the Federal laws that govern management of clinical trials for protection of entered patients.

I then briefly summarized the nature of our therapy, the history of the clinical trial, and my concerns about the study's mismanagement:

> we believe that Dr. Chabot at Columbia repeatedly accepted into the study for treatment by us patients who did not meet the entrance criteria, and who were so ill they could never possibly follow our regimen.

> Though we protested each time Dr. Chabot approved a patient we believed did not meet the study criteria, our concerns were either discounted or ignored. Because of such inaction, not once but twice I wrote directly to Dr. Andrew von Eschenbach, then Director of the NCI, who did nothing except refer my complaints back to the study supervisors—the source of the problem. In August of 2005, in desperation over the ongoing mismanagement of the trial we approached Congressman Dan Burton of Indiana, a long time supporter who was himself involved with the initial discussions of the project in 1998. In November of 2005, Congressman Burton wrote to Dr. Elias Zerhouni, Director of the National Institutes of Health, expressing his grave concerns over the mismanagement of the trial. However, Dr. Zerhouni, without performing due diligence, without reviewing our extensive documentation, and without even contacting us to hear our side, supported completely Dr. Chabot's claim that the study had been flawlessly managed.

> In January, Congressman Burton's staff asked that I document in writing each and every protocol violation and episode of mismanagement by Dr. Chabot and the other study supervisors from the NCI and NCCAM. I recently completed this manuscript, which runs approximately 400 typed pages. Congressman Burton is so concerned about the situation that last week he again wrote to Dr. Zerhouni requesting an in-depth investigation.

> I want to make it clear that over the years, Dr. Isaacs and I have voiced our concerns about obvious protocol violations repeatedly to the appropriate in-

dividuals within the NCI and NIH hierarchy, right up to the Directors of the NCI and NIH. . . .

I then discussed several specifics, beginning with those patients admitted into the study without evidence of signed informed consent, and our frustrating efforts over 2½ years trying to learn what happened to the missing documents in two cases. I also catalogued more briefly the other trial subjects Dr. Chabot approved for treatment with us whom we believed did not meet the entry requirements of the written protocol. Further on in the letter, I described Dr. Chabot's potential conflict of interest that should have precluded him from serving as Principal Investigator of the study. I followed this section with an analysis of the April 22, 2006 data sheet and its many unexplained changes.

Several days later, I sent Dr. Borror a copy of my detailed response to Dr. Zerhouni, and shortly thereafter OHRP opened a formal investigation into the trial's management based on the evidence we had provided. At that point, I spoke directly to Dr. Dahlberg of ORI, who informed me that his staff would await the OHRP findings before taking any action.

During one of our subsequent conversations, Dr. Borror advised me that based on her initial review, an evaluation of the pertinent issues in this case most likely would require a minimum of six months, perhaps even a year or two, depending on the evidence Dr. Chabot provided in his defense against my allegations. Should Dr. Chabot and Columbia vigorously oppose my charges, her office might request I provide additional documentation. Nonetheless, for the first time I felt somewhat optimistic that our concerns would be taken seriously within what had previously seemed to be an indifferent and impenetrable government hierarchy. While Dr. Chabot might split hairs and argue about some of the issues I had raised, according to what Dr. Borror told me the missing consent forms seemed more clear-cut. Either the forms existed, or they didn't, and if they didn't Dr. Chabot had violated strict federal regulations.

Chapter 23

The Attempted Publication by Chabot et al.

D espite the OHRP investigation, we still faced a serious risk to our reputations and our years of work if the Columbia team succeeded in publishing an article heralding chemotherapy as victorious, using what we believed to be meaningless data from a poorly managed study. By that point, we assumed Dr. Chabot and Dr. Grann from Columbia, Dr. White and Dr. Smith from the NCI, and Dr. Killen of NCCAM knew that I had criticized the study's management right up to the director of the NIH. In his letter to Congressman Burton, Zerhouni acknowledged his office had been in contact with NCCAM and NCI personnel to discuss my many allegations, so my dissatisfaction with the trial's course was hardly a secret. All of them must also have been aware that Congressman Burton and Senator Harkin had requested Zerhouni's office review the project's oversight. We suspected that the group would shortly learn of the OHRP investigation, brought on at my urging.

I was sure none of the Columbia or government personnel, particularly Dr. Chabot, could be very pleased with us. For all we knew, they might try and publish an article without informing us, hoping to be in print before the completion of any federal investigation. In this way, the team might neutralize my complaining and justify their management of the trial in the public forum of a medical journal. I could even conceive Dr. Killen finally getting his wish, an official NIH press release denouncing my treatment and countering at long last the "positive data of the pilot study."

A June 22, 2006 e-mail from Dr. Wendy Smith of the NCI to the various supervisory personnel, with a copy sent to us, made our concerns about publication very real. In this brief communication, she announced the next staff meeting for the trial would convene June 26, 2006 at Dr. Chabot's Columbia office—and mentioned as well a proposed article:

> To all:
>
> The next research team meeting is scheduled for Monday, June 26, 2006 from 2:00pm until 4:00pm in Dr. Chabot's office. There are two items on the agenda:
>
> 1. Update on status of subjects in the chemotherapy arm
>
> 2. Discussion of data analysis and the preparation of the study manuscript.

Several days later, via regular mail we received a letter from Dr. Smith dated June 22, 2006, the same date of the e-mail, but specifically addressed to us. In her note, Dr. Smith referred to her e-mail of "June 2," though the document was actually sent June 22. I assumed the error represented just a simple mistake.

Though we had no intention of attending the June 2006 session, Dr. Isaacs and I knew we must address the proposed publication. So four days after the scheduled meeting presumably took place but before we received the official minutes, I composed a letter addressed to Dr. Chabot, with copies sent to Dr. Victor Grann of Columbia, Drs. Wendy Smith and Jeff White of the NCI, and Drs. Linda Engel and Jack Killen of NCCAM. This note, dated June 30, 2006, read in part:

> Dear Dr. Chabot:
>
> I am writing in response to your letter from April 22, 2006, and Dr. Smith's letter of June 22, as well as the e-mail sent by Dr. Smith in preparation for the June 26, 2006 meeting.
>
> I gather that you, Dr. Grann, Dr. Smith, Dr. White and Dr. Killen continue to believe the clinical study progressed under your direction as an appropriately managed effort, yielding valid and valuable data. From the recent e-mails and

Dr. Smith's letter I also understand that you are all determined to publish the results of the study in a peer reviewed journal quickly.

For your own benefit, and for the benefit of the others involved from the NCI and NCCAM, I strongly suggest that you withhold any publication. Though you may all believe the study has been appropriately managed, I have been in discussion with a number of regulatory agencies who do not share your perspective. I am aware that shortly, two very serious investigations into the management of the trial, and those involved with it, will be beginning.

You continue to deny that you admitted any patients into the nutrition arm who did not meet the explicit entrance criteria of the study and continue to position yourself as the defender of the written protocol. In fact, the situation is quite different from what you claim; you have already admitted to us in e-mails and at the group meetings as the minutes confirm, that you accepted and sent to us for treatment at least two patients as if they had been properly consented when in fact no signed consent forms had been obtained. Though you, and the other supervisors seemed remarkably unconcerned about this oversight, the written protocol for this study, NCI regulations, and as I have been told, Federal law require that all subjects entered into clinical trials such as ours must sign informed consent. Oral consent is not a valid substitute, and I have been clearly and strongly told that no IRB can, years after the fact, declare the oversight inconsequential. Not only did you enter patients without the required documents, but you seemed reluctant to give us an explanation as to what happened despite our repeated e-mails regarding the matter sent over a two year period.

As another illustration of management lapses and protocol violations, you entered two patients into the nutrition arm long after the eight week window from biopsy despite our complaints, and despite the clearly written protocol requirements.

I could go on, as you might surmise, for many pages. However, at this point, I do not believe this letter to be the appropriate place to detail each and every management failing. Suffice it to say that Dr. Isaacs and I find the indifferent attitude of some of the government scientists toward obvious violations of the written protocol and the conduct of the trial rather astonishing, since it was their responsibility, not ours, to follow up and intervene to correct such problems when they became evident. While you, Dr. Smith, Dr. White and apparently Dr. Killen see no problem with repeated and serious protocol violations occurring under your supervision, including the failure to obtain informed consent, the regulatory investigators with whom I have been in communication, I assure you all, see the situation much differently.

With serious government investigations about to begin, it would be very unwise to attempt publication. . . . Other than violating Federal law, I can see no greater career debacle than to be in the sorry position of being required to retract a published article because of obvious protocol violations, general mismanagement, and/or invalid data.

In the above, I referenced only the two patients lacking evidence of informed consent whom Dr. Chabot had, according to our understanding, counted as "Gonzalez patients" for nearly the entire study. I did not mention the one he himself had disqualified in 2002, when he realized the patient had never signed the required document.

Not long after I sent off my warning to Dr. Chabot and team, the brief minutes of the June 26, 2006 meeting—the last that would be held—arrived, consisting of a single page. Below I excerpt the section related to the planned publication:

Regarding the submission of the manuscript, plans are to have this submitted shortly. In terms of plans to present the data at a scientific meeting, plans will be considered after the publication of the paper. . . .

Although there have been several attempts to communicate with Drs. Gonzalez and Isaacs by both email and post, there has been no communication from them since an email March 26, 2006 requesting the most recent staging breakdown of the chemotherapy patients and when they were entered. Dr. Chabot supplied this information to Dr. Gonzalez in a letter dated April 22, 2006.

Clearly they were moving fast. And after reading the notes, I thought that the official written record was deftly creating a picture of calm propriety on the part of Dr. Smith and the other supervisors, in contrast to our difficult and indefensible behavior. In truth, we had received only three communications from anyone involved in the study after our March 2006 e-mail sent to each of the supervisory personnel, and none of these requested a response.

Nonetheless, I had actually reacted to the team activities in multiple ways, completing my lengthy manuscript to counter Dr. Zerhouni's denials, filing formal complaints in June 2006 with the OHRP and ORI, and then sending my

June 30, 2006 letter warning them all not to publish with federal investigations about to begin.

Overall, I found Dr. Smith's statements both misleading and absurd. For all of her allegations of our unresponsiveness, Dr. Isaacs and I had waited nine months for her and the others to address, finally, the multiple errors in the minutes of the June 20, 2005 group meeting. And when weeks passed and none of the team responded to my June 2006 letter, Dr. Isaacs and I assumed the proposed publication had sensibly died its well-deserved death, at least pending the outcome of the OHRP investigation.

On another front, Dr. Zerhouni never did acknowledge receipt of my May 16, 2006 letter to him and the monograph sent with it. However, he did in a manner of speaking reply to Congressman Burton in a brief note dated August 4, 2006 signed not by him but by Norka Ruiz Bravo, Ph.D., identified as Deputy Director for Intramural Research. The Congressman's aide Monica Knab e-mailed me a copy of the document the day she received it. As I reviewed this letter, I could not understand why Dr. Zerhouni had passed off the responsibility of answering the Congressman's serious questions, but regardless, Dr. Ruiz Bravo wrote:

> Dear Mr. Burton:
>
> Dr. Elias Zerhouni, Director of the National Institutes of Health, asked me to respond to your letter dated June 13, 2006, regarding a supplement to an NIH center grant (P50-CA-013696) that supports a study on the use of nutritional treatments for pancreatic cancer. This study is currently under way at the Irving Cancer Research Center, Columbia University.
>
> We wish to assure you that all appropriate actions are being taken to address the concerns raised in your letter. These actions may include a review by the Office of Research Integrity, the Office for Human Research Protections, the NIH Office of Management Assessment, and other components of the Department of Health and Human Services. We will not have additional information until these reviews have been completed.
>
> We appreciate the information provided in your letter and your interest in the matter.

So, in response to allegations of serious mismanagement and possible misconduct, Dr. Rulz Bravo could write only vaguely "These actions may include review," nowhere saying with certainty what the NIH actually intended to do. I was once again not impressed.

In my subsequent conversations with Ms. Knab, I learned that Congressman Burton likewise thought the NIH response to his note and accompanying documentation completely unacceptable. To my relief, in a subsequent letter dated August 24, 2006, he expressed his dissatisfaction yet again to Dr. Zerhouni:

> Dear Dr. Zerhouni:
>
> I received your office's response to my letter of June 13, 2006 reiterating my serious concerns about the handling of the nutritional pancreatic supplement treatment protocol currently underway at Columbia University (A supplement to NIH Center grant P50-CA-013696). It has now been eight months since my initial letter asking for you to investigate these concerns; and in my most recent correspondence, (June 13, 2006), I respectfully asked you to provide a detailed response to the issues raised. A one page letter from the Deputy Director of Extramural Research which only suggests that these issues may be referred to several other entities for investigation is, in my view, an insufficient answer. I am disappointed that the Department does not appear to take credible allegations of research misconduct much more seriously. Consequently, I would once again, respectfully ask you to clarify for me precisely what the Department is doing to investigate and deal with this issue. Obviously, I do not wish to compromise any investigation which may in fact be ongoing but I would specifically like to know:
>
> 1. Have you referred the concerns raised to the Office of Research Integrity for investigation? If not, why not?
> 2. Have you referred the concerns raised to the Office of Human Research Protection for investigation? If not, why not?
> 3. Have you referred the concerns raised to the National Institutes of Health (NIH) Office of Management Assessment for investigation? If not, why not?
> 4. Have you referred the concerns raised to other components of the Department of Health and Human Services for investigation? If so, specifically what 'other components'?
> 5. Given that these issues were first raised some eight months ago, why has the Department not considered investigating this matter until now?

6. If the allegations prove to be true, any data or conclusions published about this trial may do a disservice to pancreatic cancer patients who are looking for quality information to assist them in their treatment decision-making. Do you intend to prohibit the researchers and staff from publishing or speaking about any studies or other information related to this trial until all questions about the possible ethical and research improprieties have been completely resolved? If not, why not?

As these questions are fairly straight forward, I would greatly appreciate your written response by closed [sic] of business on Friday, September 8, 2006.

I thought, as I read the Congressman's strong response, at least Dr. Isaacs and I were not alone battling the entrenched interests of the Washington scientific community. Mr. Burton clearly was in the battle to the end.

To my surprise, Dr. Zerhouni responded to the Congressman relatively quickly, in a note dated September 12, 2006. In his reply he included the Congressman's specific questions, with his answers placed alongside, as reproduced below:

Dear Mr. Burton:

I wish, once again, to assure you that we take all allegations involving National Institutes of Health (NIH)-conducted or -supported research extremely seriously and pursue them through established processes that may involve multiple Department of Health and Human Services (HHS) Agencies and/ or Offices. Protection of human research participants is among our primary concerns. It is also of utmost importance that we protect the reputations of innocent parties. In addition, we must promote the progress of meritorious research while simultaneously participating in thorough investigations into allegations of wrongdoing.

These investigative processes are conducted carefully with attention to all of these important issues, and necessarily take time. We share your goal to not compromise ongoing investigations and provide the following answers to your questions.

1. *Have you referred the concerns raised to the Office of Research Integrity for investigation? If not, why not?* Yes, we referred these concerns to the HHS Office of Research Integrity (ORI); ORI staff have been in communication with Dr. Gonzalez.

2. *Have you referred the concerns raised to the Office of Human Research Protection for investigation? If not, why not?* Yes, we referred the concerns to the HHS Office for Human Research Protections (OHRP) for investigation; ORI [sic] staff have been in communication with Dr. Gonzalez.

3. *Have you referred the concerns raised to the National Institutes of Health (NIH) Office of Management Assessment for investigation? If not, why not?* Yes, we referred these concerns to the NIH Office of Management Assessment.

4. *Have you referred the concerns raised to other components of the Department of Health and Human Services for investigation? If so, specifically what 'other components'?* These concerns have not been raised to other components of the HHS.

5. *Given that these issues were first raised some eight months ago, why has the Department not considered investigating this matter until now?* The NIH responded immediately upon receipt of these concerns and handled them using established procedures to address complaints.

6. *If the allegations prove to be true, any data or conclusions published about this trial may do a disservice to pancreatic cancer patients who are looking for quality information to assist them in their treatment decision-making. Do you intend to prohibit the researchers and staff from publishing or speaking about any studies or other information related to this trial until all questions about the possible ethical and research improprieties have been completely resolved? If not, why not?* We are committed to providing the public with accurate and timely information regarding the results of NIH-funded research. If some or all of the allegations are found to have merit, HHS will determine the appropriate methods for the responsible institution to alert the patient-subject community.

I appreciate the opportunity to provide additional information.

Sincerely,
Elias A. Zerhouni, M.D.
Director

As I read Dr. Zerhouni's words, I laughed to myself. The OHRP and ORI investigations began only after I had contacted each of these two offices, not due to any effort on the director's part. Nevertheless, we hoped that with Congressman Burton's support, Dr. Zerhouni and staff would no longer brush aside my well-documented allegations.

Over the next few months, I communicated on occasion with Dr. Borror, who assured me the OHRP investigation continued on its slow but steady course. I heard no more from Dr. Chabot or any of the other supervisory staff, not one of whom would ever respond to my June 30, 2006 letter warning them not to publish.

Autumn began and proceeded quietly, with no further drama. But then on Sunday, December 3, 2006, at about 10:35 at night as I was preparing to retire, my answering service contacted me, informing me a Dr. Boris Pasche from Chicago had called my office number insisting he needed to speak to me as soon as possible regarding an urgent issue. My office receives dozens of calls from all over the world every work day and often on weekends, from active patients needing advice but also from those, including professionals, seeking information about my work. When calls come in during off hours, my excellent service long ago mastered the art of distinguishing truly important messages from the more mundane, those that might wait until my office reopened. On this occasion, the woman on the other end of the line—though she wasn't sure who Dr. Pasche was—advised I should return this call immediately.

I myself had no idea who Dr. Pasche might be or why he had called late on a Sunday evening, but I dialed his number thinking perhaps he was a physician with information about one of my patients. The man who answered the phone immediately identified himself as Dr. Boris Pasche before expressing his gratitude that I had returned his call at such an inconvenient time. He then explained he was an oncologist living in Chicago who had worked at Sloan-Kettering for years, knew my mentor Robert Good, and had followed my own career for some time with interest, including my efforts to have my treatment methods evaluated in clinical trials. Currently, he was affiliated with the medical school at Northwestern University, while also serving as Oncology Editor at *The Journal of the American Medical Association (JAMA)*. In this latter capacity, he had before him on his desk a manuscript submitted for publication at

JAMA, authored by John Chabot, Robert Fine, Karen Antman, Victor Grann and others associated with Columbia University and entitled, as he read to me, "Pancreatic proteolytic enzyme therapy vs. gemcitabine-based chemotherapy for the treatment of pancreatic cancer (PANCAM)." The paper had been tentatively approved for publication, pending his final personal review. So, as I was to learn that Sunday night, Dr. Chabot and friends had attempted to publish an article about the study in a major medical journal, without my knowledge and despite the federal investigations.

Dr. Pasche summarized the report, which claimed that in patients with advanced pancreatic cancer, my therapy had shown no effect whatsoever in contrast to the GTX chemotherapy regimen which had provided significant benefit. Surprisingly, the data presented indicated patients treated with my nutritional program not only failed to respond in terms of their cancer but also experienced a significantly worse quality of life than those receiving GTX.

Dr. Pasche explained that as he studied the manuscript carefully, he had grown increasingly concerned by possible significant problems with the trial. As a start, it appeared to him that two experimental regimens were being compared, my nutritional treatment versus the still unproven GTX. This odd situation, he said, essentially invalidated the data. In an appropriately designed clinical study, he continued, the new treatment under scrutiny must go up against the best standard therapy, which in this case would have been the single agent Gemzar.

He was also most perplexed that I had not been listed as one of the co-authors. For some time he had been aware of the clinical trial, which he knew had been funded to test the efficacy of my treatment. The paper itself, he said, made clear that I had been in charge of treating the nutrition patients. But in an addendum of sorts appearing after the main text, the authors claimed that I had withdrawn from the study and refused to cooperate with the preparation of the manuscript. This statement, Dr. Pasche said, left him only more bewildered. Why would I quit a trial testing my therapy and not participate with publication of the data unless there had been some sort of conflict between the study supervisors and myself?

After pondering the situation, he told me he decided to call one of the Columbia team to ask why I wasn't a co-author on a paper discussing a multi-year investigation of my regimen. This individual, according to Dr. Pasche, insisted that I had withdrawn from the study, refused to cooperative with manuscript preparation, and furthermore, that I had "disappeared" and couldn't be found.

Thinking this explanation less than believable, Dr. Pasche decided to find out for himself if I had indeed strangely vanished without a trace. He obtained my office phone number easily enough, then deliberately called late on a Sunday night to discover how hard I might be to locate. He remarked, laughing, that I had returned his phone call within five minutes.

I agreed that I was pretty easy to track down, was not in hiding, and that the extraordinary explanation given him was most likely intended to discourage him from seeking me out to learn my version of the clinical trial—which he seemed very anxious to hear. I then said contrary to what had been written in the postscript, I had not resigned from the trial, had never seen the manuscript in question, didn't know it existed, and had not refused to cooperate with its writing. In fact, I told Dr. Pasche that because of what I believed to be Dr. Chabot's serious mismanagement of the project, I had instigated at least one federal investigation at OHRP, with another possibly in the works—about which Dr. Pasche knew nothing.

I mentioned that months earlier I had written all supervisory personnel involved in the trial, warning them not to try and place an article with two government evaluations in progress. When I heard nothing back, I assumed, evidently incorrectly, that Chabot et al. would not try and publish the results of a tainted effort.

At Dr. Pasche's urging, I summarized the various problems associated with the study's management, particularly the numerous patients admitted who did not meet the entry criteria. I mentioned the three lacking evidence of signed informed consent, those admitted beyond the eight-week cut-off from biopsy, patients accepted for our therapy who could not eat, study candidates Dr. Chabot qualified despite psychiatric illness, etc., etc., etc. I explained that so few nutrition patients actually complied with the prescribed regimen, the study's data really had no meaning, as confirmed by Dr. Engel's official NIH letter—which I learned was not referenced in the manuscript, and about which Dr. Pasche until that point again had known nothing. He also seemed concerned when I described Dr. Chabot's direct participation with Dr. Fine's research, a conflict of interest not disclosed in the article.

Dr. Pasche expressed some unhappiness that Dr. Chabot never informed any-one at *JAMA* about Dr. Engel's letter or the OHRP involvement. Under this cloud, Dr. Pasche believed the paper should never even have been submitted and would be rejected by *JAMA*. He assured me he would write Dr. Chabot with his decision, at the same time advising him not to seek publication else-where. He also promised to e-mail a copy of the article to me in the morning. I thanked him for his candor, and as we said our goodbyes, I felt I had just encountered someone with enormous integrity.

After I hung up, I was so livid with Chabot, and White, and Smith, and Killen, that I couldn't fall asleep for hours, but I was also extremely grateful that Dr. Pasche had chosen to inform me about the paper. He didn't have to track me down, he could easily have taken the authors at their word and approved the article for publication. In his position, as an esteemed conventional oncologist, why not? After all, Dr. Chabot was at that time Chief, Division of General Sur-gery at a major Ivy League medical center, his co-authors included colleagues at Columbia as well as Dr. Karen Antman, the first woman President of the American Society of Clinical Oncology and by that point dean of a medical school. On the other hand, Dr. Isaacs and I were always the outsiders on the fringe of the academic world, controversial alternative practitioners providing an unconventional nutritional therapy.

As promised, the following day Dr. Pasche e-mailed as an attachment a copy of the manuscript, running some 26 pages including graphs. What I read left me somewhat dumbfounded.

The article began as per usual in medical journals with an abstract preceding the main body of the paper, summarizing the trial's purpose, methodology, results, and the conclusion which Dr. Pasche had read to me the night before.

> **Context:** Median survival among patients with inoperable pancreatic adeno-carcinoma is close to 6 months. Until recently, conventional medicine had little to offer such patients and many sought alternative treatments.
> **Objective:** To compare the outcomes of proteolytic enzyme therapy and gem-citabine-based chemotherapy
> **Design, Setting, and Patients:**
> The NCI in 1998 sponsored a phase III randomized controlled trial of proteo-lytic enzyme therapy vs. chemotherapy. Because eligible patients refused ran-dom assignment, the trial was changed in 2001 to a controlled observational

study. Enzyme therapy patients were seen by Dr. Gonzalez and all patients by one of the investigators at Columbia University. All patients had to meet strict clinical criteria for eligibility. Of 58 patients with inoperable pancreatic cancer who agreed to participate, 23 elected chemotherapy and 35 enzyme treatment.

Intervention: Treatment included orally ingested pancreatic enzymes, nutritional supplements, detoxification, and an organic diet, or gemcitabine-based chemotherapy.

Outcome measures: Primary outcome was overall survival and secondary, quality of life.

Results: At enrollment, the treatment groups had not [sic] statistically significant differences in age, sex, weight, performance status, stage of disease, pathology, quality of life, or clinically meaningful laboratory values. . . . At 1 year, 55% of gemcitabine patients were alive, but only 14% of enzyme therapy patients remained alive. The quality of life ratings were better in the chemotherapy than the enzyme treated groups (p<0.001).

Conclusion: Among patients with pancreatic cancer, those who chose gemcitabine-based chemotherapy survived nearly twice as long as, and with better quality of life than those who chose proteolytic enzyme treatment.

From the first sentences of the abstract I found the paper to be unscientific. As a start I questioned the statement in the "Context" section that "Until recently, conventional medicine had little to offer such patients and many sought alternative treatments." Though assuredly some patients diagnosed with pancreatic cancer seek out "alternative treatments," I knew then and know now of no reference to support the claim, no objective epidemiological evidence, that "many" do so. During the time of the trial, approximately 38,000 patients were diagnosed with the disease yearly in the U.S., and of these, I suspect only a very small percentage pursued a therapy that would be considered "alternative."

Further on, I immediately identified an obvious factual error. The study changed design not in 2001 as reported here, but in April 2000, as Dr. Zerhouni had correctly stated in his December 22, 2005 letter to Congressman Burton. I was also somewhat surprised that now Chabot counted only 35 nutrition patients, not the 37 listed in his April 2006 data sheet, nor the 39 that had actually been admitted by our accounting. Once again, without explanation, he had eliminated another two subjects from the study.

Following the abstract, the text of the paper itself began with a lengthy introduction, describing my involvement with enzyme therapy along with some background information about Dr. Beard and the pilot study data. The authors did see fit to reference briefly Dr. Pour's positive results in the nude mouse model for pancreatic cancer—then dismissively reported in bolded print:

> but **the rationale for the purported anti-cancer effect of this treatment is unknown.**

Of course, in his 1911 book Dr. Beard in great elegant detail provided the scientific basis for the therapy along with the impressive laboratory and preliminary clinical results.[9] To date I have uncovered no legitimate evidence disproving the basic tenets of his hypothesis or his experimental findings.

The subsequent paragraphs described the study design, followed by a section entitled "Recruitment":

> **Recruitment:**
> This study was widely publicized through the NCI. All patients who were interested were reviewed by the study chair or one of the co-investigators. If they wished to be entered in either the control or experimental arm, they filled out a detailed questionnaire. All laboratory, radiological, and pathologic findings were reviewed at Columbia University Medical Center.

Since the NCI never sent its completed letter to oncologists encouraging their cooperation and never took out the promised ads in journals, I was unaware that the NCI "widely publicized" the trial. Yes, as Dr. Zerhouni had claimed in his December 22, 2005 letter to Congressman Burton, at our urging the NCI did include a summary of the project on its website, amidst the descriptions of many other research efforts it actively supported. But a mention on a website hardly translated into a study being "widely publicized."

The second sentence I found misleading. Beginning in July of 2000 and for the greater part of the trial, as far as I knew Dr. Chabot alone reviewed all patient records and he alone determined eligibility. No "co-investigator" (as defined by the official protocol) assisted in the process beyond the first 20 months of this seven-year adventure.

The next paragraph read:

> **Eligibility criteria:**
> The enrollment criteria were carefully defined. To be eligible study patients had to have signed a consent form that was both witnessed and dated; to be

greater than age 18; to have a histologically confirmed adenocarcinoma of the pancreas that was inoperable with either an advanced primary tumor or metastases (stages II-IV); to have no prior treatment except surgery with non-curative intent; and to be within 8 weeks of diagnosis. . . .

Enrollment restrictions for the study took into account the stringencies of pro-teolytic enzyme therapy; patients and their families had to be willing to under-take and be able to administer the treatment at home, needed to be able to eat solid food with no allergy or intolerance to pork (pancreatic enzymes used in the protocol are pork derived). . . .

I thought it ironic that Dr. Chabot would so carefully enumerate the entry re-quirements which he had repeatedly violated. Even in this cataloguing he did not get the criteria right. His statement "needed to be able to eat solid food" reports only half of what actually appeared in the relevant section from the written protocol:

Non pregnant, non lactating
Able to eat solid food, three meals per day . . .
Supportive live-in spouse or other family member

The phrase "three meals per day" is hardly trivial. And as stated earlier, the official consent form for the study restated this requirement quite bluntly, to avoid any confusion about its intended meaning:

Seventy to ninety patients will participate in this study. You were selected as a possible participant because you have been diagnosed with adenocarcinoma of the pancreas and have not previously received chemotherapy or radiation. Furthermore, you are able to eat normally and care for yourself, both require-ments for entrance into the study.

The next section of the article described the study design in detail, the essentials of the nutritional and chemotherapy treatments, and the statistical methods used to evaluate the data. This was followed by the crux of the matter, the section titled "Results" that began on page 20 of the manuscript. The first paragraph read:

Of 70 patients with pancreatic cancer who expressed interest in the study, 8 did not meet the eligibility criteria. Of the first four eligible patients, three re-fused to be randomized and withdrew. One additional patient signed a consent form, which was misplaced due to a change in staffing. No differences were noted in the analyses with or without this patient.

I had no idea where the number 70 came from, but knew the third sentence did not conform to our records. As I have earlier shown in some detail, Dr. Chabot sent to us for treatment as if properly admitted not one, but three patients for whom no evidence of a signed consent form existed. Furthermore, his explanation here contradicted his own statements made at the March 20, 2006 group meeting as recorded in the official minutes. At that time, he claimed that two patients had "walked off" with the forms—not that any had been "misplaced due to a change in staffing." His story here had completely changed from the version previously told for the study record.

Returning to the paper, in the "Results" section two paragraphs down, Chabot et al. wrote:

> Table 1 presents the demographic and clinical characteristics of the participating patients, by treatment group. The patients in both the control and experimental arm were carefully **enrolled** according to **strict** entry criteria.

The bolding appears in the original manuscript, for obvious emphasis. In this paragraph, Dr. Chabot completely disregarded his already documented mishandling of informed consent in the three cases sent to us for treatment in violation of the "*strict* entry criteria." And though earlier, under "Eligibility criteria," he specifically and correctly stated that all patients were to be admitted within eight weeks of biopsy—under "Results" he completely ignored those he had approved who failed this rule. I thought this omission particularly striking since I had referenced these patients in my June 30, 2006 letter to him.

As per usual in medical journals, the "Comment" section appeared towards the end of the paper. Traditionally, here the authors of a research report discuss the data, its validity, any problems with the study's management, and the conclusions that can be drawn from the results. In this case, the authors wrote:

> **Comment:**
> This report may be the first controlled cancer trial to compare allopathic treatment to an alternative medicine program consisting of proteolytic enzymes, diet, nutritional supplements, and detoxification procedures for a hard endpoint such as survival. Other studies have investigated mixtures of herbal or vitamin therapies or compounds isolated from natural substances. Many

conventional chemotherapeutic agents come from plants; the vinca alkaloids come from a common shrub; paclitaxel is derived from the bark of the Pacific yew tree, and docetaxel from the needles of the English yew tree. Palitaxel [sic] has had a major impact on the treatment of breast, ovarian, and lung cancer. Less successful herbal treatments include PC-SPES which in Phase II trials among prostate cancer patients lowered PSA levels and improved abnormal bone scans, but was withdrawn from the market after certain batches were found to be contaminated by prescription drugs and beta-carotene which in Phase III trials for the prevention of lung cancer showed an increase in deaths among male smokers who received it compared to a placebo control group.

The difference in survival between patients who chose gemcitabine-based chemotherapy and those who chose enzyme treatment was statistically significant. . . .

In these paragraphs, I thought Chabot and his co-authors had compiled a badly organized hodgepodge consisting of completely irrelevant statements about naturally derived standard oncology drugs and an unrelated bogus alternative cancer treatment. The references to paclitaxel and PC SPES, all mixed together with the survival results of this study and its methodology, made no sense to me.

I wasn't at all surprised by the meager median and mean survival for the nutritional group as reported, since at most only 8 of the 39, or 37, or 35 patients ultimately entered—the numbers of qualified subjects varied depending on which Chabot document one read—adhered to the prescribed regimen to any extent, and only one completely. But nowhere in the article did Dr. Chabot mention the compliance issues so clearly identified in Dr. Engel's January 2005 letter.

This section continued with an out-of-sequence and in my opinion gratuitous paragraph on complementary medicine, along with an enthusiastic summation of the particular Columbia chemotherapy regimen serving as the control treatment in our study:

Most patients with cancer use some form of *complementary* medicine, such as vitamins, nutritional supplements, diet, exercise, or prayer, *in addition to* their cancer therapy. Many studies have been published on the merits and dangers of these additional remedies. Little is known, however, about either the prevalence, or the benefits and harms of *alternative* medicine used *in place of* conventional evidence-based treatments.

> The experimental arm in this study failed to show any advantage over the control arm. . . .

> The chemotherapy chosen for the control arm was the best reported when this study was initiated in 1998. Since that time additional agents have been added, such as both xeloda and taxotere [sic], which is currently being studied in a Phase II trial at our institution.

The last sentence above confirmed the Columbia connection to the GTX regimen, once again bringing to mind Dr. Chabot's evident conflict of interest. But nowhere in the paper did Dr. Chabot acknowledge that he worked closely with Dr. Fine at Columbia over the years, helping to develop the very complex multi-agent treatment approach used in our clinical trial.

The final two sentences of the **"Comment"** section read:

> Pancreatic cancer is the fourth major cause of cancer death. Our findings suggest that recent advances in conventional treatment have the potential to improve survival and offer new hope to pancreatic cancer patients. Hopefully, these observations should spark additional clinical research in this relatively neglected disease.

As I studied the article, in one sense it seemed, at least to me, constructed to answer precisely my specific complaints about the study's management. Chabot completely disregarded those nutrition patients who failed to meet the entry criteria, and nowhere referenced, even in passing, the many—we estimate at least 30—who could not or did not pursue the prescribed treatment appropriately. He chose to ignore Dr. Engel's January 27, 2005 official NCCAM letter, written at a time 38 nutrition patients had already been entered, in which she astutely warned:

> In spite of everyone's best efforts, it appears as if the current design and implementation of the study may have resulted in accrual into the two study arms of patient populations that are not comparable. As a consequence, it is very difficult (if not impossible) to ascertain treatment effect with certainty. . . .

We discussed at considerable length his concerns about the probable accrual of patients unable to comply fully with the nutrition arm of the protocol. It was our impression that everyone in the room basically agreed that, despite best efforts, there is in fact, reason to be concerned about this issue, and that it clouds interpretation of the data. Even if we assume, however, that this is the explanation for the disappointingly poor outcome of patients on the nutrition arm, accrual of 15 or 20 additional patients to the nutrition arm of <u>this comparative study, as it is designed and currently being implemented</u>, would only be appropriate if there is a chance that the interim results would change.

These statements weren't written by me, or Dr. Isaacs, but by the Program Officer for the study. Reading Chabot's paper, one would only assume that under his supervision all patients accepted into the nutritional arm met all entry criteria, complied with the therapy completely, and simply failed to respond to our treatment.

The addendum Dr. Pasche had mentioned in our discussion the night before followed the **"Comment"** section as a free-standing asterisked paragraph:

> The Pancam study was proposed to the National Institutes of Health by Dr. Gonzalez and Dr. Wynder in 1997. In 1998, Columbia University's Herbert Irving Comprehensive Cancer Center was awarded a supplement to its National Cancer Institute Cancer Center Grant to implement Dr. Gonzalez's study protocol. Over the subsequent 7 years, Dr. Gonzalez served as a coinvestigator, attended all quarterly research team meetings at Columbia (in person or by telephone), and played an active role in study implementation, admitting and following all the patients accepted to the enzyme arm. In 2005 after the study was already closed to enrollment, Dr. Gonzalez expressed concern related to patient selection and elected not to continue participating in the study or its research meetings. Although repeatedly invited to discuss the manuscript and to serve as co-author, Dr. Gonzalez declined to participate in manuscript preparation.

In the first sentence of the above paragraph I discovered yet another error I would have been happy to correct had Chabot contacted me before submitting the paper. My mentor Dr. Wynder, as supportive of the trial as he may have later been, was not involved with any proposal to the NCI or the NIH related to my therapy, nor did he help earn the grant ultimately awarded.

I identified at least two significant mistakes in the third sentence. Never did Dr. Isaacs or I participate in any group meeting "by phone." We were there in person in every instance from the beginning of the trial until the June 2005 session. After that point onward, since we no longer trusted the official record keeping, we attended none of the scheduled conferences in person or by phone.

Dr. Chabot and his co-authors also erred by claiming that I played "an active role in study implementation, admitting and following all the patients accepted to the enzyme arm." Of course Dr. Isaacs and I treated all approved nutritional patients, and true, for the first 20 months of the project, including the disastrous first year of its randomized incarnation, Dr. Isaacs and I could veto patient entry. During this period only four patients had been qualified for treatment with us, and after July 2000 Dr. Chabot alone would manage all aspects of patient evaluation and approval. No one from my office could even discuss our treatment or the study with any patient seeking information about the project. Though the above sentence implied that I participated in the selection process throughout the trial's history, in truth for most of the time neither Dr. Isaacs nor I had "an active role" in patient "admitting."

The next statement, "In 2005 after the study was already closed to enrollment, Dr. Gonzalez expressed concern related to patient selection and elected not to continue participating in the study or its research meetings" seemed reminiscent of Dr. Zerhouni's claim in his December 2004 letter to Congressman Burton, that I complained about the study's management only at its end. Regardless, the statement here is completely inaccurate, as can be easily verified. The records of the project definitively show that over a period more than two years preceding 2005, Dr. Isaacs and I repeatedly advised in writing that Dr. Chabot had admitted multiple patients into the nutrition arm whom we believed did not meet the eligibility criteria, including the two for whom we discovered no evidence of signed consent existed. Our first written queries to his office regarding this specific issue date to the fall of 2003, and multiple subsequent e-mails over the years confirmed our concern with this issue.

Dr. Isaacs and I also repeatedly warned long before the study closed that so many patients had been admitted into the nutrition arm who either could not or would not comply with the prescribed regimen that the data had been rendered meaningless. My lengthy January 7, 2005 letter sent to all supervisory personnel catalogued in detail this problem, long before the study would close to accrual in October 2005.

Dr. Engel's January 2005 letter addressed to Dr. Chabot, written directly in response to my concerns, supported my allegations, particularly regarding the entry of so many patients who had not to that point complied with the prescribed treatment. She also immortalized in the official record that we had been discussing these issues for some time:

> There have been numerous and very difficult scientific, operational, and procedural challenges in carrying out this trial. These have been well documented and frequently discussed.

Furthermore, at no point did Dr. Isaacs and I elect "not to continue participating in the study" though after June 2005 we did, for very good reasons as previously described, decline to attend further group sessions. Since we could no longer depend on the minutes to be accurately transcribed, from that point forward we chose to communicate with the study staff only in writing, not verbally. But never in any written document or in any phone conversation did I state that Dr. Isaacs and I were officially withdrawing from the trial. Quite the contrary, I expected to remain fully engaged so I could monitor with appropriate diligence Dr. Chabot's activities, any instances of mismanagement, and possible efforts to promote useless data as meaningful.

Ironically, Dr. Chabot's own words as recorded in official study documents created throughout 2005 and 2006 contradicted his claim that in 2005 I "elected not to continue participating." The minutes of the December 12, 2005 group meeting—which Dr. Isaacs and I did not attend—included a statement attributed to Dr. Chabot in which he himself considered us to be active participants in the trial:

> Dr. Gonzalez has not attended the last two meetings. Dr. Chabot continues to consider Dr. Gonzalez a part of the research team. Unless he hears differently from Dr. Gonzalez, Dr. Chabot plans to continue to invite him and Dr. Isaacs to future meetings and to assume Dr. Gonzalez will participate in the development of the manuscript as originally planned.

The minutes of the March 20, 2006 conference similarly recorded Dr. Chabot's correct belief that we were still involved:

> Dr. Chabot has not heard anything from Dr. Gonzalez but again welcomes his participation and continues to consider Dr. Gonzalez a part of the research

team. Unless he hears differently from him, Dr. Chabot plans to continue to invite him and Dr. Isaacs to future meetings and to welcome Dr. Gonzalez' participation in the development of the manuscript as originally planned.

To clarify a point here, the phrase "Dr. Chabot has not heard anything" was misleading. At that time I still awaited a reply from him regarding those patients he had admitted whom I believed did not meet the written entry criteria. Nonetheless, by late March 2006 Dr. Chabot considered me "part of the research team," nowhere mentioning for the record that I had "elected not to continue participating in the study."

Dr. Chabot's April 22, 2006 letter addressed to me further acknowledged I was actively engaged with the trial—why else send it? In this communication, Dr. Chabot defended his supervision of the study, particularly his oversight of "patient selection," but nowhere did he even imply that I had withdrawn from the trial. On the contrary, his words reflected his belief that by late April 2006 I was still a member of the team:

> It is my understanding that you are waiting for a written response to several issues that you have been concerned about over the past year. I hope the following satisfies those concerns.

Three months later, in her June 22, 2006 letter addressed directly to Dr. Isaacs and myself, Dr. Wendy Smith, one of the NCI supervisors, also treated us as active participants. She cheerfully invited us to the next meeting scheduled for June 26, 2006, mentioning nothing about either of us having quit:

> As you know from my reminder email, June 2, the next research team meeting is scheduled for this Monday, June 26, 2006 from 2:00pm until 4:00pm in Dr. Chabot's office. There are two items on the agenda:
>
> 1. Update on status of subjects in the chemotherapy arm
> 2. Discussion of data analyses and the preparation of the study manuscript. . . .
>
> Please let me know if you have any questions.

Had we resigned from the study, we find it hard to believe Dr. Smith would not have referred to that fact.

Though we did not attend, Dr. Smith sent us the minutes of the June 2006 meeting promptly—another indication to us that in the minds of the NCI personnel, we remained part of the "research team" and should to be treated as such. Once again, this official record makes *no mention* of our having "elected not to continue participating in the study."

The last sentence of the *JAMA* submission was perhaps the most inaccurate of all: "Although repeatedly invited to discuss the manuscript and to serve as co-author, Dr. Gonzalez declined to participate in manuscript preparation." At no time did anyone involved in this study invite me to review any manuscript that had been prepared for publication, nor did I even know a completed paper existed. We had learned from Dr. Smith's June 22, 2006 e-mail announcing the next scheduled meeting that Dr. Chabot and the team intended to *discuss* a proposed article about the trial. The subsequent minutes of that session confirmed that Dr. Chabot and the others did plan to publish and publicize the data.

With the OHRP investigation in progress, in late June 2006 I sent my letter to Dr. Chabot with the others copied, advising strongly against submitting any article. In this note nowhere did I say I had withdrawn from the study or that I would refuse to cooperate with manuscript preparation. Nor did I expect at any future time to be excluded from discussions related to the data or any planned publication. When not one of the study supervisors responded—as would have been appropriate—we assumed they all had enough sense to put a hold on their plans. I learned a finished paper existed and had been sent off for review only when Dr. Pasche called me that Sunday, December 3, 2006.

So the document came to its end. Sadly, the errors and the tone hardly surprised me, after all we had witnessed during the years of the study. Even putting aside for a moment the misstatements, I thought this was one of the most poorly organized, badly written scientific papers I had ever read.

But with an article like this, if published in a highly regarded medical journal, what better way to counter my serious allegations that had already reached up to the directors of the NCI and the NIH? Should this paper see the light of day, I could envision a media circus of such intensity, a backlash against me and my treatment so strong that my legitimate complaints about the study's management would be lost in the fray. My concerns, up against a peer-reviewed article in *JAMA,* would seem inconsequential and self-serving, of little import compared to the opinions of the academic experts from the esteemed institutions of Columbia, NCCAM, and the NCI.

I knew the stakes were high for Dr. Chabot's academic career. Should Dr. Isaacs and I ultimately be vindicated and our charges validated, Dr. Chabot's standing at Columbia might be jeopardized, as well as his chances of ever securing another government grant—the kiss of death for an academic physician whose position and prestige rise and fall depending on such funding. We knew from what he had told us that this was his first federally funded research effort, so a grand misstep here would not be viewed very favorably within his own institution or at the NIH, particularly if the failure proved to be due to mismanagement. I also suspected that for the various government officials assigned to the project, a controversial clinical trial that disintegrated on their watch, the $1.4 million wasted on nothing over eight years, and the questions about my treatment that would remain unanswered, would hardly represent a big career boost within the bureaucracy of the NCI and NIH.

I also knew I needed to protect our reputations, the future of this valuable therapy, and most importantly, the truth. First, I sent copies of the Chabot paper to Dr. Borror at OHRP and Dr. Dahlberg at ORI, along with cover letters, explaining in some detail the blatant inaccuracies. Then I spent the next week constructing a letter of complaint alleging what I believed to be scientific misconduct on the part of Dr. Chabot, addressed to Dr. Lee Goldman, the Dean of Columbia University College of Physicians and Surgeons. In this and in great detail, I countered the false assertions in the *JAMA* submission, including the statement that Dr. Isaacs and I had withdrawn from the study. When finally completed, the letter ran 14 pages, single-spaced, with many pages of additional supporting documentation:

I began by identifying myself, before describing in detail my recent conversation with Dr. Pasche. Below I provide a much shortened, edited version:

Dear Dr. Goldman:

I am a physician practicing in New York City who employs an aggressive nutritional program in the treatment of advanced cancer. As you may know, since 1998, my colleague Dr. Linda Isaacs and I have been collaborating with Columbia investigators on an NIH funded, NCI supervised clinical trial comparing my approach to chemotherapy in the treatment of patients with inoperable pancreatic adenocarcinoma. Dr. John Chabot, Chief of General Surgery at Columbia, has served as Principal Investigator.

Though I remained a co-investigator throughout the duration of the study, on Sunday, December 3, 2006, I became aware in a phone call from Dr. Boris Pasche, the Oncology Editor of the Journal of the American Medical Association, that without my knowledge or approval, Dr. Chabot and the other Columbia investigators were attempting to publish a paper about the trial. Furthermore, as Dr. Pasche and I talked it became clear that the article, to my astonishment, contains within it false information. . . . Dr. Pasche, unaware of an ongoing Federal investigation of Dr. Chabot's role, was concerned enough by our conversation that he told me he intended to write Dr. Chabot rejecting the paper and advising against publication anywhere else. The following day, Dr. Pasche e-mailed the article to me, a copy of which is attached. In consequence of my conversation with Dr. Pasche and my detailed review of Dr. Chabot's written report, I am contacting you now to file a formal complaint of scientific misconduct. . . .

As you may also know, many problems have plagued the project since its inception, including what we considered inappropriate study design, slow accrual and the reluctance of oncologists to refer patients into the study. In more recent years, Dr. Isaacs and I uncovered serious flaws related to the management and implementation of the study under Dr. Chabot's direction that rendered the data meaningless. Though we have documented numerous such examples, far more than appropriate for this letter, some more telling illustrations should suffice to make the point.

I then described, in summary fashion, many of the patients Dr. Chabot admitted into the nutrition arm who did not meet the protocol requirements for entry, including those three for whom no evidence of signed consent existed. I outlined the multitude of patients entered who could not or would not comply with the prescribed treatment, as well as Dr. Chabot's clear conflict of interest:

Overall, we estimate of the 39 patients Dr. Chabot ultimately approved for the nutrition arm, only 6-8 at most liberal analysis actually followed the regimen as prescribed to any significant degree. . . .

We also later learned that Dr. Chabot was hardly a disinterested third party referee of the study, as clinical trial ethics demand for a Principal Investigator. On the contrary, Dr. Chabot had worked closely with Dr. Robert Fine at Columbia developing and testing the drug regimen being used in most patients assigned to the chemotherapy arm of our clinical trial—as multiple publications attest. His involvement with Dr. Fine's research represented and represents today a clear conflict of interest which Dr. Chabot never revealed to us.

Despite the many problems we observed, my colleague, Dr. Linda Isaacs and I continued to participate in the study, hoping that Dr. Chabot would, as he repeatedly promised, correct the project's direction and work toward a fair, equitable and scientifically valid outcome. However, when the problems continued unchanged, on January 7, 2005 I wrote a 29 page letter detailing my concerns about the management and progress of the project, sent to all scientific staff from NCCAM (NIH), the NCI and Columbia. In response, Dr. Linda Engel of NCCAM wrote an official NIH letter to Dr. Chabot dated January 27, 2005 that in essence confirmed my complaints. In her letter, a copy of which I have enclosed. . . .

I included lengthy quotes from Dr. Engel's letter, before continuing my discussion:

I want to emphasize that in her thoughtful, official NIH statement, Dr. Engel did not counter a single fact or point discussed in my earlier 29-page document, but specifically and in essence affirms them all—and documents prior agreement with my claims among all those involved, including Dr. Chabot.

After January 2005, Dr. Isaacs and I continued to cooperate with the project when Dr. Chabot promised once again to correct previous shortcomings, such as the admission of patients unable to follow the nutritional regimen. However, as time passed, we came to realize that the promises were empty, that corrective action would not be appropriately implemented, that Dr. Chabot would continue to ignore or dismiss our concerns—despite their NIH validation—and that the trial was not headed toward an equitable or scientifically valid conclusion.

I then discussed the history of Congressman Burton's involvement, and my complaints filed with OHRP:

In June 2006, I learned Dr. Chabot, despite the many documented problems with the study, and despite the NIH's own opinion of the data as expressed in its official letter of January 27, 2005, intended to write and publish a paper about the project and its alleged "results" as if it had been a legitimate and properly supervised clinical effort. In response, on June 30, 2006, I wrote to

Dr. Chabot again, expressing my grave concern over the study, its management and the data, as well as my belief that with two active Federal investigations in progress, publication was unwise. I have enclosed a copy of that letter for your use.

I received absolutely no response from that letter, nor have I heard from Dr. Chabot or anyone else involved with the study since, not via phone, e-mail, regular mail, certified mail, Federal Express, or any other commonly or uncommonly available mode of communication. I assumed that Dr. Chabot had taken my advice and would not seek to publish data that the NIH itself has identified as most likely meaningless.

I want to emphasize that neither Dr. Isaacs nor I have ever resigned from the study, nor did we ever express disinterest in any intended publication. On the contrary we expected as per appropriate procedure to be included at every step as the project wound down, and to be informed of any attempt to publicize or publish the study's very flawed data. It is true that we did stop attending the regularly scheduled group meetings after June 2005 for very specific and valid reasons, as detailed later in this letter. But we never resigned from the study.

I then described my phone conversation with Dr. Pasche, my own review of the paper and the multiple errors contained within. I concluded with a lengthy analysis of the asterisked paragraph at the end of the paper:

Since I have never resigned from the study, I remain now eight years still involved. Though Dr. Isaacs and I attended all team meetings from the study's inception through June 2005, we thereafter did not attend any further meetings for reasons that are clearly documented. First, we did not find these time-consuming sessions productive in any way, nor did they seem to have any impact on the disastrous direction of the project. More importantly, as the September 2005 meeting approached, the official minutes of the June session had strangely not yet been prepared for review, so no valid documentation existed to confirm what had been previously discussed. Without an ongoing record, we felt it inappropriate to attend since we had no evidence our statements were being properly recorded. We decided all future communication needed to be in writing and only in writing. We most assuredly did not resign from the study as Dr. Chabot claims, but did inform all involved we would no longer be attending and the reasons why. I would add that never at any time did we participate in any planned formal group session "by telephone."

In great detail I then debunked the claim that I had "withdrawn" from the study, using the official meeting minutes and Dr. Chabot's April 2006 letter as evidence that he himself considered me "a part of the research team" right up until the end.

I then concluded:

> The last sentence of the paragraph reads "Although repeatedly invited to discuss the manuscript and to serve as co-author, Dr. Gonzalez declined to participate in manuscript preparation." This statement is false . . . an excuse to publish, without my knowledge, data that the NIH has previously identified as meaningless. . . .
>
> After my June 30, 2006 letter to Dr. Chabot advising against publication with two Federal investigations underway, I never heard from Dr. Chabot or anyone involved with the study again, in any way or in any form, either by phone, via e-mail, by regular mail, by certified mail, by Federal Express, etc. He did not respond in any way to my June 30, 2006 letter, and at that point no paper had been written, only planned. When I heard from no one, I assumed that appropriately no paper would be written. I had no knowledge of any "manuscript preparation" in progress, I was never invited to discuss the manuscript during its preparation, and I never heard from anyone about a manuscript until Dr. Pasche of *JAMA* called me on December 3, 2006. . . .
>
> You will see, as you investigate the matter, that my version of manuscript preparation is the true version.

I sent the letter off to Dr. Goldman, along with the supportive documentation, and copied Dr. Chabot, who never did respond.

Meanwhile, I didn't hear again from Dr. Pasche, whom I assumed had followed through as promised and rejected the paper. On Tuesday, December 12, the day after I sent my letter to Columbia Dean Dr. Goldman, in the late afternoon my staff informed me that Dr. Catherine DeAngelis, the Editor-in-Chief of *The Journal of the American Medical Association*, was on the phone, wishing urgently to speak with me. I immediately took the call.

At first, somewhat to my surprise, Dr. DeAngelis seemed very stern, even hostile toward me, in complete contrast to Dr. Pasche's attitude of a week earlier. She clearly did not believe I knew nothing of the Chabot article until my conversation with Dr. Pasche. At one point, when she bluntly suggested that I must have been aware of the paper, I repeated the truth, that I had no knowledge of its existence until I spoke with Dr. Pasche. She grew silent for a moment, before saying, again in a somewhat cold tone, that after Dr. Pasche reported our conversation to her, she had called both Dr. Smith at the NCI and Dr. Grann at Columbia, both of whom insisted I had been fully informed about the finished article but had refused to cooperate with its writing.

I suspected that she had believed whatever Drs. Smith and Grann had told her, without question. I tried to remain calm, explaining that their statements as described were inaccurate, and asked her if either of them had mentioned the federal investigation into the trial's management currently in progress. Since I had discussed OHRP's involvement at length with Dr. Pasche I assumed he had shared the information with her.

Dr. DeAngelis acknowledged that neither Grann nor Smith had referred to the OHRP in their respective conversations with her, then requested I describe the exact nature of the investigation, and how it came to be. I started by relaying in some detail the history of the study and its many problems, and my turning in frustration to Congressman Burton, OHRP and ORI when the management issues remained unresolved. As we talked, I thought that her opinion of me might be changing, to the point she actually might be accepting my version of events as true, particularly when I provided the details of my complaints to OHRP and ORI. Eventually, as her attitude toward me softened, she expressed a growing anger with Chabot et al. She repeated what Dr. Pasche had told me, that with two federal investigations in progress, the article should never have been submitted to *JAMA* or anywhere else.

Precisely for that reason, I explained, I had actually written a letter in June warning Chabot not to try and publish at this time. Since I had heard nothing back, I assumed he and his colleagues had wisely taken my advice, so I was taken off guard the evening Dr. Pasche alerted me to article's existence. I offered to send her a copy of my letter, which she in turn said she wanted to see as soon as possible.

I also told her that after reading the *JAMA* submission I had filed a written, formal complaint of misconduct against Chabot with the Dean of Columbia, a copy of which I also offered to send her, along with the supporting documentation. She seemed anxious to have that information as well, and then said she was so annoyed with Chabot, Smith, and Grann she might herself file a complaint of misconduct with Columbia.

When I got off the phone, I thought that perhaps I had just done Dr. DeAngelis a favor. Had *JAMA* unwittingly published the Chabot article with the OHRP investigation just beginning, Dr. DeAngelis could have looked foolish—particularly if my complaints were eventually vindicated. In any event, that afternoon I e-mailed Dr. DeAngelis my June 30, 2006, letter warning Chabot against publication. She responded with a simple "Thank you." At the same time, via FedEx I sent her a copy of my lengthy complaint to the Columbia Dean along with a mass of supporting documents.

Later that evening, with my patient responsibilities for the day ended and my curiosity about Dr. DeAngelis growing, I decided to look into her background. Up to that point I really did not know much about her, other than that she served as editor of one of the most influential medical journals in the world. Now that we had spent considerable time talking on the phone about the Chabot article, I wanted to learn more.

My search on the Internet very quickly yielded considerable information about Dr. DeAngelis, who like myself had followed an unusual course into medicine. She originally dreamed of a career as a physician-missionary, but due to financial constraints chose instead to pursue training as a nurse, a less expensive route into the medical field. According to the online biographies, she never gave up her dream of becoming a doctor, and after a stint at Columbia Presbyterian she entered Wilkes University in Pennsylvania to begin her premedical studies. She subsequently attended the University of Pittsburgh Medical School, and completed a residency in pediatrics at Johns Hopkins. Later, she earned a Master's Degree in Public Health at Harvard, served on the faculties of Columbia and the University of Wisconsin Medical School, and eventually returned to Johns Hopkins. There, she quickly ascended to full professor in Pediatrics, only the twelfth woman in the institution's history to achieve that rank. In 1994 Dr. DeAngelis was appointed vice dean for academic affairs, a position she held for five years before leaving Johns Hopkins in 1999 to assume her position as Editor-in-Chief of *JAMA*.[40]

Having studied her background, I had only more respect for Dr. DeAngelis, for whom a medical career had not come easily. She seemed driven by a fundamental idealism; for example, throughout her career, she had shown considerable interest in social issues related to health care, even setting up clinics in under-served areas.

Over the next several weeks, Dr. DeAngelis and I exchanged several e-mails, all friendly in nature. Before Christmas, she wished me a wonderful holiday, and I the same to her.

In mid January 2007, I received a brief note from Dean Goldman of Columbia, in which he reported:

> We have an institutional policy regarding the evaluation of such complaints, and your allegations will be investigated in the same way that any such complaints are evaluated.

I thought the response a little too curt and far too vague, so I wrote back, asking him to be more precise, and questioning what he meant by the "institutional policy." Dr. Goldman replied in early February 2007, informing me that my second letter had been forwarded to Dr. David Hirsch, executive Vice President of Research.

During that period I also received a copy of correspondence between Naomi J. Schrag, Director of Research Compliance and Training at Columbia, and Dr. Susan Garfinkle of the Office of Research Integrity. The two had evidently discussed my allegations, as indicated in the second paragraph of the document:

> As we also discussed, Dr. Gonzalez's research misconduct allegations appear to rest on human subjects protection allegations currently being investigated by the Office of Human Research Protections ("OHRP"). As you advised, Columbia will await the outcome of OHRP's investigation before proceeding with Dr. Gonzalez's research misconduct allegations. In the meantime, as we also discussed, we will remind Drs. Chabot, Fine and Grann that they must preserve all document [sic] relevant to Dr. Gonzalez's allegations, and, in particular, any such documents concerning the drafting of the paper at issue.

In the earlier written exchanges between Congressman Burton and Dr. Zerhouni, the NIH director reported he would similarly await the OHRP findings before taking any independent action against those supervising the study. Evidently, much hinged on the thoroughness and integrity of the OHRP investigation.

Chapter 24

The OHRP Investigation Continues

On February 28, 2007, my staff put through a phone call from Dr. Patrick McNeilly, who had identified himself as an OHRP staffer. I hadn't heard his name before, but he quickly explained to me that he had taken charge of the Chabot investigation and in that capacity had been in repeated communication with Columbia. According to what Dr. McNeilly said to me, Chabot apparently now claimed in his defense that I had assisted with patient selection throughout the study, so if any subject failed to meet the entry requirements, the fault was mine.

I replied with the truth, stating that when the study first began in 1998, Dr. Antman agreed Dr. Isaacs and I should participate with the evaluation and approval of patients seeking entry into the trial. Even in those days, we were told Dr. Chabot's office would conduct the initial review of all study candidates. Only after he tentatively qualified a patient could we then veto his decision based on the written entry criteria. But I explained to Dr. McNeilly that in July 2000 the NCI insisted we be completely excluded from the process, leaving Chabot in complete charge of patient selection for both the chemotherapy and nutrition arms. During the first 20 months of the trial when we could veto patient entry, we assessed a grand total of 10 patients, six of whom we approved, but only four of whom actually joined the nutritional arm. From July 2000 onward, Dr. Chabot alone determined eligibility for the remaining 35 subjects admitted for treatment with us, often despite our documented concerns that many did not meet the entry requirements.

I suggested to Dr. McNeilly that by shifting his responsibility to us, Chabot might be hoping to avoid criticism, but his assertion that we collaborated with patient admission—except for the first 20 months—was simply incorrect.

As we talked, I was surprised to learn that Dr. McNeilly seemed unaware of my lengthy response to Dr. Zerhouni, though I had sent a bound copy to his colleague Dr. Borror at OHRP. At that point, I offered to send him a manuscript for his own use.

Later that afternoon, I put together a package of documents for Dr. McNeilly, including a bound Zerhouni manuscript along with copies of my complaint addressed to the Dean of Columbia and Dr. Engel's January 2005 letter to Dr. Chabot acknowledging, as the official NIH spokesman, that the large number of non-compliant nutrition patients had left us with essentially meaningless data. In my cover letter accompanying the materials I specifically addressed Chabot's alleged latest defense:

> In terms of the specific issue you raised today, Columbia's . . . assertion that we were involved with patient selection, Dr. Isaacs and I were very frustrated from the onset of the study. . . . So thoroughly were we excluded that, as you will see in the document, when prospective patients called our office seeking information about the trial, we had been instructed not to say a word about the project but immediately refer the patient to Dr. Chabot's office. We were forbidden from discussing the project with any patient. To us, it made as much sense for Dr. Chabot to have such authority as to put me in charge of a study selecting patients for new brain surgery technique. I am not a brain surgeon and not suitable for that role.
>
> So it was quite disconcerting to hear that now Columbia, or Chabot, now claims we were involved in patient selection, therefore if inappropriate patients were entered it now becomes my fault. . . .Yes, we did repeatedly complain about patient selection, to him directly and during the meetings, but his attitude never changed. Only during the last meeting we attended, in June 2005, after all nutrition patients had been entered, did Dr. Chabot—knowing Congressman Burton was not happy with the way the study was moving—suddenly announce that we would be allowed input into patient selection. A

few weeks later he told us no new patients would be entered into the nutrition arm.

When I didn't hear back from Dr. McNeilly after sending off the documents, I assumed he was pursuing his investigation at the usual slow bureaucratic pace.

Chapter 25

HIV-Nevirapine: An Example of Government Science Run Amok

I n early 2007, as I awaited the next move from OHRP, through a series of serendipitous events I learned of another highly publicized and mismanaged government-funded clinical trial, this one with international implications. The details of this rather extraordinary situation came my way during a conversation with my friend Robert Scott Bell, host of a weekly national show devoted to alternative medicine issues, particularly the politics of the field. Robert and his guests frequently delve into the powerful influence wielded by pharmaceutical company lobbyists in Washington, the often oppressive stance of the drug-oriented regulatory agencies in regard to nutritional therapies, and the typical indifference of the academic research community toward promising unconventional treatments.

In recent years, I had appeared on Robert's show several times to discuss my approach to cancer, and more recently, my disappointment with the progress of my NCCAM-NCI clinical trial. That spring of 2007, Robert, who normally hosted his show from a studio in Florida, happened to be in New York attending an alternative medicine conference at the Hilton Hotel in midtown Manhattan. He had set up a booth outside the main lecture hall complete with microphones, so he could interview convention speakers on his Sunday show live from the hotel. Though I wasn't a lecturer myself, Robert had asked me to come by in the afternoon to talk about my therapy, especially the current status of the clinical trial. Arriving early before his show had gone on the air, I had time to regale him with recent events including the ongoing OHRP investigation. Robert, who from our prior conversations already knew the study had not gone well, was disappointed though not surprised that the project had essentially fallen apart under the guidance of the academic experts from Columbia, the NCI and the NIH.

As we talked, he asked me if I had been following recent scandalous revelations about the U.S.-supported HIV-Nevirapine clinical trial conducted in Africa. I had actually heard of this highly funded, highly lauded NIH effort, set up to evaluate the protease inhibitor nevirapine in the prevention of HIV transmission from infected pregnant women to their babies. I also remembered reading that the study had been mismanaged, though I had not followed the issue too closely.

Robert now elaborated, explaining that from its inception the trial had been so poorly supervised by NIH personnel the lives of both the women entered into the project and their infants had been placed at serious risk. However, the wrongdoing by NIH scientists had been deftly covered up, right up the line at the NIH. When a government whistleblower, Dr. Jonathan Fishbein, tried to expose the incompetence and dishonesty to his NIH superiors, they responded by firing him. Robert informed me that fortunately, Congress had listened to Fishbein, taken up the cause, and in its own investigations vindicated his allegations. As a result, Fishbein had been reinstated at the NIH at Congressional insistence. Though the NIH had worked hard to hide the scandal, word eventually leaked out to the press, who then had a field day with the story.

Robert, who had been following the situation, explained Dr. Fishbein had appeared several times on his show, creating great interest in listeners about the case. In some ways my situation, Robert said to me that Sunday afternoon, paralleled that faced by Fishbein, who found the regulatory agencies slow to act in response to complaints of mismanagement. Unfortunately, before we could talk more about Dr. Fishbein and his troubles, we had to begin my broadcasted interview.

Spurred on by Robert's revelations, over the next few months I began my own investigation into the HIV-Nevirapine study and its rather strange history. The information I collected left me questioning whether any oversight office within the Department of Health and Human Services (DHHS) or the NIH had the motivation to pursue aggressively allegations of scientific misconduct.

The Division of AIDS (DAIDS) within the National Institute of Allergy and Infectious Diseases, itself a division of the NIH, directly supervised the HIV-Nevirapine trial in Uganda from 1997–1999, with the cooperation of an esteemed group of international researchers. During and after the project's completion, U.S. government spokespeople touted the trial as a shining example of U.S. efforts to stem the tide of AIDS in Africa. In an unusual move, the NIH, encouraged by the preliminary findings, even released the data before its publication in the peer-reviewed literature. Excited government scientists claimed a 47% decrease in the risk of HIV transmission with nevirapine compared to women receiving a short course of the control, AZT, the previous standard approach to the problem of mother-infant co-infection. Not only did the new regimen prove more effective, it was, according to reports, easily administered and inexpensive, with few reported side effects.

On September 4, 1999, in the prominent international journal *Lancet*, the HIV-Nevirapine team formally published the results to great acclaim, ushering in, it was thought, a new era in HIV prevention and perhaps finally slowing the massive epidemic in Africa.[41] As a result of the study's data and the *Lancet* article, in January 2001 Ugandan authorities approved the drug as a preventative against transmission of the disease from HIV-positive women to their babies. Subsequently, in July of 2001 nevirapine's manufacturer Boehringer Ingelheim sought FDA approval in the U.S. for use of the drug in the same context.

However, by early 2002 scientists outside the NIH began to question the initial enthusiastic reports of a great new advance against HIV. In preparation for an upcoming FDA review, researchers at Boehringer conducting an internal audit uncovered evidence of numerous and significant protocol irregularities which violated the integrity of the data already published in *Lancet*.[42] In response to Boehringer's concerns, the Office for Human Research Protections launched its own investigation of the trial's management.

An article appearing in *USA Today* in December 2004 entitled "U.S. officials knew of concerns with AIDS drug" described these early questions raised about the trial's legitimacy:

> Boehringer Ingelheim, the Connecticut-based company that makes nevirapine, told NIH it identified at least one "critical compliance issue" that compro-

mised the integrity of the study and more than four dozen issues it described as "serious" and "major."

Boehringer and NIH auditors cited concerns such as failing to get patients' consent about changes in the experiment, administering wrong doses and delays and underreporting of "fatal and life threatening" problems.[43]

The *USA Today* writer then quoted from an official analysis compiled by a private firm, Westat, contracted by Boehringer Ingelheim to evaluate the project:

It appeared likely, in fact, that many adverse events and perhaps a significant number of serious adverse events for both mother and infant may not have been collected or reported in a timely manner. . . .

Westat reported there were 14 deaths not reported in the study database as of early 2002 and that the top two researchers in Uganda acknowledged "thousands" of bad reactions that weren't disclosed.[43]

As reported by *USA Today*, in March of 2002 NIH officials began meeting for apparent damage control:

NIH officials reviewed the bad news in early March 2002.

Meeting minutes, written in shorthand, raised broad concerns: Half the babies in the study were also enrolled in a vitamin A study that could have affected the outcome, and medical staff running the trials didn't follow procedures for divulging serious adverse events (SAEs).

"No mtg minutes, no training doc(umentation), site used their own criteria for grading SAEs. No lab normal values & serious underreporting of SAEs," the minutes stated.

The minutes quote an NIH official who visited Uganda as saying, "The site staff doesn't know what they don't know." . . .

In January 2002, Boehringer sent NIH an early copy of its report. But the drug maker, fearing publicity about the report might destroy its chance to get the FDA approval of the drug for domestic use, asked NIH to destroy it before FDA regulators could learn about it.

"Sensitive information. Asked for it to be destroyed when audit is upon us," NIH official Mary Anne Luzar wrote on the cover page of Boehringer's report. . . .

> Lane [an NIH scientist] said the request to destroy the report was inappropriate and NIH never complied. But he conceded his agency inappropriately kept the audit from FDA for weeks. . . .[43]

As the evidence of mismanagement mounted, Boehringer withdrew its application for FDA approval. Nonetheless, despite the growing storm over the data, on June 19, 2002, President Bush unveiled his $500 million dollar "New Mother and Child HIV Prevention Initiative," with none other than nevirapine as the showcase intervention. Bush happily announced that the U.S. "will support programs that administer a single dose of nevirapine to the mother at the time of delivery, and at least one dose to the infant shortly after." *USA Today* reported:

> "This major commitment of my government to prevent mother-to-child HIV transmission is the first of this scale by any government, anywhere," Bush said in a Rose Garden announcement.[43]

No one at the NIH had bothered to tell the President that the study had been a shambles, its data questionable at best. On the contrary, NIH officials, fully aware of its own audits and the Boehringer findings, deliberately kept the bad news from the White House:

> But the National Institutes of Health, the government's premier health research agency, chose not to inform the White House as it scrambled to keep its experts' concerns from scuttling the use of nevirapine in Africa as a cheap solution, according to documents obtained by the Associated Press.[43]

In July 2002, less than a month after the Bush announcement, the Department of Health and Human Services notified the Ugandan government that this once praised study had repeatedly violated NIH criteria for protection of research subjects:

> NIH's nevirapine research in Uganda was so riddled with sloppy record keeping that NIH investigators couldn't be sure from patient records which mothers got the drug. . . .

> The NIH research "may have represented a failure to minimize risk to the subjects," the Office of Human Research Protections told Ugandan authorities in summer 2002.[43]

During this time, the NIH higher-ups not only neglected to inform the President about the many protocol violations, the unreported serious side effects including deaths, and the poor management of the trial, they chose not to alert the press. The catastrophic problems remained a big NIH secret.

In March 2003, the Division of AIDS (DAIDS) released its own analysis of the study's management, strangely excluding any critical statements. The media, along with the White House, seemed at the time blissfully unaware of the ongoing scandal, so successful were the efforts to hide the bad news.

In July of 2003, the National Institute of Allergy and Infectious Diseases, the parent Institute over DAIDS, contracted Dr. Jonathan Fishbein, a clinical trials expert, to serve as the first Director of Office Policy in Clinical Research Operations in the Division of AIDS. In this capacity, Dr. Fishbein "was to assure that DAIDS sponsored clinical research was in compliance with applicable regulations, guidance and policies and meets established standards of quality, integrity and ethics to protect the volunteers."[42] His superiors at DAIDS, according to published reports, advised Fishbein they wanted the office to operate like a "virtual drug company." However, in his new role Fishbein quickly learned HIV-Nevirapine had not only been grossly mismanaged, but that the study's many failings had been covered up within the NIH.

Two weeks later, as Fishbein began his own investigation, South African regulators, now aware of the troubling reports, announced they would discount the flawed HIV-Nevirapine data when assessing the drug's value as a preventive despite feverish attempts of NIH officials to gloss over the trial's problems.[42]

On September 11, 2003, *Lancet* published a follow-up article that completely disregarded the allegations of mismanagement and the subsequent cover-up, instead once again enthusiastically proclaiming the value of the drug in blocking mother-baby HIV transmission.[44] At that point, Dr. Fishbein, assuredly not much of a team player and oddly determined to take his oversight responsibilities seriously, filed a formal complaint against the Deputy Director of DAIDS, Dr. Jonathan Kagan, with the new DAIDS director, Dr. Edmund Tramont. In the tradition of great bureaucracies, Dr. Tramont responded by instructing Dr. Kagan, the subject of the complaint, to *fire* Dr. Fishbein. In turn, on March 3, 2004 Dr. Fishbein notified the Department of Health and Human Services Counsel that "on information and belief, Edmund C. Tramont, M.D., Director, DAIDS, knowingly and willfully altered conclusions in the HIVNET 012 remonitoring report to conceal serious deficiencies in the study."[42]

Four days later, Dr. Fishbein "repeats his allegations of scientific misconduct in the HIVNET 012 remonitoring effort to officials of the U.S. House of Representatives, Energy and Commerce Committee, Subcommittee on Oversight and Investigations."[42] Finally, in May 2004, in conjunction with NIH officials the subcommittee arranged for a formal review of the study, its management and data, by the Institute of Medicine (IOM), a non-governmental organization in Washington charged with assessing and mediating scientific controversies. In addition, NIH Director Zerhouni's office began its own investigation, the results of which were released in July of 2004.

The NIH report, highlighted in an Associated Press article, provided a very unflattering picture of the Division of AIDS:

> The government's AIDS research agency "is a troubled organization," and its managers have feuded, used sexually explicit language, and engaged in other inappropriate conduct that hampers its global fight against the disease, an internal review has found.
>
> The review for the director's office of the National Institutes of Health substantiates many of the concerns that a whistle-blower, Dr. Jonathan Fishbein, raised about the agency's AIDS research division and its senior managers.
>
> The division suffers from "turf battles and rivalries between physicians and PhD scientists," and the situation had been "rife for too long," the report concluded.
>
> Nonetheless, the NIH formally fired Fishbein on Friday, over the objections of several members of Congress. The top Republican and Democrat on the Senate Finance Committee are protesting, saying the firing was an example of whistle-blower punishment. . . .
>
> Fishbein, a private sector safety specialist, was hired by the NIH in 2003 to improve the safety of its AIDS research. He alleges that he was fired because he raised concerns about several studies and filed a complaint against one of the division's managers alleging sexual harassment and a hostile workplace.
>
> In a series of developments relevant to the internal review, the news media have reported that:
>
> An NIH AIDS study in Africa violated federal safety regulations.

Senior NIH managers engaged in sexually explicit pranks and sent expletive-laced e-mail messages to subordinates. . . .

An internal report, written on Aug. 9, 2004, by a special adviser to NIH chief Elias A. Zerhouni but never made public, raised concerns that the NIH's efforts to fire Fishbein at the very least gave the "appearance of reprisal."[45]

Surprisingly, at times truth does come out on top in government circles. As the DAIDS scandal erupted in the press and as the government investigations continued, finally, in 2006 the NIH hierarchy forced DAIDS to reinstate Dr. Fishbein, as reported in an AP story at the time:

A medical safety expert whose firing drew national attention to the lack of whistleblower protections in some areas of federal research is back on the government payroll.

The National Institutes of Health's reinstatement of Dr. Jonathan Fishbein settles a two-year battle that prompted investigations into allegations of scientific misconduct and sexual harassment in federal AIDS research.[46]

After I had studied the HIV-Nevirapine fiasco in some detail, I spoke to Robert Scott Bell several times about Dr. Fishbein and the harassment he had endured. Though Robert described Dr. Fishbein as a man of great idealism and obvious honor, the vicious attacks he experienced at the hands of his colleagues and superiors at the NIH had left him disillusioned and discouraged. The NIH not only ignored his honest and well-motivated concerns, but had sought to punish him for being so relentless in pursuit of the truth. According to Robert, after his firing Dr. Fishbein doubted he would work productively in medicine again, so determined was the NIH to destroy his credibility as a scientist. Despite Fishbein's reinstatement, Robert thought he would be viewed always as a pariah to be avoided at all costs, that strange creature who put honesty and integrity above convenience, career advancement, and the status quo. New NIH job or not, Dr. Fishbein's future at the NIH could hardly be a happy one.

In the HIV-Nevirapine affair, Dr. Isaacs and I saw a warning of NIH incompetence and blatant corruption, a morality play of sorts about the perversion of scientific truth for personal and political gain at the highest levels of the federal research community. But as we were to learn, the HIV-Nevirapine trial would have a far more personal meaning to us than just an instructive cautionary tale.

Chapter 26

A Closer Look at the NCI and NCCAM Supervisors

I had the fortunate experience, in my previous life as a journalist, to have studied and worked under several of the best editors in New York, who taught me the traditional and honorable profession of reporting, driven, as it was in those days, by an absolute obsession to find the truth wherever it may lie and whatever the personal and professional risks. In my first job after college at Time Inc., I had been assigned to work in the Books Division under Byron Dobell, who appeared to me, youngster that I was, to be a very serious and formidable personage. As I quickly learned, other staffers considered my boss Byron to be one of the most esteemed magazine editors in the country. Before his stint at Time Inc., he had served as Managing Editor at *Esquire* during its glory days in the late 1960s, publishing legions of notable writers, from Truman Capote to Tom Wolfe.

Byron's Rolodex, which on his instruction I had at times searched looking for the phone number of some luminary whose input we needed for one of our projects, contained the contact information of just about every major and minor writer not only in New York, but it seemed in the universe. I heard from old Time-Life hands I befriended that Byron had aided many a starving writer and shaped more than one major literary career. Legend had it that Byron helped keep Mario Puzo financially solvent by giving the struggling author books to review for a couple hundred dollars a shot while he completed his epic *The Godfather*. That novel made Puzo a multimillionaire, but without Byron's ongoing help, I was told, the writer would have been unable to pay his mortgage or feed his large family.

Byron eventually left Time Inc. to serve as Executive Editor of *New York Magazine*, which he helped convert from a local publication into a well-respected national venue for top-notch political writing and investigative journalism. While at *New York Magazine*, Byron actually published my first major cover piece when I was only 24 years old, an article which created quite a stir at the time.[47]

Early on in my career Byron taught me that as a good first principle of investigative journalism, if there is a problem on the surface of a situation—whatever that situation might be—usually the problem beneath is ten times worse. A true journalist, he said, would keep digging until the last layer of the last problem had been unearthed. Some 35 years later I remembered Byron's adage, as I pondered my current situation facing a failed clinical trial, eight years of work wasted, and my early hopes for the study long gone.

So with Byron's rule in mind, in the spring of 2007 I began systematically investigating the various personnel assigned to our trial, particularly Dr. Jeff White and Dr. Wendy Smith of the NCI, and Dr. Killen of NCCAM. I decided to concentrate on these three since in the first paragraph of his December 22, 2004 letter to Congressman Burton, NIH Director Zerhouni clearly stated that he had based much if not all of his defense of the study's management on information provided to his office by NCI and NCCAM staff. Since we assumed, at least for the sake of argument, that all three had taken Chabot's side against us, we wanted to know as much as we could about them.

Of course we were familiar with the trio to some degree, since we had worked with them for years. Dr. White had been on board almost from the study's inception, when in 1998 he became the first director of the NCI's newly created Office of Cancer Complementary and Alternative Medicine (OCCAM). Dr. Smith, also of OCCAM, joined the project in 2000, Dr. Killen in late 2004.

I first met Dr. White in 1995 or 1996, long before the pilot study had reached its end, and long before the Columbia trial had come into existence. At the time he was on leave from the NCI, serving as a consultant to the then fledgling Office of Alternative Medicine (now the National Center for Complementary and Alternative Medicine), headed by Dr. Wayne Jonas, whom I had known for some years. Dr. White and Dr. Jonas had traveled to New York to meet with my mentor, Dr. Ernst Wynder, who at the time was lobbying the NIH to support studies of promising alternative treatments for cancer such as mine. We lunched together in the cafeteria of the elegant Ford Foundation building on Manhattan's East 43rd Street, where Dr. Wynder rented space for the executive offices of his own organization, the American Health Foundation. During our cordial and informal meal and meeting, Dr. White asked a few questions about my Kelley study completed under Dr. Good, with which he was familiar. He then explained he was himself a vegetarian, I suppose to demonstrate some personal interest in nutrition and create professional camaraderie. I subsequently ran into him on occasion at conferences in Washington, but we never talked much until the NCI later assigned my study to his office at OCCAM.

When the NCI appointed Dr. White as its liaison for our clinical trial, Dr. Isaacs and I assumed someone in his position would have a strong interest in nutrition and alternative medicine issues as well as great competence in clinical trial management. We looked forward to working closely together, presumably as colleagues with a common goal of a rigorous evaluation of my treatment. However, from our earliest interactions at group meetings, and in our phone conversations as we labored to get the study up and running, he appeared to me very detached and lacking any real enthusiasm for the project he was supposed to help manage.

Later, as the trial moved along, from our perspective Dr. White did not follow up on promises made, though he always provided reasons for his lack of action. It was he who assured us that the NCI intended to send out an official letter to all U.S. oncologists urging them to cooperate with the study, though the document was never sent. He agreed with me that official advertisements in medical journals announcing the project would be helpful in terms of patient accrual, but the advertisements never appeared.

In early 2004, exasperated by the various and seemingly endless managerial lapses, particularly the entry of so many patients who couldn't comply with our treatment, I called Dr. White at his NCI office. I remember very well how annoyed he seemed with me, as he dismissed my criticisms of Dr. Chabot offhand. In that conversation, I realized Dr. White did not intend to champion what I thought were very legitimate concerns.

About a year later, as the study came to its end, I had several lengthy and troubling phone conversations with two individuals who were at that time scientists within the NIH system. Both had followed my work for some time, both knew of the early promising pilot study data, and both hoped at its inception that the NCI effort would proceed fairly and honorably. But now each independently of the other warned me that the NIH and NCI senior staff had little respect for my work or this clinical study. I was also told that the NCI had set up its Office of Cancer Complementary and Alternative Medicine more for reasons of political expediency, to appease Congressmen and Senators like Dan Burton and Tom Harkin, rather than out of some new attitude of openness toward alternative outsiders like myself. I had no way to verify any of this information, but with two different NIH insiders telling me the same story, I couldn't help but wonder if OCCAM staff would supervise the study with the appropriate interest or diligence.

Now, in 2007, I had begun to believe my two supporters within the Washington bureaucracy were on target, that the NCI and NIH hardly approached our trial with any real seriousness or a vigilant concern for doing the job right. Perhaps senior management at those institutes, who in a sense had inherited this study from a now-departed Dr. Klausner, wished it would simply dry up and go away.

By the time I began to look at Dr. White more closely, with the study collapsed and the federal investigations in progress, I had already learned quite a bit about him over the years from my casual review of various government websites. I knew that he completed his undergraduate work at Cornell and medical school at Howard University in Washington, D.C., followed by subsequent specialty training in medicine and oncology. Dr. White was a NCI "lifer" having joined the institute after completing his post-graduate training.

The official NCI biography described his career rather briefly:

> he performed pre-clinical and clinical immunology research with a focus on monoclonal antibody therapies for leukemias and lymphomas. . . . In 1997, he became the director of the Branch's Clinical Trials and Clinical Care Program. . . .

> In 1995, Dr. White became an oncology consultant to the NIH's Office of Alternative Medicine. In October 1998, he was named the director of the new NCI Office of Cancer Complementary and Alternative Medicine.[48]

In 2007, and more recently in preparation of this manuscript, I conducted literature searches on PubMed seeking out articles Dr. White might have authored or co-authored in the peer-reviewed journals. Prior to 1998, I found only several papers related to his immunology research. For the years 1998 and 1999, I could find nothing, but from 2000 to 2010, I located a total of twelve articles with his name attached, all dealing with alternative medicine topics. The majority appeared to be the same general article, rewritten and repurposed over and over again, with slightly different titles, discussing NCI research approaches to complementary and alternative medicine (CAM):

Complementary/alternative medicine and cancer research. A national initiative (2000)[49]

Comprehensive cancer care: integrating alternative, complementary and conventional therapies (2000)[50]

Complementary and alternative medicine in cancer: a National Cancer Institute perspective (2001)[51]

Cancer: current research in alternative therapies (2002)[52]

The National Cancer Institute's perspective and agenda for promoting awareness and research on alternative therapies for cancer (2002)[53]

Complementary and alternative medicine research: a National Cancer Institute perspective (2002)[54]

Research-design issues in cancer-symptom-management trials using complementary and alternative medicine: lessons from the National Cancer Institute Community Clinical Oncology Program experience (2005)[55]

Exceptional disease courses after the use of CAM: selection, registration, medical assessment, and research. An international perspective (2006)[56]

Survey of cancer researchers regarding complementary and alternative medicine (2008)[57]

Survey of complementary and alternative medicine practitioners regarding cancer management and research (2009)[58]

National Cancer Institute Best Case Series program (2010)[59]

Herbal use by cancer patients: A literature review on case reports (2010)[60]

Other than the article on herbal use, from my reading I thought the first article from 2000 seemed hardly different from the others in subject and in tone. To me, for a long time NCI scientist his bibliography seemed rather thin, basically the same summary paper resurfacing multiple times.

As I remember, in late 2000 Dr. Wendy Smith joined Dr. White's group, subsequently serving as the NCI co-supervisor of our clinical study. We first interacted during one of the group meetings which she and Dr. White attended via conference call from Washington while Dr. Isaacs and I, along with the Columbia team, met in person at Dr. Chabot's office. I remember Dr. White introducing "Wendy" whom he explained had just recently come over to his group from the National Institute for Alcohol Abuse and Alcoholism, though he did not say much else about her academic pedigree. I assumed she must be a physician or a basic scientist, perhaps a biochemist, but I still couldn't understand why someone from the National Institute for Alcohol Abuse and Alcoholism would be assigned to a NCI clinical trial evaluating a nutritional approach to pancreatic cancer.

At subsequent meetings, I began to suspect that though she talked like an expert in clinical trial management, her training and background might be somewhat different from what I had initially believed. Some time after she joined the study I learned from a friend at the NIH who knew Dr. Smith that her degree was not in medicine or some basic science like biochemistry or cell biology, but psychology—a revelation that left me ever more baffled. Then when I searched for information via the Internet, I found numerous references to her but not one—until she joined OCCAM at the NCI—even remotely related to cancer or nutrition.

A brief biography of her appeared at the time on the official OCCAM website:

> The Research Development and Support Program (RDSP) is directed by OCCAM Deputy Director Dr. Wendy B. Smith, M.A., Ph.D., B.C.I.A.C., a research psychologist with advanced training in hypnosis and a nationally certified biofeedback therapist. Dr. Smith joined NIH in 1990 as a research psychologist with the Anesthesiology and Neurobiology Branch of the National Institute of Dental and Craniofacial Research. She came to OCCAM in 2000 to lead RDSP.[61]

Oddly, the reference left out any mention of her stint at the National Institute on Alcohol Abuse and Alcoholism, where she served apparently not as a researcher, but as the contact person for grant applicants.

I have searched PubMed on several occasions, most recently in January 2011, looking for any articles with her name attached. I located an early publication dating from 1987, entitled "Biofeedback and relaxation training: the effect on headache and associated symptoms."[62] I could find only one paper from her pre-OCCAM days with a subject related to alcohol abuse; "Women and alcohol problems: a critical analysis of the literature and unanswered questions."[63] From my own review, since joining OCCAM in 2000, it appeared Dr. Smith had co-authored a total of six articles, all dealing with alternative and complementary medicine subjects, three written with Dr. White, three bearing her name but not his.

Dr. Smith's publication history hardly seemed impressive to me, and I found no evidence in the titles or article abstracts of any expertise whatsoever in cancer in general, pancreatic cancer in particular, nutrition, or clinical trial management. I began to wonder why Dr. Smith had transferred from the National Institute on Alcohol Abuse and Alcoholism to OCCAM at the NCI. What skill set did she possess that justified the switch?

As I studied the backgrounds of both Dr. White and Dr. Smith, I couldn't understand why, with all the talented scientists supposedly working within the NIH hierarchy, the NCI management had assigned to our clinical trial two people without much of a publishing history, and one in particular who seemed to have no training in a field related to oncology or cancer research.

We met the third member of the government triumvirate, Dr. Killen, at the contentious December 13, 2004 group meeting held at Columbia. By that time, Dr. Isaacs and I already suspected that both the NCI and NCCAM lacked a real commitment to our study's original intent, a fair and rigorous evaluation of my treatment, and Dr. Killen's behavior at that session did nothing to lessen our concerns. Only recently assigned to our trial, he had no prior direct experience with its problems and tribulations. Yet once Dr. Chabot reported that chemotherapy appeared to be proving far more effective than my treatment, Killen wasted little time announcing we needed to send out the press release countering the "positive results of the pilot study."

After the December 2004 meeting, I went to the NCCAM website, hoping to learn more about this new face assigned to the study. In typical government style, Killen's official biography seemed overblown, but despite the laudatory flowery prose his career seemed fairly mundane for an NIH lifer. He completed his undergraduate education at Kenyon College, medical school at Tufts, residency and oncology fellowship at Georgetown, before joining the NIH. In his long government career he appeared to have moved from one office to another within the NIH oligarchy, from one mid-level managerial role to the next. Based on what I read on the site, I didn't find any particularly worrisome information.

Whatever Killen's motives may have been, my January 7, 2005 letter effectively put a stop to any thoughts about press releases. After all, Dr. Engel's subsequent correspondence with Dr. Chabot had vindicated my main allegations, that the entry of so many nutrition patients who could not or would not comply with the prescribed treatment had rendered the data to that point meaningless. And Dr. Killen's brief February 2005 letter to me did, I thought at the time, seem conciliatory in tone compared to his brash statements made the previous December. So in early 2005, with Killen backing down and our major concerns officially acknowledged, Dr. Isaacs and I agreed we would give everyone involved, including Dr. White, Dr. Smith, and Dr. Killen the benefit of the doubt, hoping we might still turn the study around.

When I reread Dr. Killen's letter some two years later in 2007, my optimism long gone, I thought it considerably less conciliatory than I had remembered:

Dear Dr. Gonzalez:

I am writing in response to your letter to me dated January 7, 2005. I was dismayed to discover that you apparently misunderstood my intentions at our meeting on December 13, and also that I did not have an opportunity to talk with you about these matters in real time. Your letter prompted the letter from Linda Engel to Dr. Chabot addressing your major points of concern (copy attached), but I want to convey just two additional thoughts to you directly.

First, as a medical oncologist who trained at an institution that specialized in treatment of patients with GI cancer (Georgetown), I have always believed that the promising results of the pilot study merited investigation. . . . I have watched this study with considerable interest (albeit from a distance) for years before joining NCCAM. Now, having learned about its implementation and progress, I also understand that the trial has presented many big challenges from many directions, and my respect and admiration for the team that has worked with such extraordinary diligence and care on this study has grown immensely.

Second, I assume that my direct, "devils' [sic] advocacy" style of questioning created confusion about my motives. . . . My primary focus at this juncture is in identifying a clear, scientifically sound plan for this study that derives from the data available to us today and all that the team has learned in the process of carrying it out. . . .

I hope this helps clarify for you my fundamental position about this study, and I look forward to the opportunity to continue this important discussion when we meet on March 7th.

Though I had originally accepted his note as an apology of sorts, upon reread-ing it seemed far less repentant than I had remembered. I now thought Killen had shifted the blame from himself and his statements to me for having "mis-understood" his intentions, and for my apparent state of "confusion" about his "motives." Dr. Killen's words at the December 13, 2004 meeting couldn't have been clearer nor more forcefully spoken, allowing for no misunderstanding or confusion.

Dr. Killen skipped the March 7, 2005 meeting at Columbia, though Dr. Engel did make her way from Washington. Before we addressed the business at hand, Dr. Engel announced to the group that Dr. Killen felt somewhat uncomfort-able being present because of my January 2005 letter. I thought her statement somewhat surprising, since in his note to me Dr. Killen claimed he looked "for-ward to the opportunity to continue this important discussion when we meet on March 7th."

Dr. Killen did not attend the June 20, 2005 meeting in person, though he linked up by conference call from some southern island where he was vacationing. The brashness gone, he said nothing about press releases, and in fact he did not say much at all. Since that meeting was the last for Dr. Isaacs and myself, Dr. Killen and I never had the "opportunity to continue this important discus-sion," as his letter suggested he wished to do.

By late spring 2007, I had reviewed the backgrounds of Dr. White and Dr. Smith, and had also carefully studied the HIV-Nevirapine fiasco, an example of mismanagement reaching right into the highest levels of the NIH. But neither Dr. Isaacs nor I had really seen any connection between that scandal and our own study, only a warning to us of NIH indifference to corruption within its ranks. That is, we had not seen any connection until Dr. Isaacs, to her credit, began her own Internet investigation of Dr. Killen.

One afternoon that June of 2007 she pulled up Dr. Killen's official biography on the NCCAM site, which I myself had reviewed in late 2004 after our first meeting with him. The document actually appeared in the form of a press release dated September 8, 2003, announcing Dr. Killen's appointment to NCCAM.

This time around, Dr. Isaacs read it with renewed interest and with considerable care, an effort that yielded great reward.

> Bethesda, MD—Following a nationwide search, John Y. Killen, Jr., M.D., has been appointed director of the Office of International Health Research (OIHR) of the National Center for Complementary and Alternative Medicine (NCCAM).
>
> Established in 1998, NCCAM is 1 of 27 Institutes and Centers that make up the National Institutes of Health (NIH), an agency of the U.S. Department of Health and Human Services. NCCAM is the lead Federal agency supporting scientific research on complementary and alternative medical (CAM) practices, training CAM researchers, and disseminating research findings to the public and health professionals.
>
> OIHR was created in 2001 to identify promising international CAM practices and encourage their rigorous scientific assessment and development through international scientific collaborations, training of researchers, and dissemination of authoritative information to the public and health professionals.
>
> In announcing this new appointment, Stephen E. Straus, M.D., NCCAM Director, said "Dr. Killen's global experience in the study of HIV/AIDS and cancer make him the ideal person to take on this job. NCCAM, its fellow NIH Institutes, and the entire CAM research community are fortunate to have Dr. Killen assume this new role." . . .
>
> "It was my distinct pleasure to work with Dr. Killen when he directed the Division of AIDS at National Institute of Allergy and Infectious Diseases (NIAID), and more recently in his position with the Office of Biodefense," said Margaret Chesney, Ph.D., NCCAM Deputy Director. "In both capacities, he demonstrated his deep respect for multidisciplinary research, as well as his sensitivity and compassion to cultural and clinical issues faced by patients confronting debilitating chronic conditions."

Dr. Killen's 21-year NIH career has focused on designing, implementing and managing multidisciplinary research programs in cancer, HIV/AIDS and other infectious diseases, and on the ethics of clinical research. Most recently (2002–present) he was head of the Office of Biodefense Research at NIAID. Prior to that, he served as Associate Director for Research Ethics, NIAID, and also headed the International Research Section in the Department of Clinical Bioethics (2001–2002) at the Warren Magnuson Clinical Center of the NIH. *From 1993 through 2001, Dr. Killen served as director, after serving as deputy director (1987–1993), of the Division of AIDS, NIAID.* [italics mine] In this position he was responsible for a broad array of scientific, ethical, regulatory, and policy issues that emerged in domestic U.S. and international research programs during the early years of the epidemic. At a global level, this involved collaborative projects with the World Health Organization, the Joint United Nations Programme on HIV/AIDS. . . .[64]

Dr. Isaacs asked me to read very carefully the NCCAM biography/press release of Killen sitting in front of her on our computer screen, advising me to pay special attention to the information relating to his tenure at the National Institute of Allergy and Infectious Diseases. There, as Dr. Isaacs pointed out, Dr. Killen served as director of the "Division of AIDS" from 1993–2001, right during the time that particular office supervised the tarnished HIV-Nevirapine study which ran from 1997–1999. We couldn't believe what we were reading, that Killen headed the very division responsible for one of the most bungled studies in the history of the NIH. As we sorted out the chronology, only after HIV-Nevirapine's completion, but before the scandal broke in the press, had he been transferred to NCCAM and ultimately to our study.

As I reread the official biography, I was surprised that during my review of newspaper articles written about the HIV-Nevirapine trial, I hadn't come across his name, which I presumably would have noticed. To my recollection, none of the media reports specifically mentioned him, but now, since his involvement with that trial seemed likely, Dr. Isaacs and I began looking for the connection we suspected might exist. It didn't take long, thanks to the Internet, to find the missing link putting him at the center of the study's action—an interview with Killen that appeared as a CNN "chat," broadcast on July 15, 1999. That same day, the NIH first released the project's data to the press in anticipation of its formal publication two months later in *Lancet*. In this conversation, Killen talked excitedly about the project without referring to any of its problems.[65]

After a brief introductory statement identifying Dr. Killen as director of the AIDS division of the National Institute of Allergy and Infectious Diseases, the CNN correspondent described the study in enthusiastic terms, as if nevirapine's benefits were now definitively proven. Then the actual interview segment began, with Dr. Killen summarizing the alleged results of the project:

> "HIVNET 012 compared two different regimens of antiviral drugs given late in pregnancy. . . . A single dose of nevirapine to the mother and to the infant resulted in a 48 percent decrease in transmission compared to a short course of AZT. The regimen is very easy to administer and very inexpensive and will hopefully make a major contribution to stemming the HIV epidemic in the developing world. . . .
>
> "there is every reason to believe that the cost and simplicity of this regimen will make it a real option and will lower one of the big obstacles to effective control of the epidemic in children."[65]

When a "Chat Participant" asked pointedly about side effects, Killen responded:

> "The side effects seen in this study were very few and very mild, mostly mild anemia and skin rashes in the infants, all rare."[65]

The discussion as posted goes on for seven pages, during which Dr. Killen promoted the treatment as cheap, safe, non-toxic, easy to administer, and undoubtedly destined to usher in a new era of HIV control.

With this interview in hand, Dr. Isaacs and I pieced together the timeline of Killen's career at NIAID as the scandal unfolded. He remained director of the Division of AIDS at NIAID until 2001, when he assumed the role of "head of the Office of Biodefense Research at NIAID," a position he held until his move to NCCAM in 2003. By 2001, while Killen still served as the director of the Division of AIDS, the NIH audit of the study was already in progress, with its first highly critical report completed in early 2002. The NIH successfully kept this information from the press until 2004 with the onset of the Fishbein fiasco. In fact, the NIH honchos successfully kept even President Bush in the dark at the time of his 2002 speech on AIDS, when he unwittingly lauded this very effort.

So as far as we could tell Killen moved over to NCCAM some two years before the story first became national news. But how, we wondered, did Killen's transfer to NCCAM actually happen? How did he end up at NCCAM just in time to avoid the media onslaught of HIV-Nevirapine?

We searched for clues, once again turning to the Internet, beginning with Dr. Stephen Straus who first came on board as NCCAM's director in 1999. We quickly located the NIH press release announcing Straus' appointment on October 6, 1999—just as the HIV-Nevirapine study drew to its close.

Right in the headline, we saw a connecting link between Straus and Killen:

NIAID's Stephen Straus To Direct NCCAM

Dr. Stephen E. Straus was named Oct. 6 as the first director for the National Center for Complementary and Alternative Medicine. An internationally recognized expert in clinical research and clinical trials, he has served since 1991 as chief of the Laboratory of Clinical Investigation at the National Institute of Allergy and Infectious Diseases.

Straus has basic and clinical research experience related to many diseases for which there are alternative remedies, including chronic fatigue syndrome (CFS), Lyme disease, AIDS/HIV, chronic hepatitis B virus and genital herpes infections. . . .[66]

After listing Straus' many achievements, the writer then quoted an enthusiastic Dr. Harold Varmus, at the time NIH Director:

"The American public is increasingly interested in complementary and alternative therapies, and it is critical that NIH put its scientific expertise to work to help determine which therapies are safe and effective," said NIH director Dr. Harold Varmus. "The appointment of Dr. Straus, with his experience in alternative therapies and his expertise in clinical evidence, will result in significant expansion of clinical research in this field. He brings to this position a clear sense of leadership, strong management and organizational expertise, and superb communication skills."[66]

The press release then described Dr. Straus' stellar academic background, undergraduate degree from MIT, medical degree from Columbia, residency at Barnes Hospital in St Louis, followed by his long and illustrious career at the NIH.

As an aside, from what I have read, prior to his appointment as NCAAM director Dr. Straus never acknowledged an interest in any aspect of alternative medicine, contrary to Dr. Varmus' statements.[67]

Though the headline and the first paragraph indicated he and Killen had been colleagues at NIAID, Dr. Straus supervised a separate laboratory during his tenure there and we could not directly link him to the HIV-Nevirapine study. Nonetheless, as the NIH audit and the OHRP investigation into HIV-Nevirapine revved up in 2001 and 2002, Dr. Straus must have known what was going on, and what was about to happen. Then a year after Killen joined NCCAM the scandal exploded in the media, and by its zenith in 2005 with the Fishbein firing, he would have been long gone from NIAID.

As we were to learn, at least one other NCCAM employee seemed to have migrated with Killen from NIAID. In the laudatory press release announcing Killen's arrival at NCCAM, Dr. Margaret Chesney, the Center's deputy director, stated:

> "It was my distinct pleasure to work with Dr. Killen when he directed the Division of AIDS at the National Institute of Allergy and Infectious Diseases (NIAID), and more recently in his position with the Office of Biodefense."[64]

As we reviewed the situation, Dr. Killen's transfer to NCCAM in 2003 hardly seemed the result of any intense, meticulous, high level "nationwide search" as claimed. Dr. Straus' "search" I suspect didn't extend beyond his circle of friends.

Chapter 27

NCCAM—Its Origins and Mission

From its earliest incarnation as the Office of Alternative Medicine (OAM), controversy has followed NCCAM at every step. Congress initially mandated OAM's creation in October 1991 in response to public pressure, the growing national interest in alternative medicine, and the conviction that government research institutions traditionally refused to investigate promising unconventional and nutritional treatments because of an inherent pro-drug bias. OAM formally began operations in 1992 as a small NIH branch office allocated a meager $2 million—a miniscule amount compared to the more than $30 billion annual total NIH budget. Despite such humble beginnings, I remember well that OAM fostered considerable enthusiasm among alternative medicine leaders, who spoke of a new era of open-mindedness within the Washington scientific establishment.

According to the NIH website chronology, Stephen C. Groft, Pharm.D., whom I never knew, served as OAM's Acting Director, succeeded in October 1992 by Joseph Jacobs, M.D., M.B.A., the first permanent Director of OAM. I always thought Dr. Jacobs, whom I did meet several times at NIH conferences in Washington, well intentioned, but with his very limited budget, somewhat powerless. I hardly envied his position; shortly after OAM came into being, word of a NIH backlash against the office surfaced in the media and by word of mouth within the alternative community, this being in the days before the Internet and e-mail. During Dr. Jacob's tenure, I remember reading the words of one critic who complained quite angrily that the NIH, bending to political pressure, saw fit to waste valuable resources investigating "quackery" instead of legitimate science. I heard through my sources that the NIH Director at the time, Dr. Varmus, had vigorously opposed OAM, which he felt had been forced upon him by Congressional meddling. I thought the criticisms somewhat odd, since valid new ideas in science always seem initially bizarre, and I knew of no way to separate legitimate science from "quackery" without conducting appropriate clinical studies. Nonetheless, despite the hostile climate OAM survived, its budget growing substantially throughout the 1990s, though the Office still earned little respect from the mainstream scientific community.

In 1995, Dr. Varmus appointed Dr. Wayne Jonas to run the Office. Trained as a family practice physician with very conventional credentials, Dr. Jonas, prior to accepting the OAM post, had served in the military, reaching the rank of Colonel and supervising research training at the Walter Reed Army Medical Center. In addition to his academic accomplishments, Dr. Jonas had long been a serious student of alternative practices, particularly homeopathy, even publishing a book on the subject.

I had long held Dr. Jonas in great esteem, ever since we first met when he visited my office in 1990 to discuss my treatment approach. At the time, he was still in the Army and at Walter Reed. Since then, we had talked about my work periodically over the years, both by phone and in person when we would see each other at various conferences in Washington. I thought he seemed a perfect fit for OAM, with his combination of traditional academic training and scholarship in unconventional therapies.

Once in charge at OAM, against extreme odds and with little support from his superiors, Dr. Jonas tried valiantly to turn OAM into a legitimate, serious research arm of the NIH, supporting valid investigations of promising alternative approaches—its actual defined Congressional responsibility. Unfortunately, with his arrival antagonism toward the office seemed only to worsen. His open-minded attitude provoked only more resentment and suspicion within government scientific circles, even to the point, as I have heard from several sources, that the NIH assigned a "mole" to OAM with orders to report on Dr. Jonas' activities to the NIH Director.

During his tenure at OAM, Dr. Jonas could not provide funding for specific projects without approval from higher up in the NIH bureaucracy, a requirement he believed hampered his Office. Too often, I have heard, the NIH used its veto power over OAM to block research efforts Dr. Jonas thought worthy of support. I know during his early days at OAM, Dr. Jonas wished to fund a large-scale clinical study of my treatment but found his efforts stymied at every turn.

In October 1998, despite opposition within the NIH, Congress designated OAM as a free-standing "Center" within the Department of Health and Human Services, the umbrella organization that oversees the NIH and its many individual Institutes. In its new incarnation, OAM, now to be called the National Center for Complementary and Alternative Medicine (NCCAM), would be free from direct NIH control. It would have its own independent director with a budget provided directly by Congress, not by the NIH. And during the first year, Congress proved to be quite generous, raising NCCAM funding to a respectable $50 million for 1999.

This change was, in institutional terms, a major promotion. But despite increasing Congressional support, in late 1998 Dr. Jonas left OAM in frustration over the endless political battles he found himself fighting. For a time he returned to the military, before assuming the executive leadership of a private non-profit foundation based in Washington, where he remains to this day.

In January 1999, Dr. William Harlan, a highly regarded career NIH scientist, previously Director of the NIH Office of Disease Prevention, succeeded Dr. Jonas, serving as the OAM interim director until a permanent replacement could be appointed. My friend and mentor Dr. Wynder told me the choice for Dr. Jonas' successor, even if only temporary, couldn't have been better. He respected Dr. Harlan enormously as a seasoned, thoughtful researcher within the NIH universe, appreciated by colleagues for his superb managerial skills as well as his fair and open mind.

In February 1999, shortly after Dr. Harlan's arrival at OAM, the Secretary of the Department of Health and Human Services signed the provision formally converting the Office of Alternative Medicine into the free-standing and prosperous NCCAM. The official NIH history of the transformation reads as follows:

The U.S. Secretary of Health and Human Services (HHS) signs the organizational change memorandum creating NCCAM and making it the 25th independent component of the NIH. The NCCAM Director is vested with broad decision-making authority, especially concerning financial and administrative management and fiscal and review responsibility for grants and contracts.[68]

I first met Dr. Harlan in the spring of 1999 shortly after he assumed the helm at NCCAM. Along with other researchers, Dr. Harlan and I had been invited to speak at a Congressional hearing on alternative medicine organized by Representative Burton, at the time Chairman of the House Committee on Government Reform, one of the most powerful committees in Congress. In his talk, Dr. Harlan argued eloquently that the government should look more closely—and more fairly—at potentially useful unorthodox and nutritional therapies. Several of the other presenters referred to my pilot study as an example of a well-conceived and appropriately managed evaluation of an alternative treatment. After the session, I talked at some length with Dr. Harlan, who as it turned out had been following the progress of my research, particularly the pilot study, with some interest over the years, even before his appointment as OAM-NCCAM director in 1999. He was fully aware of the developing Columbia-NCI trial, and told me he hoped NCCAM might become involved in some way, either financially or in a supervisory capacity, or both. The partnership seemed logical to him, since the Center existed to develop and fund trials of unconventional treatments for disease including cancer. I found his manner and suggestion, to say the least, most refreshing.

When our pilot study results appeared in the June1999 issue of *Nutrition and Cancer*, I sent Dr. Harlan a copy of the journal He responded with a note dated July 13, 1999:

Dear Nick:

Thank you for the follow-up on your study and the paper that describes the results. We are pleased that the therapy is now in a randomized trial phase that should provide the data that will expand its use and benefits to patients if results are positive. I also expect that the paper will increase patient accrual to the trial. At the National Center for Complementary and Alternative Medicine, we are prepared to assist in recruitment as well as provide financial support for the study.

Your continued efforts to find better approaches to treatment of patients with cancer is [sic] both compassionate and scientific.

Sincerely,

Bill [signed]

William R. Harlan, M.D.

Shortly thereafter, Dr. Harlan formally proposed that NCCAM fund the entire Columbia investigation of my therapy, an offer the NCI happily accepted.

Dr. Harlan's strong support proved to be one of the few bright spots in the ordeal that was just then beginning to unfold. In recent years I have often thought how differently our trial might have turned out had Dr. Harlan remained at the helm of NCCAM. Unfortunately, that was not to be, and in October 1999, when Dr. Stephen Straus assumed the post of permanent NCCAM Director, Dr. Harlan returned to his previous position at the NIH.

In June 2000, not long after Dr. Straus arrived at NCCAM, the prestigious journal *Science* published a lengthy interview[69] in which the author, Eric Stokstad, lauded the new director while belittling, ridiculing, and mocking alternative medicine in general—and my study in particular.

In retrospect, with all I know today I find the article a wonderful illustration of unintended irony. The writer boasted proudly of Straus' tenure at the esteemed Institute of Allergy and Infectious Diseases, a bastion of true science, as opposed to the "witchcraft"—Stokstad actually used the word—apparently permeating NCCAM. Stokstad seemed completely unaware of the corrupt HIV-Nevirapine study that had just recently been completed at the very institution he praised and where Dr. Straus had previously worked.

The article expressed so well the prevailing attitude among scientists and the mainstream media toward "alternative medicine":

> Why in the world would a respected researcher like Stephen Straus leave a top-flight lab at the National Institutes of Health to run NIH's new National Center for Complementary and Alternative Medicine (NCCAM)? After all, the center's predecessor, the Office of Alternative Medicine (OAM), was a child of politics that was widely denounced by mainstream researchers. Conceived by Senator Tom Harkin (D-IA), a die-hard fan of alternative medicine . . . the

office was earmarked into existence in 1992. It soon gained a reputation as a counterculture enclave for pseudoscience. After just 2 years, the office's first director resigned in protest. Harkin, he claimed, had stacked the advisory board with credulous advocates and was meddling in OAM affairs.

The office's reputation didn't improve under the tenure of the next director, a homeopathic physician. High-profile scientists continued to condemn OAM for sponsoring inconclusive research and bestowing prestige on practices that sometimes resembled "witchcraft." In 1997, former presidential science adviser D. Allan Bromley and others urged Congress to abolish the office. Instead, Harkin kept boosting its budget, from an initial $2 million to nearly $70 million this year. And, in 1998, he succeeded—over the objections of then-NIH director Harold Varmus—in elevating the office to a full-fledged center. . . .

So, last fall, when Varmus recruited Straus, a battle-hardened mainstream clinical investigator, to head up the new center, even critics of OAM lauded the choice. . . .

Even so, Straus faces formidable challenges. His goal is to bring scientific rigor to a field that many of his peers would just as soon see disappear.[69]

After devoting considerable space to Straus' background, including his long-standing interest in Chronic Fatigue Syndrome, the writer eventually targeted my project:

Science or quackery?

The kind of therapies Straus is charged with investigating—from homeopathy to shark cartilage to coffee enemas—would make many of his colleagues smirk. . . .

Yet principles aside, Straus also has to follow the mandate of Congress—and some of its, well, less-than-scientific members. NCCAM is stuck funding a 5-year, $1.4 million trial of an unusual protocol designed to treat terminal pancreatic cancer by physician Nicolas [sic] Gonzalez. The so-called Gonzalez Protocol—a hodgepodge of pancreatic enzymes, coffee enemas, and up to 150 dietary supplements a day—caught the attention of Representative Dan Burton (R-IN), who in 1998 encouraged the National Cancer Institute (NCI) to study it. Even though Straus considers the evidence just an "aggregate of interesting anecdotes," he defends the trial—albeit lukewarmly.[69]

Of course Stokstad never contacted me to hear my side, or review any data I might have to support the treatment's efficacy. In any event, two specific comments warrant addressing. I have read elsewhere the story that Congressman Burton intervened on my behalf with the government scientific establishment, forcing a reluctant NCI to fund my study. I have no knowledge of any such lobbying, though Congressman Burton has long argued that the Washington academic institutions need to restrain their inherent biases and objectively investigate promising alternative therapies—not a bad bit of advice, one would think. And when I first read the piece, I thought it troubling that Straus could publicly support my study only "lukewarmly" in far contrast to the more encouraging attitude of his predecessor Dr. Harlan.

I hadn't met Dr. Straus at the time of his *Science* interview, nor had he had made any attempt to communicate with me in any way since his arrival at NCCAM. We actually did not cross paths until October 2000, a year after his appointment and four months after the *Science* interview, when each of us appeared at hearings held in Washington before the White House Commission on Complementary and Alternative Medicine Policy. During his rather dull, 15-minute talk presented in academic monotone, he read off a list the various clinical trials at the time supported by NCCAM. I thought, watching from the audience, that Straus seemed very uncomfortable, as if he would rather be somewhere else. And though my project had already generated enormous interest and controversy, he only briefly mentioned it at the near-end of his presentation, almost as an afterthought without any particular fanfare or enthusiasm.

After his presentation, during a break in the proceedings Straus headed toward the exit door as if fleeing. I managed to catch up with him, intending only to introduce myself. As he awkwardly took my extended hand, he regained his composure, scowled and said oddly, "I want you to know that from now on NCCAM will be doing *real* science," and then abruptly turned around and continued walking. He couldn't get away from me fast enough, I thought, as if I suffered some deadly communicable disease. I found his comment and behavior somewhat peculiar, a far contrast to my interaction with Dr. Harlan when we first met at Congressman Burton's hearings.

Nonetheless, in his new, highly visible role, Dr. Straus appeared quite adept at dealing with the press, which increasingly sought him out as the controversies surrounding NCCAM persisted. It seemed that the conventional scientific community and the media found him a champion of sorts, a "real scientist" who would heroically clean up NCCAM and rid the world of witchcraft medicine like my treatment.

Some months after we met in Washington, in an interview appearing in the April 3, 2001 *New York Times*, Dr. Straus talked at length about his own background, his scientific interests, and his plans for NCCAM. As had the *Science* writer nine months earlier, the *Times* reporter described Straus with great respect, a dedicated scientist faced with the thankless—perhaps *embarrassing*—job of investigating fringe medical treatments. When the *Times* writer brought up my name and study, this time around Straus offhandedly dismissed the significance of the positive pilot study data:

> Q. You've been heavily criticized for funding a study of the Nicholas Gonzalez protocol cancer therapy. His therapy relies heavily on enemas, doesn't it?
>
> A. Enemas, and a whole number of nutritional supplements. This is for an incurable cancer. The best chemotherapy for it affords an extra few months of life. The aggregate of anecdotes from Gonzalez—and that's all they are—is that in a handful of selected patients, they had an average survival of over 18 months.
>
> I don't have any reason scientifically to feel that the Gonzalez regimen should work. On the other hand, here's something that addresses an incurable disease for which the best available therapy is poor. I think we should be willing to tolerate some discord and skepticism for the sake of getting a clear answer. If it doesn't work, we have a clear answer. If it does work, we will try to figure out why. Our study is funding Columbia University to run it, not Gonzalez. I have no problem justifying this one right now.[67]

After reading that article when it first appeared, I remember my sense of renewed disappointment with his statements. He knew full well that my first study was not an "aggregate of anecdotes" but a formal Phase II clinical trial developed in cooperation with the NCI, and supervised by a team of eminent scientists. The pejorative statement "in a handful of selected patients" ignores the fact that the NCI had itself suggested that with a disease as virulent as advanced pancreatic cancer, I needn't enroll more than ten subjects to make a valid point about the therapy. Had the NCI demanded more patients be accrued, I would have done so. I also noted that Straus, as in the *Science* article, did not refer to me as "Dr. Gonzalez," only "Gonzalez," showing in my opinion the same lack of respect I felt the first time I met him in Washington.

The statement "I don't have any reason scientifically to feel that the Gonzalez regimen should work" implied once again that my therapy lacked any legitimate rational foundation. Had he called or written me, I would have happily provided him the exhaustive documentation dating back to John Beard's laboratory experiments and clinical experiences, which carefully demonstrated the anti-cancer properties of proteolytic pancreatic enzymes. I would have sent the supportive evidence from the mainstream medical literature reporting the beneficial effects of coffee enemas, which for reasons that still remain a mystery to me invariably evoke such disdain among conventional physicians and journalists. Critics, such as the reporter here, seem completely unaware that esteemed medical and nursing textbooks, including the Merck Manual, recommended coffee enemas as a treatment modality for the better part of the twentieth century. I have in my files a compilation of dozens of papers from the peer-reviewed literature describing the utility of enemas in a variety of serious clinical situations—including an article from the September 8, 1922 issue of the *New England Journal of Medicine,* in which the authors reported their successful treatment of mental disease with "colon irrigation."[70] Unfortunately, since Dr. Straus made no effort to contact me, he apparently remained to his death from brain cancer in 2007 ignorant of the evidence backing up each aspect of our treatment.

His words "I think we should be willing to tolerate some discord and skepticism for the sake of getting a clear answer" I thought most telling. He could have said, "because of the promising pilot study results this project needs to move forward, whatever the critics say," or that "we at NCCAM are behind this study 100% for the sake of science," or, as did Dr. Harlan, my "efforts to find better approaches to treatment of patients with cancer is both compassionate and scientific." Instead, he emphasized that he and NCCAM would essentially *tolerate* the project.

Dr. Harlan's kind and supportive letter of June 1999 and Dr. Straus' pejorative and dismissive words as described in the June 2000 *Science* article and the April 2001 *New York Times* interview provide an interesting contrast. Here we have two men, both highly regarded NIH career scientists, both serving, and in sequence, the same role at the same office as director at NCCAM, responding to me, my therapy, my pilot study, my life's work, in irreconcilable ways.

In my personal encounters with the two men, in each case the behavior matched their words. When I first met Dr. Harlan at Congressman Burton's hearings, he made a point of introducing himself to me in a manner both warm and gracious, expressing his admiration for my previous research efforts and for my sincere goal of testing my therapy in rigorous clinical trials. He seemed knowledgeable about my treatment approach, referencing Dr. Beard, for example, and discussing the pilot study in some detail. Not only did he wish that NCCAM be involved with my developing NCI project, he provided me with contact information for a special government office set up to help researchers patent natural products and natural treatments so that I might better protect my intellectual property. He told me he hoped that a new dawn might be breaking within government circles that would finally allow serious alternative researchers like myself the chance to work cooperatively with academic scientists. I found his words most encouraging, and in subsequent conversations at other Washington meetings, his manner and manners were no different. He treated me like an equal, as someone he respected and whose work he admired, never once making pejorative or snide comments about my therapy, the coffee enemas, or my data.

When I met Dr. Straus at the White House Commission meetings in October 2000, he made no effort to find me, but instead I had to seek him out. When I introduced myself to him, after his initial comment about "real science," he couldn't disengage fast enough, offering no suggestions, no advice, before disappearing still scowling.

I came to know both Dr. Harlan and Dr. Straus through the same route, via my determined research efforts. Dr. Harlan wasn't some personal friend of long standing or some political connection anymore than was Dr. Straus. I behaved no differently with each; only the attitude of the two men differed. Ironically, Dr. Harlan was what the media wanted Dr. Straus to be, a true scientist, though he would never boast of such—open-minded, fair, not driven by bias, able to look at data objectively and without emotional overlays.

When Dr. Isaacs and I reviewed all our old documents in 2007, hoping to understand why our clinical trial, for which we had such hope, ultimately catastrophically failed, we came across the *Science* and *New York Times* interviews in our media files. As I reread these articles, I could see, after the passage of more than six years, the harbinger of Dr. Killen's behavior and statements at the December 13, 2004 group meeting, his insistence the press be notified to "counter the positive data of the pilot study." Killen's words, I suspect, only reflected his boss's lukewarm support for the project and his belief that no real scientific evidence supported my approach.

In Straus' *New York Times* interview, I also found the premonition of what NCCAM sadly became under his direction. As quoted above, Dr. Straus made it clear to the *Times'* readers that "Our study is funding Columbia University to run it, not Gonzalez."

First of all, as I earlier explained the truth is a little more complicated than what Straus here implied. In 1998 the then NCI director Dr. Klausner pledged his Institute's backing before NCCAM existed as such, during the days of the old OAM. In the summer of 1999, only after the NCI had approved support for the project did Dr. Harlan offer staff and funding from his own office. With the newly revamped OAM—or as it was now called NCCAM—on board, the NCI informed us that all monies would be channeled through Columbia, the institution directly supervising the study. But I earned the original NCI grant.

Secondly, the sentence itself seemed to me totally out of place. The reporter hadn't asked about the recipient of the funding, but Straus nonetheless felt the need to reassure the world that the money was not going to me, the alternative fringe guy, but to the eminent institution, Columbia.

The point made here was neither casual nor insignificant, but reflected, I believe, Straus' fundamental philosophy. For during his tenure at NCCAM until his death, Dr. Straus made sure that the rapidly growing budget at NCCAM would be channeled to conventional medical centers and their conventional researchers, the very people who had resisted the creation of OAM and had approached any form of non-traditional medicine as "witchcraft." The money most assuredly has not gone to the alternative practitioners for whom Congress created OAM in the first place.

As our study collapsed in 2005, I began to search the Internet hoping to learn how NCCAM allocated its budget—estimated today in the range of over $150 million a year, a respectable piece of change, and growing annually. I found the task somewhat formidable since the NCCAM website listed grants awarded, but not necessarily the amounts. With some work, I pieced together enough information to get the general picture, an orgy of gift-giving to academic institutions around the country.

For example, a press release dated 2003 revealed NCCAM awarded Massachusetts General Hospital, the main Harvard teaching hospital, $5.9 million to study acupuncture. That same year, Oregon State received $5.8 million to investigate, once again, acupuncture. An announcement sent out in the fall of 2005 from the University of Maryland proudly reported that NCCAM had approved a *$10 million* grant for the institution to study, yes again, acupuncture. I found the acupuncture theme common, the amounts extraordinary. I suspected that acupuncture, neither threatening nor in this day and age particularly controversial, seemed like an acceptable target for Straus' largess that would not raise anyone's hackles. But $21 million spread over three mainstream institutions to evaluate the same treatment? (Note that during the final editing of this manuscript, I learned that a total of *$150 million* was in the works just for acupuncture research.)

Others recipients included Johns Hopkins, Columbia for $7.8 million, the University of California at San Francisco, and the University of Kentucky, all funded to establish centers for "Alternative and Complementary Medicine."

In April 2008, I reviewed the section on the NCCAM website reporting all projects approved by the office for 2007. The list went on for some 14 pages, with about 28 individual grants described per page, with the recipient institution identified. This information confirmed that NCCAM's bounty seemed destined for mainstream research centers and mainstream academic scientists. For example, on the first page the lucky winners included investigators affiliated with the University of California, San Francisco (two individual grants), Temple University, Oregon State University (hitting pay dirt yet again), McLean Hospital (a Harvard teaching hospital), Massachusetts General Hospital, University of Maryland, University of North Carolina, Mount Sinai School of Medicine, and on and on and on.

Many of the grants did seem supportive of what might be considered alternative medicine subjects, at least judging by the titles. For example, several projects focused on stress reduction, an acceptable area of academic research; some appeared to be more esoteric with headings such as "Neuroimaging Acupuncture Effects on Human Brain Activity." Many seemed to be typical basic science projects related to nutrition of the type already supported within other NIH Institutions, i.e., "Chromium Enhances Insulin and Glu14 Action via Lipid Rafts." But regardless of the grant titles, all the recipients were researchers at traditional institutions, not practitioners or scientists one might consider "alternative." I thought it ironic that as his final legacy, Straus assured the world that the growing NCCAM budget would serve as a lucrative cash cow for these hallowed academic medical centers and their staff. Apparently, the $30 billion annual NIH budget and the $6 billion available from the NCI for the usual medical research isn't enough. But, having witnessed first hand how the government and a major medical center working together could invest eight years and $1.4 million in grant money without coming up with a legitimate answer about my treatment, I am not very confident much useful data will come out of this latest spending spree.

I still find Straus' strong belief that only academic centers like Columbia could conduct legitimate scientific investigations perplexing. Apparently, he learned little from the HIV-Nevirapine debacle, still believing, even as he faced terminal illness, in the righteousness of academic authority.

One final comment about the late Dr. Straus: we will never know the ultimate effect on our study of the *Science* article from 2000 and the *New York Times* interview appearing in 2001, widely disseminated as they were. But I think it useful to ponder Straus' statements for a moment. The research community holds *Science* in high esteem, and scientists, physicians, and lay people generally respect the quality of medical writing in the *Times*. In truth, why would any reasonable oncologist reading either or both of these pieces encourage any of his or her patients diagnosed with pancreatic cancer to consider our trial as an option, or stay on if already entered? After all, the director of the very government center responsible for funding and supervising the study had little apparent regard for the project, which at best he supported "lukewarmly." As for my treatment, he could only say with little enthusiasm "I don't have any reason scientifically to feel that the Gonzalez regimen should work," before dismissing my pilot data as "the aggregate of anecdotes from Gonzalez." If I were in an oncologist's shoes, reading all this, I would not have wanted any patient of mine to join this study, nor remain in it if admitted. On the contrary, I would have done everything in my power to encourage him or her to find another treatment somewhere else, and as quickly as possible. In the final analysis, I wonder if Straus ever realized the potential damage resulting from his statements.

In his December 22, 2004 letter to Congressman Burton, NIH Director Zerhouni denied my claim that the negative attitude of oncologists had helped undermine the study, insisting with great conviction that no prejudice existed within the conventional medical world toward me or the project. In retrospect, Zerhouni didn't have to look further than the published comments of his own government colleague Dr. Straus to find evidence for the bias I alleged.

Chapter 28

My Report to Dr. McNeilly

T hroughout late spring of 2007, Dr. Isaacs and I enjoyed a respite from
the battleground of the clinical study, concentrating on our practices,
on our patients, and on running our office. Then in June 2007, a year
since I had first contacted the OHRP and four months after our earlier conversation in February, Dr. McNeilly called me unexpectedly. He seemed cheerful
as he reported that in his latest communications with Columbia, Chabot had
now countered my various allegations with three main points: first, that as far
as he knew, no trial candidate had been admitted who did not meet the entry
criteria; second, that I had participated with the approval process throughout
the entire project so if there were any errors in judgment the fault was mine;
and third, that during the trial neither Dr. Isaacs nor I had ever expressed a
reservation about any patient accepted into the nutrition arm.

I was somewhat dumbfounded once again. When I explained the evidence
proved otherwise on each point, Dr. McNeilly suggested that I put together all
the documents, whether e-mails, letters, statements in patient charts, etc. showing that first, patients had been qualified for the study who failed to meet the
entry criteria; second, that Chabot was solely in charge of the evaluation process at least for the greater part of the study; and third, that we had questioned
or objected to the admission of study subjects. He also requested detailed documentation regarding two specific patients, identified in our charts as Patient #9

and Patient #16, for whom the consent forms had not been "identified," to use Chabot's terminology in his October 2005 e-mail to us.

As we were talking, I realized McNeilly's proposed undertaking would require yet another major investment of time. For an appropriate response, Dr. Isaacs and I would need to review all our notes in every patient chart, all our e-mails and letters spanning a period of years, and essentially all documents related to the study. When I mentioned that this project might take many weeks if not months, he responded by telling me that there was no rush, as long as I got the job done.

After I got off the phone, I felt somewhat disappointed that after a year, OHRP still seemed to be in the middle of its investigation. And once again, I had to answer the same refrains first presented in one form or another in Dr. Zerhouni's letter of nearly two years earlier. When later that day Dr. Isaacs and I discussed my conversation with Dr. McNeilly, we tried to look at the positives, agreeing we now had the chance to prove, finally, all our points in detail, using the study's own documents in our defense.

So I dove into this new project, devoting to it every free moment between patient visits, during my lunch break, in the evenings after finishing with the day's responsibilities, and always on the weekends. As the days passed, we decided that to help Dr. McNeilly sort through the mass of documents we were collecting I would create another narrative, akin to my response to Dr. Zerhouni, describing and cataloguing the supporting evidence which clearly disproved Chabot's latest allegations.

The effort eventually took three months, pursued and written without a break through the summer. The final lengthy narrative exhaustively and in my mind unassailably answered Dr. McNeilly's questions and validated our claims regarding Chabot's management of the study. Though after my conversation with Dr. McNeilly the previous June I had dreaded the task before me, the investment in time proved to be invaluable. As Dr. Isaacs and I reviewed trial documents going back to the beginning ten years earlier, we realized more than ever how poorly supervised the study had been, how serious the managerial lapses.

I divided the manuscript into 12 chapters, as defined in the "Table of Contents":

Table of Contents

As the headings above indicate, in the first chapter I described in detail the history of the two patients #9 and #16, of particular concern to Dr. McNeilly, both sent to us for treatment without evidence of signed consent. I also included a very lengthy history and analysis of the informed consent issue within the second chapter, "Admission of Patients Who Did Not Fulfill Protocol Requirements at Time of Entry." Overall, I exhaustively answered Chabot's three main defenses: first, that no one had been admitted who failed to satisfy the entry requirements; second, that I assisted directly in the evaluation of prospective study candidates throughout the trial; and third, that Dr. Isaacs and I never complained about his approval of any individual patient. To defend my position, along with the text I sent OHRP copies of relevant supporting records such as biopsy reports to substantiate my claims.

In the chapters that follow, I have extracted and condensed the information I provided Dr. McNeilly and the OHRP. I realize I have already covered similar material to some extent in my earlier "Chapter 3: Failure of Handling Informed Consent" and "Chapter 12: Admission of Patients Who Did Not Fulfill One or More Entry Criteria," both based on my response to Zerhouni. For Dr. McNeilly I expanded many of my points considerably, particularly my discussion of Chabot's handling of informed consent. I have decided to present this more thorough—though here edited—exposition of the same issues from my McNeilly monograph to demonstrate the detailed nature of the evidence sent to OHRP.

Note that when I refer to my "Zerhouni monograph" in the following chapter I mean the lengthy manuscript I had previously created to answer the NIH director's litany of denials in his December 2005 letter to Congressman Burton.

Chapter 29

Admission of Patients Who Did Not Fulfill Protocol Requirements at Time of Entry (As Adapted from my McNeilly Manuscript)

In the following section, I list each category of protocol violation, accompanied by a discussion of the various patients we believe appropriately fall within each classification. To fulfill HIPAA requirements, I have redacted the actual names and any identifying information such as addresses, and provided our number identifiers.

Patients entered more than eight weeks after biopsy confirmation of diagnosis. The written protocol simply and bluntly stated that in order to qualify patients must be admitted to start treatment within eight weeks of biopsy:

3.1 . . . No prior treatment, except surgery with noncurative intent (such as biopsy or palliative bypass).

Diagnosis within 8 weeks of beginning therapy.

I have identified three patients Dr. Chabot qualified for the nutritional arm of the study more than eight weeks after biopsy diagnosis: Patients #14, #16 and #34. Note that I describe Patient #14 and Patient #16 in detail within the category "Patients entered with psychiatric illness." However, since both Patients #14 and #16 did not qualify under criteria 3.1 as above, I have included brief summaries of each here.

Patient #14: I am surprised that Dr. Chabot not only entered this patient into the study, but continued to count her as appropriately admitted in his last data chart from April 2006.

Though Patient #14 underwent a biopsy on November 8, 2002, the formal report confirming pancreatic adenocarcinoma was dated November 11, 2002. Dr. Isaacs subsequently met with Patient #14 on December 18, 2002, but Dr. Chabot did not approve her until January 24, 2003—77 days, or 11 weeks, after the actual biopsy and 74 days after the date of the biopsy report. At that point, since her window of eligibility from diagnosis had long passed, she should have been disqualified. To make matters worse, between her first consultation with Dr. Isaacs on December 18, 2002 and Dr. Chabot's decision on January 24, 2003, she had followed no portion of the prescribed regimen. So five valuable weeks of treatment time had been lost, a potential disaster for a patient diagnosed with pancreatic cancer.

Patient #16: Patient #16 underwent exploratory surgery and biopsy proving pancreatic cancer on December 20, 2002 but I did not meet with him in my office for his initial consultation until February 6, 2003, nearly seven weeks after his diagnosis. Dr. Chabot had scheduled his intake interview several days later, but then withheld his final decision about eligibility until the Columbia pathologists reviewed the biopsy slides. By March 5, 2003, nearly a month after our first meeting and nearly 11 weeks since the biopsy, Dr. Chabot still had not come to a conclusion about the patient's status. By that point, the patient no longer qualified.

Patient #34: Dr. Isaacs and I first learned of this trial candidate during the third week in August 2001 after she had contacted Dr. Chabot's office expressing an interest in entering the clinical trial. As instructed, she had sent her medical records to Columbia, but when she didn't hear back after several weeks, she then faxed the relevant documents to us on August 24, 2001. As I studied the file, I realized her biopsy date of June 28, 2001, some 57 days earlier, already placed her one day outside the eight-week window for eligibility—and she still had not been evaluated formally by Dr. Chabot or by my office.

The day I first read through her records, August 24, 2001, I e-mailed Dr. Chabot, relaying my observation that she was no longer qualified:

> Right before she left [for vacation], Michelle [Gabay] called and let us know about the status on a few patients, since they have a tendency to contact us right after she leaves. Later the same day, we got an 80 page fax from [Patient #34] who, Michelle told us, hadn't sent in repeat labs. The patient said in her material that she had sent in 80 pages of material to your office, but never heard back. Perhaps the fax never went through to your office, and she apparently did not call to confirm that her fax was received. . . .
>
> Her biopsy was June 28, which I believe puts her outside the time limit for the trial.
>
> Anyway, she's waiting to hear about her status.

Dr. Chabot chose not to reply. And, though at that point the patient should have been disqualified because of the eight-week rule, Dr. Chabot did not immediately reject her from consideration. Instead, he set up an appointment for his intake evaluation, which did not take place until September 6, 2001, nearly two weeks after my e-mail when to our surprise Dr. Chabot approved her for the nutrition arm and instructed us to begin the treatment process.

Patients who could not eat adequately at the time of entry as required for the protocol. The protocol defined the appetite requirements as follows:

> 3.5. Non pregnant, non lactating
> > Able to eat solid food, three meals per day. . . .
> > Supportive live-in spouse or other family member

Though this statement, as written, might seem somewhat vague, in our many discussions as Dr. Antman, Dr. Wynder and I wrote and rewrote the initial drafts of the protocol, we all intended that patients must be able to eat *normally* to qualify for entrance into the study. And the final version of the official consent form, written in 2000 after the design had changed from randomized to matched cohort, made this point even more clearly on the first page under "Study Purpose."

Seventy to ninety patients will participate in this study. You were selected as a possible participant because you have been diagnosed with adenocarcinoma of the pancreas and have not previously received chemotherapy or radiation. Furthermore, you are able to eat normally and care for yourself, both requirements for entrance into the study.

This statement could not be clearer.

I would now like to discuss in some detail each of the patients Dr. Chabot admitted into the nutrition arm whom we believe could not eat adequately at the time of his intake evaluation. In my Zerhouni monograph I had identified ten such patients that should have been excluded for this reason, though I kept my discussions brief except in the cases of Patients #8 and #9 whom I described at some length.

As we reviewed our files to satisfy McNeilly's request, Dr. Isaacs and I thought that several trial candidates may have misrepresented their status in order to gain entry. In the following discussion, I identify those patients who may have been less than candid about their food intake.

I also described two patients, Patients #22 and #32, I did not include in my Zerhouni monograph as trial subjects we believe should have been excluded. Upon reviewing all our office records for McNeilly, Dr. Isaacs and I realized neither could eat adequately at the time of admission and should have been rejected. In the case of Patient #22, the written records indicated we had questioned Dr. Chabot's decision bluntly. In the second of these two, though Dr. Isaacs did document Patient #32's poor appetite in her intake record, we did not object to her admission into the trial.

Patient #2: Dr. Isaacs met with Patient #2 for her initial consultation on December 18, 2002, before he had been evaluated by Dr. Chabot and approved for entry. In her note from that day, Dr. Isaacs described the patient's contradictory answers to questions about his appetite:

> In USOH [usual state of health] until April 02 when developed diarrhea—had loose malodorous stools multiple times during day and also at night awakening him from sleep. He also developed wt loss, despite good appetite + food intake.

> Currently, he feels fairly well. . . . He eats 3 meals/day, fills up fast, appetite is "not great." He lost 40 lbs [when] diarrhea developed, but reports wt is stable since surgery.

The 40-pound weight loss, even in the context of diarrhea, indicated this patient wasn't eating adequately. Nonetheless, Dr. Chabot qualified him and Dr. Isaacs proceeded with the treatment process. Unfortunately, upon returning home Patient #2, with a long history of diabetes, required hospitalization because of erratic blood sugars. After his discharge he attempted to begin the regimen, but when he developed symptoms of a gastric outlet obstruction, he was readmitted to his local hospital.

On December 27, 2002, Dr. Isaacs e-mailed Dr. Chabot, describing the recent developments:

> Patient #2 wound up in the hospital for labile blood sugar today, apparently his blood sugar has ranged from 35 to 350 over the last couple of days. He had begun but not completed the liver flush and has not yet swallowed a capsule.

Subsequently Patient #2, who continued to deteriorate, was repeatedly hospitalized as the lengthy faxes from his daughter and Dr. Isaacs' own notes confirm. On January 6, 2003, 19 days after the initial consultation in our office, Dr. Isaacs informed Dr. Chabot via e-mail of the patient's declining condition and inability to pursue the treatment plan:

> Patient #2 tried to start his pills over the weekend, but promptly started throwing up. He stopped them on Saturday but still lost his dinner on Sunday. He was seen by his gastroenterologist today and an UG was done. He has narrowing of the pylorus and the duodenum. . . . I am holding off having him start his pills.

Patient #2 eventually died on February 12, 2001, never having followed the prescribed regimen.

In this case, the patient reported a failing appetite and a 40-pound weight loss during his intake interview with Dr. Isaacs on December 18, 2002. His attempts to begin treatment on December 24, however determined, failed because of nausea and vomiting. Dr. Isaacs documented his inability to comply in her office notes and in e-mails to Dr. Chabot dated December 27, 2002 and January 6, 2003.

Patient #3: Dr. Isaacs first met with Patient #3 on November 26, 2002, before she had been seen by Dr. Chabot for his assessment. During this initial session with Dr. Isaacs, the patient reported an improving appetite since a laparoscopic procedure performed November 21, 2002. She did complain of constipation, perhaps brought on by pain medication prescribed by her local doctors, but otherwise to us Patient #3 seemed suitable for entry.

However, after Dr. Chabot approved her, Patient #3 returned home and quickly deteriorated. A note in Dr. Isaacs' chart dated December 1, 2002, only six days after her first office visit with us, described an "emergency" call from the patient's husband, who expressed concern because of his wife's worsening constipation despite the use of stool softeners:

> severely constipated, took Senokot 2 last night w/ minimal result—a little stool w/ AM enema.

A note dated December 4, 2002 documented her declining situation:

> She has been nauseated, afraid to eat because of the nausea.

The following day, December 5, 2002, Dr. Isaacs recorded her further deterioration:

> She threw up breakfast + lunch when she started her pills. She has lost most of the pills she took today. She has an Rx [prescription] for an anti-nausea medication.

Dr. Isaacs spoke to the patient again on December 6, 2002, as documented in the chart:

> she is in excruciating pain. For lunch she had 6 almonds + 6 grapes, took her pills + then threw them up. She is taking anti-nausea Rx. I told her husband to go ahead and give her another. . . . Also told him to contact LMD to discuss hospitalization for pain control and medical evaluation, since her pain has rapidly exacerbated in a short period of time. I told him if she continues to vomit she will have to go to the ER. He understood. . . .

The patient was then hospitalized. A note by Dr. Isaacs dated December 10, 2002 summarized a phone conversation with the patient's husband, who reported the local doctors were urging her to begin chemotherapy and radiation:

> No intestinal or biliary blockage. . . . They have informed him that the only way the pain can be managed is to get chemotherapy and RT [radiation]. So this is what is going to happen. She is currently down in surgery getting a catheter installed for chemotherapy.

After the call with the patient's husband, Dr. Isaacs e-mailed Dr. Chabot, describing the situation:

> [Patient #3] ended up in the hospital for pain control over the weekend. Her MS [morphine] usage doubled over the space of less than a week and she was vomiting as well. She got down 3 days of supplements. The day before she started them, her son told me that "she is so nauseated she is afraid to eat."

That same day, December 10, 2002, Dr. Isaacs contacted Dr. Chabot a second time, expressing her concern that yet another patient approved for the nutritional arm had been unable to comply with the prescribed regimen:

> I spoke with Patient #3's husband today. . . . She is getting ready to start chemotherapy and radiation, which her doctors said is absolutely essential for pain management. . . .
>
> They want to get back on their supplements at some point, but my guess would be that she never will. We are, of course, more than a bit frustrated. I find it hard to believe that she was really eating OK at the time she saw us when, 5 days later, her son reports she can't eat at all because of nausea. . . .
>
> Any possibility of getting her switched to the chemo arm since that is what she actually will be doing? She took 3 days of supplements.
>
> Our frustration again, as we've discussed before, we don't have a washout period and we've had a number of patients who just didn't do the therapy, and yet will be called "Gonzalez failures."

Though this patient should not have been admitted, in retrospect Dr. Isaacs and I believe that she overstated her food intake during the first visit in our office on November 26, 2002.

Patient #4: In my Zerhouni monograph I included this patient as one "who could not eat adequately at the time of entry." In retrospect she might just as appropriately have classified among "Patients entered with psychiatric illness."

Dr. Isaacs first met with Patient #4 on July 5, 2000, after Dr. Chabot had already formally approved her entry into the study. During the initial session with Dr. Isaacs, the patient described a recent history of anxiety and depression, as documented on page 1 of the note from that day:

In 5/00 she saw her MD c/o cough and CP [chest pain] in epigastric area, radiating around her side. She was felt to have anxiety + placed on Paxil. . . .

She has stayed on Paxil, which was first prescribed 5/00 when sx [symptoms] were felt due to anxiety.

Dr. Isaacs also described the patient's declining food intake:

Appetite is less, but eats 3 meals/day.

In the "Assessment" section at her note's end, Dr. Isaacs reported as one of the patient's problems "Anxiety/depression," but since she had already been qualified, we decided to proceed with the treatment process as instructed. Subsequently, Patient #4 discontinued treatment after only eight days because of rapidly declining clinical status requiring multiple hospitalizations. She never did resume her therapy.

I acknowledge that the documentation arguing for exclusion to be less strong in this case than perhaps for some of the others. In retrospect, I believe her anxiety, severe enough to require Paxil, probably made her ineligible more so than her diminished appetite. In my Zerhouni monograph I used this case as an example of a patient who, deteriorating very shortly after beginning treatment, would have been excluded had a lead-in period been written into the protocol.

Patient #5: Dr. Chabot had already approved this patient when Dr. Isaacs first met with him on September 20, 2001. During that initial session, Patient #5 reported a 12-pound weight loss as documented in Dr. Isaacs' note, but claimed to be feeling "fairly well."

After returning home, Patient #5 attempted to begin the regimen. However, by October 4, 2001, 14 days after his first meeting with Dr. Isaacs and after completing only seven days of supplements, he reported a significantly declining appetite, as Dr. Isaacs documented in the patient's chart:

Spoke [with him]—appetite is poor, he reports. On day 7 of supplements. Eating OK, just no appetite.

A note from October 8, 2001, four days later, described a phone conversation:

Spoke w/ [with] him—poor appetite, pain, gas, bloating, on day 10 of supplements.

Thereafter, when the patient's condition worsened to the point he could not continue treatment, he entered a hospice program.

We suspect this patient may have misstated his clinical status during his initial visits with both Dr. Chabot and Dr. Isaacs. Though he reported a recent 12-pound weight loss, he also claimed to be feeling "fairly well." His rapid subsequent deterioration suggests a patient already in severe decline at the time of his trip to New York. I included him in my Zerhouni monograph as another illustration of a patient admitted who, unable to proceed with treatment beyond a week or so, would have been disqualified had a lead-in provision been allowed. However, without this safeguard in place, Dr. Chabot considered Patient #5 a properly qualified treatment failure.

Patient #6: Though in my Zerhouni manuscript I discussed this patient as one who should have been declared ineligible because of poor appetite, his serious bipolar illness may have been a more legitimate reason for exclusion.

I first met with Patient #6 on September 5, 2002, before he had consulted with Dr. Chabot or been approved for the study. During this session he reported trouble eating, along with a 12-pound weight loss over a six-week period, as described on page 2 of my consultation note:

> His appetite is down. He has had a weight loss of about 12 pounds in the last six weeks.

On page 3, under the section "Past Medical History," I recorded that his diagnosis of bipolar illness might "preclude him from entry into the clinical trial." Further along in the "Assessment" section on page 4, I questioned his suitability because of the psychiatric history.

> History of metastatic pancreatic cancer. . . . I am not sure that he is completely eligible. The bipolar illness may preclude him. He is going to see Dr. Chabot next week.

In an e-mail sent to Dr. Chabot the day of my initial consultation, I discussed the patient's long history of active bipolar episodes. I advised Dr. Chabot, who had not yet evaluated Patient #6, that he had downplayed his psychiatric history during our conversation, a history which his wife more candidly discussed. In this note, I emphasized the psychiatric issue, rather than his poor appetite, as grounds for exclusion:

> I spoke to Michelle about [Patient #6], whom I saw for the first time today.
> . . . It turns out as we talked and I probed he has a long history of bipolar ill-
> ness, with according to his wife obvious manic episodes, when he then down-
> played. His wife says he tends to deny the seriousness of his illness. He is on
> Welbutrin [sic] now but not lithium. Again, in our experience, and as you
> know this program requires such focus, patients with psychiatric problems
> just don't do it. Certainly, he seemed nice enough, and was grateful but the
> last thing we need is another non complier. I didn't discourage him because
> ultimately I know it's your decision, but I wanted you to be informed.

I would like to add that patients diagnosed with bipolar illness commonly deny
the seriousness of their disease. Also, note in the above that I once again acknowledged Dr. Chabot's unilateral authority over patient entry. Nonetheless,
despite the psychiatric history and poor appetite, Dr. Chabot approved Patient
#6 for treatment with us.

Although Patient #6 tried to follow the prescribed regimen, his rapidly declining appetite made good compliance impossible—as I documented in a note
dated October 17, 2002:

> I spoke to Mr. and Mrs. [Patient #6]. . . . He is having trouble eating, trouble
> doing the carrot juice, and trouble getting the pills down.

After another phone conversation with the patient on October 28, 2002 I recorded a worsening situation along with my belief he should not have been
admitted into the study:

> [Patient #6] is having trouble with nausea, and he is not able to get his pills
> down. I think he is just too sick. I do not think he should have been entered
> into the trial.

Two days later, on October 30, 2002, I described a discussion with the patient's
wife:

> [Patient #6] is not doing well. He spent the day in bed. When I talked to him,
> he is overdosing himself on pain medication. He barely could talk. I spoke to
> his wife. He was slurring his words. He is on OxyContin. He was not sure of
> the dose. He is on some other pain medication; he was not sure of that. . . .
> He is not able to do this part of the program now, so we are headed for this
> downward spiral where the patient cannot do it.

On November 1, 2002, I documented yet another phone call from the patient's wife:

> I spoke with Mrs. [Patient #6]. . . . a local internist wants to hospitalize [Patient #6]. He is not able to eat. It sounds like he is obstructing. She wanted reassurance, and I said he has to go into the hospital.

On November 6, 2002, I e-mailed Dr. Chabot, questioning his approval of this patient:

> [Patient #6] is not doing well. He could never be stabilized in terms of his pain, nerve block didn't work, very quickly ended up with ascites. . . . He's not able to eat, hasn't been able to eat.
>
> This is part of our frustration which we expressed to you in our meeting, when patients just can't do the therapy properly. Some of these patients are just so sick, beyond what we would ever attempt to treat in our private practice. A patient like this would as you know would not have been entered on the Gemzar study because he could never be stabilized. . . . Is it out of the realm of possibility to have a least a one week lead-in written into the protocol . . . ?

As the excerpts from the chart indicate, I detailed in writing my belief Dr. Chabot had entered yet another patient too ill to follow through with the treatment, and my disappointment over the lack of a lead-in period.

Patient #7: Dr. Isaacs first met with Patient #7 on March 16, 2004, after she had already been qualified by Dr. Chabot for entry. During that first visit, Patient #7 acknowledged a severely diminished appetite, as Dr. Isaacs carefully documented on page 1 of her record from that day:

> She reports she has long standing intermittent nausea x 1 year . . . her appetite is diminished, she eats [approximately] ½ of what she used to. Has lost 10 lbs in 8 weeks.

Though already approved, Patient #7 admitted she was not even sure she wanted to proceed with our treatment, as Dr. Isaacs wrote in the "Plan" section at the end of her note:

> Pt is considering whether to proceed w/ [with] clinical trial. I told her that this is of course her decision.

Based on her own statements, Patient #7 should have been excluded since her ambiguity about joining the trial violated the requirement that trial candidates and their families must be fully committed to the therapy. I excerpt the relevant paragraphs below:

> 3.3. Since the Enzyme-Nutritional Therapy will be administered by the pa tients at home, they and their families must be willing to undertake the required work . . .

> 4.2 All prospective patients must undergo extensive interviewing to determine their willingness to follow, and their suitability for Enzyme-Nutritional Therapy, a complex dietary program that involves major changes in lifestyle and it is not suitable for all patients.

During the second session with Dr. Isaacs the following day, March 17, 2004, Patient #7 again discussed her diminishing food intake:

> Pt seen. She reported nausea and difficulty eating breakfast this AM but moderately good intake yesterday at lunch.

> She has decided she wants to proceed w/ [with] trial. . . .

Because of her eating difficulties, after returning home Patient #7 could never fully comply with the prescribed regimen. By March 20, only 13 days after her second visit in our office, her oral intake had declined to such a point her local physicians prescribed prednisone as an appetite stimulant, as Dr. Isaacs noted in the chart:

> Saw oncologist today—they suggest Prednisone 20 mg QD to help w/ [with] appetite and nausea. I suggested trying only 10 mg per day. . . .

In a series of phone conversations, all documented by Dr. Isaacs, the patient and her husband reported a relentless worsening in her condition that prevented any degree of compliance with our treatment.

A note from April 19, 2004 summed up the patient's ongoing difficulties:

> Spoke w/ [with] her—she was slow to resume her protocol . . . only doing 4 doses of PGT [pancreas enzymes] day [secondary] to nausea. She feels her intestinal tract is moving slowly. She wants to know what the most important pills are. So after one pill cycle completed, essentially she can't do the whole protocol.

After another phone conversation on April 27, 2004, Dr. Isaacs recorded the patient's inability to continue the prescribed regimen:

Not doing mealtime pills.

Her oncologist suggested transdermal Scopolamine for nausea. I suggested she go ahead + try it. She sounds sedated. I suggested backing off on Methadone a little. She is not able to do her protocol.

Two days later, Dr. Isaacs e-mailed Dr. Chabot, alerting him to the latest developments:

[Patient #7]'s husband called yesterday to say that she has been hospitalized for dehydration. The nausea that she reported when she was here has steadily worsened and she hasn't been able to do her protocol for the past ten days or so.

On April 30, 2004 Dr. Isaacs contacted Dr. Chabot again, this time describing the patient's latest crisis, a newly diagnosed small bowel obstruction. Some three weeks later, Dr. Isaacs again e-mailed Dr. Chabot to report that after intestinal bypass surgery, Patient #7 could not resume her nutritional regimen:

I heard from [Patient #7]'s husband today, she underwent laparoscopic gastrojejunostomy on 5/3/04 but was never really able to start eating again afterwards. She was discharged yesterday, is at home, barely eating, unable to do any aspect of the protocol. She has been off it altogether since 4/21 and had only been able to be partially compliant before that.

On June 17, 2004, Dr. Chabot's assistant, Michelle Gabay, e-mailed Dr. Isaacs to let us know that the patient's husband refused to send some required insurance forms, claiming his wife had not been on the trial:

on [Patient #7]. do you have her insurance address. Her husband refuses to send it to suzanne [sic]. He keeps stating that she was never on the trial.

Apparently, even this patient's spouse understood that she was not a suitable candidate nor could she comply adequately. Nonetheless, in his last data chart from April 2006, Dr. Chabot continued to count Patient #7 as appropriately admitted and fully treated, though she could never follow the prescribed regimen adequately because of poor appetite.

Patient #8: In my Zerhouni monograph, I devoted considerable space to this patient's history since in my mind his entry represented such a glaring violation of the written protocol, and because in his April 22, 2006 letter to me Dr. Chabot strongly defended his decision to approve him. For McNeilly, I again retold the story in some detail.

When I first met with Patient #8 on January 16, 2001, before he had been seen by Dr. Chabot for his intake evaluation, I very quickly realized he was unsuited because of his very poor appetite. When I discussed my reservations openly with the patient and his wife, she began to cry thinking he would not be able to receive my treatment. I then explained I would treat him for free even if Dr. Chabot excluded him from the study.

Beginning on page 3, I described the situation in my note from that day:

> The patient reports that his surgeon, Dr. M—also told him that chemotherapy would not be particularly helpful and actually suggested he think of alternatives. One of the biggest problems is that the patient's appetite has been "terrible." A week ago one of his doctors (and he's not sure which one) started him on Megace 2-tsp day. With this his appetite has improved although it's still down. He reports a 20–25 lb. weight loss.

After the consultation, I immediately called Dr. Chabot, arguing that Patient #8 did not meet the eligibility criteria, a conversation I reported in the "Assessment" section of the chart record:

> The patient was tentatively approved for the clinical trial but he doesn't meet the criteria at this point. . . . He has no appetite and he's on Megace for appetite. An inability to eat precludes his entrance into the trial. I discussed this with Dr. Chabot.

In the "Plan" section I wrote:

> I am willing to start the patient on a program but I'm going to have to discuss with the various investigators whether he's appropriate for the clinical trial.

In this single initial note, before Patient #8 had been seen or approved by Dr. Chabot, in three separate places I documented his "terrible" appetite, and in two places my belief he was not suited for entry.

I e-mailed Dr. Chabot that same day, documenting my belief that this patient failed to meet the explicit entry criteria:

Since then he's lost 25 pounds, admitted he wasn't eating, couldn't eat and had no appetite until his Local MD put him on Megace a week ago. He is eating some now, but we have never had any success with a patient staying on the program who had to be put on Megace because of appetite. . . . I know from my experience he's already missed his window and I doubt he will stay on the program ten days.

Dr. Chabot had scheduled his intake interview for the following day, January 17, 2002, before Patient #8 returned to my office to review the prescribed protocol. After his meeting with the patient, Dr. Chabot called me, stating he would order additional blood work before making his final determination about eligibility. Since the written protocol required that certain laboratory parameters fall within a specific range, Dr. Chabot wanted to make sure the patient's results met the entry criteria. In my mind, the blood counts and chemistries, whatever they might be, had nothing whatsoever to do with the patient's poor appetite, which in and of itself disqualified him.

Dr. Chabot instructed me nonetheless to proceed with my second session as if Patient #8 had been formally admitted. In my note from that day, I indicated my willingness to treat Patient #8 regardless of his status on the trial:

> [Patient #8] came in with his family. We spent 2 hours reviewing his protocol. I spoke with John Chabot as well regarding his eligibility for the protocol.
>
> Dr. Chabot agrees that we need to check his blood work and have more recent blood work. I explained this to [Patient #8]. He wants to do the program regardless. I won't charge him, if he's not eligible.

When five days later the lab results came back within the accepted range, I suspected Dr. Chabot would approve this patient despite his poor appetite.

I reported the latest series of events in the patient's chart:

> [Patient #8]'s blood work came in. It actually looks within the parameters of the clinical trial.
>
> I called Mrs. [Patient #8] and told her that we don't have a final decision. I'm waiting on Dr. Chabot . . . he is eating.

By my comment "he is eating" I did not mean to imply a normal food intake, only that he was getting some food down, or at least according to what his wife reported to me.

Two days later, on January 24, 2002, I recorded that Dr. Chabot had not yet notified the patient or me of his decision:

> His wife called wondering whether he had been formally approved for the clinical trial. I have not heard from Dr. Chabot although I faxed the blood work and have called 3–4 times. I told her I would let her know as soon as possible.

Between January 17, 2002, when I completed my second in-office session with Patient #8 and April 23, 2002, I documented in writing 12 individual phone conversations with either the patient or his wife. In the earlier calls, I answered simple questions about the mechanics of the program. In my note from January 24, 2002, I indicated he had complained of severe diarrhea. A week later, on January 31, 2002, he posed a simple question about water filters, but thereafter the record is one of a terminal cancer patient in rather rapid decline.

On February 7, 2002, the patient's wife informed me that her husband had been hospitalized with dehydration, treated, and discharged. My note reported "He is eating," and "To me, it sounds like he's doing better," but these remarks must be seen in the context of a patient so debilitated by dehydration and poor food intake he had to go to the local emergency room. After returning home he began eating, but only minimally as opposed to not at all.

On February 28, 2003, his wife and I again talked. She reported that Patient #8 had resumed the Duragesic patch, a very powerful synthetic morphine derivative usually reserved for terminal cancer patients experiencing intense pain. I documented in my note:

> The last couple of days she said he's struggling. He's having trouble getting all the pills down.

After another phone call from the patient's wife three weeks later, I wrote in the chart:

> He's doing much better. I spoke with his wife. She said over the last few days, he really seems to have turned a corner.

Here I transcribed a discussion with his wife and not the patient, who was still too weak to come to the phone to speak for himself. So this comment, as the others, must be seen in context.

My note dated March 27, 2002 recorded:

I spoke with Mrs. [Patient #8].

[Patient #8]'s generally doing okay. He seems to be doing his program.

Once again I spoke only with the wife of the patient, who himself was too debilitated to talk with me. Twelve days later, on April 7, 2002, Patient #8's wife called to alert me that her husband was declining rapidly:

His local doctor is taking care of the low potassium. He hasn't been doing well. He's been off his program for 10 days. He has ascites. They think he has an intestinal infection. They took him to the emergency room 2 nights ago. They let me [sic] out today. So he hasn't been on his program at all and he's not feeling well. He just wasn't suitable for the protocol. He couldn't eat when he started.

The following day, Patient #8's wife called me again:

I had a long talk with Mrs. [Patient #8]. His family had sent me a note.

They're very concerned that the pain isn't being managed properly locally. The pain doctor that they had been seeing was away for 2 weeks. He's back tomorrow. He's not eating. His gut seems to have shut down. The workup of stool specimens was all negative. . . .

They're very concerned about him.

On April 10, Patient #8 experienced a brief respite when he seemed to improve somewhat:

I called [Patient #8] because I was worried about him. I spoke with his wife.

She said he's really turned around. He started getting the enzymes down again a couple of days ago and she said he just perked up. His appetite improved. His energy improved.

As before, I discussed the situation with the patient's wife, not the patient himself. Though she optimistically reported that his appetite had improved and overall he seemed better, her statements must be seen in light of his recent decline when he could not eat at all. Regardless, shortly after this conversation he quickly deteriorated. Only five days later, on April 15, 2002, Patient #8 was hospitalized once more, this time with a life-threatening pulmonary embolus, a blood clot that had traveled from the veins in his left leg to one of his lung arteries.

I documented the situation in my notes:

> They thought he might die this weekend but they got him home. He's actually home and he's back on his enzymes, so he's certainly trying.

> The problem is he hasn't been able to eat since he started the program and he just wasn't really a suitable candidate for the protocol. That's the problem he never was able to do it.

That same day, April 15, 2002, I e-mailed Dr. Chabot, expressing my concern that he had approved yet another patient unable to comply with treatment:

> Not unexpectedly, [Patient #8], though well meaning, has not been able to follow the diet virtually from day 1, and has been living on milk shakes. I am amazed he has lasted nearly four months since diagnosis with his stage IV disease and doing half the protocol. You may remember that he was on Megace when seen in your office because he couldn't eat, and hasn't been able to eat. . . .

> We are concerned that another two patients haven't been able to do it. . . . Maybe we should have a meeting to discuss all this?

I have no record of any response, but two days later, on April 17, I wrote in the chart:

> [Patient #8]'s not doing well. He's almost comatose. He has a visiting nurse every day so he's comfortable.

> The family was very grateful. His wife said it just took them too long to diagnose him and he was too sick and I agree.

On April 23, the patient's wife called to inform me her husband had died four days previously:

> I spoke with Mrs. [Patient #8].

> [Patient #8] passed away on April 19. He died at home. The family was extremely grateful. He had been off his program for a number of weeks at the time he died.

Though on April 10 the patient's wife reported he was doing better, only nine days later he died in a coma.

Four years after the fact, in his April 22, 2006 letter to me Dr. Chabot continued to defend his approval of this patient:

Other concerns that have been raised by you at investigative meetings include three particular patients that you imply should have been excluded from entry into the study. I have carefully reviewed the three charts that I believe you are referring to, and upon review, I believe our inclusion criteria were met. . . . An additional patient was being treated with Megace as an appetite stimulant. There is nothing in the protocol that specifically would exclude a patient who is being treated with Megace. Both you and I saw the patient on several occasions and note that his appetite was improving steadily over the initial phases of our contact with him. Your office notes *suggest* [italics mine] significant improvement in his appetite and ability to eat.

Earlier, I responded in some detail to Chabot's claims in the above paragraph about the patient's general condition and appetite. In my Zerhouni manuscript from 2006, I had also countered at length the same Chabot argument:

Nowhere in my notes do I once say his appetite "was improving steadily over the initial phases of our contact with him," as Dr. Chabot claims in his letter. Nowhere do my "office notes suggest significant improvement in his appetite and ability to eat." Had Dr. Chabot actually read my extensive medical chart for this patient, he would have seen the careful documentation of exactly the opposite of what he puts to paper.

Until his April 22, 2006 communication to me, written after I had complained about the study's management up the NIH chain of command, Dr. Chabot had never previously disputed in any note, e-mail, or phone conversation my facts about this case, or my belief that this patient should not have been admitted.

Patient #9: I first met with this patient on February 5, 2003, before Dr. Chabot had interviewed or approved him for the trial. In my note from that day I documented my belief that Patient #9 could never possibly comply with our regimen because of his eating difficulties and his significantly debilitated overall condition.

Currently, he does not seem to be doing well. Frankly, I think he is too sick to enter into the clinical trial. He has developed chronic, dull lower back pain that is resolved with Darvocet. His appetite is down. He lost about 20 pounds in the last six weeks. . . . His appetite is very poor and it sounds like he is starting to deteriorate.

In the "Assessment" section at the end of my report, I repeated my concern:

> Widely metastatic pancreatic cancer. He [sic] last blood work is already a
> month old. I suspect it is much worse that it was. Liver function tests were
> elevated at the time. In the last week, there has been significant deterioration
> in his clinical status. I do not believe he is going to be strong enough to do the
> program. I think it is too late. I think he is probably not going to last very long.
> I will e-mail Dr. Chabot at Columbia and let him know about my feelings on
> this patient.

That afternoon, I e-mailed Dr. Chabot, expressing my reservations about this
patient's eligibility:

> I saw [Patient #9] today for his first session, you will be seeing him Friday.
> . . . However, he looked like a patient who is about to crash very soon. From
> my experience, I know he isn't going to make it. Over the past week, he and his
> wife both said there has been a significant deterioration, he is having trouble
> eating, he is getting pale, he gets short of breath going up stairs (his lung
> sounded clear on exam so I suspect it's anemia). His window of opportunity
> has passed.

The following day, February 6, 2003, as per Dr. Chabot's instructions I met
with Patient #9 to review the prescribed program, though he had not yet been
to Columbia for his intake interview. After the session with me, in the chart I
again clarified my position that this patient did not qualify, though I offered to
treat him off protocol and for free:

> My feeling is that he is too sick and I suspect his liver functions tests will have
> worsened since they were done a month ago. He is going to discuss these issues
> with Dr. Chabot. He wants to do the program regardless of whether he is on
> the clinical trial or not and I agreed of course to do that.

Nonetheless, despite my objections Dr. Chabot later informed me that he had
accepted this patient for treatment with us. He justified his position by telling
me Patient #9 had been able to "walk up and down the hallway without any
problem," an accomplishment I thought irrelevant to the issue at hand, his
inability to eat.

Though Patient #9 to his credit tried to comply with the regimen, he simply
was too ill and his appetite too poor. A note from my files dated February 18,

2003, dictated just 12 days after the patient's second visit with me, described a phone conversation in which he admitted he couldn't eat:

> [Patient #9] complains he cannot eat. I thought he was far too sick to do the program. He is trying to get the pills down but it is difficult.

Two days later, on February 20, 2003, I e-mailed Dr. Chabot documenting my concern that he had admitted yet another patient unable to comply. Once again, I gave Dr. Chabot the benefit of the doubt, suggesting that perhaps study candidates like this one downplayed their true clinical status in order to gain entry:

> I am concerned about [Patient #9]. He called after five days on the supplements to tell me he has no appetite and "can't eat." This was my concern when I first worked him up. I think patients like this are so desperate to get on the clinical trial they mislead you about their eating. We've had three patients recently who couldn't do it.

In a chart note dated March 10, 2003 written in response to another phone conversation with Patient #9, I restated my opinion that he should never have been approved:

> I called [Patient #9] to see how he is doing. He is not doing well. I do not think he should have ever been entered into this clinical trial. He cannot eat. His local doctor put him on Megace because he cannot eat. His pain is poorly controlled with morphine and Darvocet. . . .

Then on April 28, 2003, I e-mailed Dr. Chabot, one again questioning this patient's acceptance into the trial:

> I had started to get suspicious about [Patient #9] from —. I hadn't heard from him for weeks. I called several times leaving messages, but no call back. Today his wife called saying he had died two weeks ago, not doing his program.

> As it turns out, for the record, within days of returning to — after his meetings with us his oncologist locally started him on Megace because he "couldn't eat." This was my concern about entering him into the study because had had lost some 20–25 pounds in the weeks before coming to New York and he and his wife said to us he couldn't eat well.

Dr. Chabot never replied, nor did he counter my charge that this patient should not have been qualified. The record clearly shows that Patient #9, because of his very poor appetite and weakened condition, should not have been admitted, and that I had strongly argued against his entry directly with Dr. Chabot to no avail. Nonetheless, Dr. Chabot continued to count this patient as properly approved—despite, as we later learned, the lack of signed consent—until we discovered he had been removed from the list of accepted nutrition patients on the data chart sent us in April 2006.

Patient #12: Dr. Isaacs met with Patient #12 and his family on January 13, 2004, before Dr. Chabot had evaluated him for the study. As documented in Dr. Isaacs' note, during this initial session Patient #12, who appeared cachectic, avoided answering questions about his appetite:

> Currently, he feels "not too bad." He did not clearly answer questions re food intake, but his wife and daughter reported he "eats something every meal." He is 15 lbs below his usual weight, but has stabilized since Amaryl was D/C'd [discontinued]. . . . On Phenergan for nausea.

Though initially he described no psychiatric history, in the chart record Dr. Isaacs included among his current prescriptions Valium, an anti-anxiety drug, and Lexapro, an anti-depressant. In her description of the physical exam, she recorded a height of 5′ 8½″ and a weight of 130 lbs., indicating he was severely underweight.

She described him as follows:

> Alert, cachectic male, NAD [No Acute Distress].

In the "Assessment," section on the last page of her note, Dr. Isaacs included "Depression" among the patient's medical problems, along with "Pancreatic ca [into] liver."

The day of her initial visit with Patient #12, Dr. Isaacs e-mailed Dr. Chabot expressing her opinion that this patient did not qualify for the trial:

> I saw [Patient #12], the patient from —— today. Given his cachexia, it is difficult for me to believe that he will be able to do the program. From our experience, he's just too sick and coming too late.

> I would appreciate hearing about the results of his bloodwork and your final assessment of his eligibility.

Note that the Webster's definition of cachexia reads "general physical weakening and malnutrition." So Dr. Chabot had been notified of this candidate's debilitated condition, his poor appetite, his overall cachexia, and the depression that became clear during the initial evaluation with Dr. Isaacs. Nevertheless, despite the evidence Dr. Chabot approved the patient for treatment with us.

On January 18, 2004, Dr. Isaacs wrote in the chart that only five days after he had been first seen and only one day after he had begun his supplement regimen, Patient #12 complained he could not adhere to the regimen:

> He is on 2nd day of supplements, having heartburn. . . . Told them to continue PPI [proton pump inhibitors], hold supplements till 1/20 to give PPI a chance to kick in.

I myself e-mailed Dr. Chabot, questioning his decision to enter this patient. I again suggested, as I had before in similar situations, that perhaps he had been misled by the patient, though the obvious cachexia reported by Dr. Isaacs clearly argued for exclusion:

> I know Linda had e-mailed you regarding the patient she saw today and I think she underplayed it. He's not eating, and we think he wasn't straightforward with you in order to get into the protocol. He's a [profession] and hasn't any money, and probably feels he wants to do our therapy regardless but couldn't afford it unless he gets into the trial. We've seen this several times, where we think that the patient is being less than candid in order to gain acceptance into the nutritional arm.

Dr. Chabot responded on January 19 with one word, "Noted," at least acknowledging my communication.

Within six days of his meeting with Dr. Isaacs, Patient #12 was hospitalized for dehydration, after which time he never pursued the prescribed nutritional regimen. Nonetheless, Dr. Chabot's April 2006 data chart listed him as properly admitted and as treated, though he should never have been approved and though he never followed the therapy beyond one or two days.

Patient #22: In my Zerhouni monograph, I did not include this patient as one who should have been excluded. However, on review of patient charts for McNeilly, Dr. Isaacs and I realized that his anorexia requiring an "appetite stimulant" at the time of entry should have disqualified him from the trial.

Dr. Isaacs first met with Patient #22 on April 2, 2003, before his appointment with Dr. Chabot scheduled for later the same day. During his initial conversation with Dr. Isaacs as documented on page 1 of her note, Patient #22 described ongoing diarrhea, along with two differing stories about his food intake, one of a "good" appetite while acknowledging a 30-pound weight loss:

> His appetite is good, especially since his LMD started him on an appetite stimulant: his food intake is limited by early satiety. His wt has gone from 190 to 160, though he feels it has been stable in the last two weeks. His diarrhea continues, slightly improved by Pancrease.

In her "Assessment," Dr. Isaacs described, as one of the patient's problems, "Early satiety, diarrhea, pain, wt loss" and in the "Plan" section immediately following she expressed her doubts about the patient's suitability for the study:

> Pt has questions re likelihood of success on program + advisability of pursuing other RX [treatment] in addition to this which I answered—reason for doing trial is to be able to answer this sort of question. I told him frankly that I had some doubts whether he would be able to do this secondary to early satiety and poor po [oral] intake for which LMD prescribed appetite stimulant. He will return tomorrow for protocol. I will verify approval for trial w/ Columbia. He also wanted to know which aspects of program are most important—I responded that they all are.

When Dr. Isaacs and I discussed Patient #22 later that day, we believed him to be ineligible for two primary reasons; first, because of his obvious poor appetite, and second, his lack of commitment. In our experience over the years, a patient who asks during the initial session about combining treatments, or who wonders which aspects of our regimen are the most important, never adequately complies.

Later that afternoon, Dr. Isaacs e-mailed Dr. Chabot:

> Did [Patient #22] meet with your approval? He is on an "appetite stimulant" presumably Megace—he left his list at home. He will let me know what it is tomorrow. He has lost 40 pounds in 3 months, so from that we put together eating is a major problem. He also had questions that typically go along with poor compliance—"what are the most important things to do" and "how do I know if I'm responding" being some of them. He also asked about chemotherapy.

The next day, April 3, 2003, as instructed Dr. Isaacs met with the patient for the second teaching session, as if he had been approved. During that visit,

Patient #22 told a somewhat different story about his weight loss, summarized in Dr. Isaacs' note:

> We reviewed his diet and protocol.
>
> On further discussion, his "early satiety" means he fills up faster than before—he used to eat an enormous amount. Now he eats as much as his wife. Wt loss probably primarily due to diarrhea.

Later that afternoon of April 3, 2003, Dr. Chabot finally responded to Dr. Isaacs' e-mail of April 2, 2003:

> I thought he was very intelligent, highly motivated and despite my challenge very committed. We are awaiting path confirmation. jc

Though Dr. Chabot believed the patient adequately motivated to follow through with our treatment, his e-mail failed to address the serious eating difficulties that alone warranted exclusion. Surprisingly, Dr. Chabot subsequently admitted Patient #22 into the trial despite his anorexia and 40-pound weight loss.

To his credit, Patient #22 did attempt to follow the prescribed regimen, though his unrelenting pain requiring multiple medications, his ongoing diarrhea, and his poor appetite, made compliance impossible. He declined rapidly before passing away on June 28, 2003, not quite three months after his first meeting with Dr. Isaacs.

In this case, we have evidence of a patient who couldn't eat "normally" at the time of entry, in fact who required an appetite stimulant because of anorexia and weight loss. We have documentation that Dr. Isaacs, in her e-mail sent the day she first met with the patient, notified Dr. Chabot of his eating difficulties and lack of motivation to proceed with our treatment. In his response to Dr. Isaacs, Dr. Chabot ignored the food issue entirely while lauding the patient's intelligence and determination, before approving him for the trial.

Patient #32: In my Zerhouni monograph I did not include this patient among those we thought ineligible at the time of entry. On review of her chart and our e-mail correspondence, Dr. Isaacs and I believe that she should not have been admitted because of her poor appetite.

Patient #32 first came to our office on March 11, 2002, after Dr. Chabot had already approved her for the nutrition arm despite a significantly reduced food intake—a problem documented on page 1 of Dr. Isaacs' note from that day:

> Currently, she reports diminished appetite, with a wt loss of 10 pounds in 6 weeks. . . . She has constipation, takes Lactulose 1x/week, and occasional nausea w/ food—uses suppositories 1x/week. She reports she "fills up fast" but is doing well w/ [with] juices.

Note that physicians prescribe the drug Lactulose for severe constipation. In any event, the following day, March 12, 2002, Dr. Isaacs proceeded with the second teaching session. Neither Dr. Isaacs nor I protested this patient's admission into the study at that time, partly because, as it turned out, she had downplayed her failing appetite. During her initial visits in our office we just didn't realize how serious this problem had been.

By March 22, 2002, just 10 days later, Dr. Isaacs spoke with the patient's daughter, who acknowledged Patient #32 could not eat adequately when she had been evaluated by Dr. Chabot, a conversation reported in the chart:

> Called—she is on the 5th day of liver flush.
>
> "No appetite"—she had no appetite when she came in and now it has gotten worse. We discussed that there is no easy solution to this one. She may have to force self to eat.

That same day, Dr. Isaacs e-mailed Dr. Chabot, to inform him of the situation:

> [Patient #32]'s daughter called me today to express her concern about her mother's poor po intake and appetite, one week after her first appointment here. She agreed that her mother's appetite and food intake is not different from when she was here. So it would seem that the patient exaggerated her ability to eat before she came in. She is on her last day of the liver flush and due to start her supplements tomorrow, so I don't yet know whether she will be able to do this or not. . . .
>
> We do know from experience that it is very common that patients exaggerate how good their appetite is before they come in, especially if they figure out that it is what they need to say to get in. Sometimes I think they think that the supplements will improve their appetite—they don't. Sometimes it helps to get specifics on what they actually eat. We usually ask specifically what the patient has actually eaten the previous day or two.

Once the daughter admitted that Patient #32 could hardly eat normally at the time of her New York visit, she should have been disqualified, though Dr.

Chabot continued to consider this patient as properly approved. Of course, as with other trial candidates we believed to be ineligible, we would have been willing to treat her at no charge off-trial in our private practice.

As her condition deteriorated over the next three months, Patient #32 struggled, though unsuccessfully, to follow the prescribed nutritional regimen. Multiple notes in Dr. Isaacs' chart documented the patient's declining clinical status, her very poor appetite, and her difficulty complying. I include selected comments from those notes below:

4/15/02

Spoke with her—gets pain from gas after eats and as a result she doesn't eat much.

4/19/02

Spoke w/ her—still having quite a bit of pain after meals. She is due to see LMD [local medical doctor] soon, suggested she be seen early next week as she may have gastric outlet obstruction—she has early satiety + some nausea.

5/20/02

They called because she has been having emesis [vomiting] when she has a bowel movement—gets that way after has bowel movement. . . .

5/31/02

[Patient #32]'s sister called up, angry and frustrated, feeling like "no one knows what's going on [in reference to the local doctors]." She was upset because [Patient #32] apparently threw up her dinner last night and has a lot of problems and setbacks. Apparently she has a lot of problems simply doing the basics of the protocol, not eating, lost a lot of weight. . . .

6/3/02

Spoke w/ her—being seen by hospice who are helping w/ pain management.

Finally, on June 26, 2002, three and a half months after her first meeting with Dr. Isaacs, Patient #32 expired. After learning of the patient's death, Dr. Isaacs e-mailed Dr. Chabot and Michelle Gabay:

[Patient #32] passed away today. She had been hospitalized Sunday for jaundice and fever, having required stent placement and replacement previously.

Her daughter called today and reported that she had been found to have pockets of infection in her liver which did not respond to antibiotics. They apparently tried several different things, but she ultimately expired.

Ms. Gabay responded as follows:

I spoke w/ her daughter last week. She told me her mother was doing well.

This comment remains to us incomprehensible; in her many conversations with Dr. Isaacs over a period of months the patient's daughter always described a worsening situation.

I would like to make a couple of points about these patients Chabot admitted who could not eat adequately. First of all, it hardly served the purpose of this trial, intended as a fair evaluation of our treatment, to enter repeatedly patients too sick to comply with the prescribed nutritional regimen—particularly in light of the intent-to-treat rule. With that provision in place, each one of these subjects, none of whom could adhere to the therapy plan, was to be counted as a treatment failure. What possible good comes from that, other than to leave us with meaningless data?

I know in multiple places in my notes I expressed my concern that Chabot had approved yet another trial subject who couldn't possibly stick to the prescribed regimen, and whom we would never have accepted into our private practice. Neither Dr. Isaacs nor I wish to appear indifferent to these desperate people or their needs as they fought to survive against overwhelming odds. But this project was a formal clinical trial that required strict adherence to its rules—as Zerhouni himself insisted. And as I previously stated, once Dr. Chabot encouraged these patients to come to New York for their final evaluation, Dr. Isaacs and I would have treated any of them for free, off trial, had they been appropriately excluded. But it made no sense to us that they be counted as part of the nutrition arm of the study.

More importantly, beyond the issues of scientific legitimacy or fairness to us, it was hardly in the best interest of these patients to enter them into this clinical trial when Dr. Isaacs and I knew, based on our years of experience, that they could not possibly comply with the prescribed therapy. How is that compassionate, or kind? All these patients would have been far better off pursuing chemotherapy, or, frankly, going into hospice and enjoying their last days with their families. But they should not have been approved for this research project.

Patients entered with psychiatric illness. The written protocol stated that any candidate with a history of psychiatric illness severe enough to interfere with appropriate informed consent *or* compliance with the treatment must be excluded:

> 3.9. No serious medical or psychiatric illness preventing informed consent or intensive treatment (e.g., serious infection).

In my Zerhouni monograph, I discussed three patients, Patient #14, #16 and #23, whom we believe should not have been approved based on this provision.

Patient #14: This patient could have been disqualified for failing to meet any one of three entry requirements, including her history of active psychiatric illness, an inadequate appetite, and a biopsy completed more than 10 weeks prior to her formal entry into the study. Previously, I discussed Patient #14 briefly as one who failed to meet the eight-week rule.

Patient #14 underwent a fine needle aspiration of a peripancreatic lymph node on November 8, 2002, though the final pathology report confirming adenocarcinoma was not issued until November 11, 2002.

On December 18, 2002, Dr. Isaacs first met with Patient #14, who reported a poor appetite, as documented in the record from the session:

> Appetite is variable, not great—eats ½ of what she used to. She lost 25 pounds, most of it at first because it "hurt to eat."

For her anorexia alone, Dr. Chabot should have excluded her. In addition, she also reported a long battle with depression, as described on page 2 of Dr. Isaacs' note:

> She finds getting cancer has actually helped w/ [with] chronic depression because of all the support she gets. She has long hx [history] of depressed thoughts at various points in menstrual cycle. Was on Prozac in 1997 and found it helped but eventually stopped it, subsequently worsened + Prozac no longer helped.

Dr. Chabot did not consult with the patient for his in-office evaluation until two days later, on December 20, 2002. During that visit, Dr. Chabot apparently learned of the patient's psychiatric issues, but instead of disqualifying her from the trial chose for reasons unknown to us to withhold his decision about her eligibility. He told Dr. Isaacs to proceed with the planned second session as if she had been approved but also instructed Patient #14, once back home, to undergo a psychiatric evaluation. When the results became available, only then would he make a final determination about her status.

Dr. Isaacs met with the patient as instructed, and as documented in the chart:

> Pt was seen by Dr. Chabot earlier today, approval for trial is pending some f/u information from her local MD's.
>
> I went ahead and reviewed diet/protocol with her . . .
>
> I told her if she is not accepted into trial and wants to pay for supplements I will continue to follow her at no cost to her. [Note that we do not sell the prescribed supplements nor do Dr. Isaacs or myself receive any commission or royalty, etc. for their sale].

Unfortunately, while she pursued the psychiatric evaluation Patient #14 chose not to begin the prescribed nutritional regimen. In view of her diagnosis of aggressive pancreatic cancer, her decision to do nothing confirmed to us she was unsuited for the trial.

To make matters worse, for reasons we never understood the psychiatric assessment was delayed for weeks, during which time the patient followed no part of the treatment and deteriorated rapidly. In a phone conversation on December 30, 2002, just 12 days after her first visit to our office, she reported a declining appetite and worsening clinical status, as documented in the chart:

> Spoke with her.
>
> A lot of trouble with nausea and has thrown up a couple of times—had increased pain medication a few days ago but not yesterday, had nausea yesterday, this AM. We discussed the impracticality of trying to do this program while having difficulties eating. She continues to work on finding a local MD to follow her.

By this point she still hadn't been formally approved.

On January 21, 2003, nearly 5 weeks after her first session with the patient, Dr. Isaacs e-mailed Dr. Chabot, asking if he had made a decision about her eligibility:

> [Patient #14] called today wondering about her status. Sounds like she saw someone locally who should have sent you a letter by now. I did not speak to

her directly. I have some concerns about her ability to eat and physically do the program—they called in early January wondering if anything in the supplements would help her keep her food down.

Let me know when a decision has been made.

To our surprise, Dr. Chabot ultimately approved this patient on January 24, 2002—77 days, or 11 weeks, after her actual biopsy, and 74 days from the date of the formal pathology report. By that point, since the eight-week window from diagnosis had long passed, she should have been disqualified for this reason if for no other. Nonetheless, Dr. Chabot informed Dr. Isaacs that since the psychiatrist who had evaluated her during *one visit* determined she was not psychotic, he had decided to admit her into the study.

We found Dr. Chabot's reasoning incomprehensible. First of all, the entry criteria for the trial, as quoted previously, did not define only active psychosis as a reason for exclusion, but any "serious medical or psychiatric illness preventing informed consent or intensive treatment." In this case, Patient #14 lost five weeks of valuable time because she chose to do no part of our therapy as she pursued the psychiatric consultation, and awaited Chabot's final decision about her status. In our opinion, whatever the psychiatrist said after a one-hour evaluation, this patient's own behavior indicated to us she could not properly follow the "intensive treatment." Furthermore, she was ineligible because of the 11-week delay from biopsy, and to add to the mix her poor appetite, described by the patient during her first session with Dr. Isaacs as "1/2 of what it had been," warranted she be rejected.

It is not surprising that numerous studies confirm that depression predicts poor compliance with dietary/nutritional treatments. I think it important to note that in all major lifestyle modification trials we have reviewed, including the Women's Health Initiative, depression counts as a reason for exclusion. So it was hardly extraordinary that the protocol for our study required candidates with a history of depression or any form of mental illness be denied entry.

Though Dr. Chabot informed Patient #14 she had been accepted into the study on January 24, 2002, she didn't begin treatment until 4 days later, on January 28, 2003. Thereafter, Patient #14 followed the prescribed regimen only partially and only briefly, before passing away in late August. Dr. Isaacs e-mailed Dr. Chabot on August 25, 2003, to inform him of her death:

> [Patient #14], the patient from —, died. . . . She had been off her program since
> June, and had found it heavy going since starting because of poor appetite and
> the side effects from the high doses of narcotics she needed for pain control.

In summary, Patient #14 should have been disqualified because of her obvious poor appetite, her psychological disability, and for the simple fact that Dr. Chabot did not approve her for admission until nearly 11 weeks had passed from her biopsy.

Patient #16: Though in my Zerhouni monograph I included this patient among those who should have been excluded for psychiatric reasons, he actually failed to meet—in our opinion—at least six separate entry criteria as documented in the records. These include: first, his poor appetite; second, his lack of motivation to follow the program, evident during the initial session with me; third, his lack of social support; fourth, his apparent psychological disability that became apparent during his first visits; fifth, the fact that Dr. Chabot did not approve him until well beyond the eight-week window from diagnosis required for eligibility; and finally, Dr. Chabot's failure to obtain the required written consent before sending this patient to us for treatment.

Patient #16 underwent exploratory surgery and biopsy proving pancreatic cancer on December 20, 2002, though I did not see him in my office for his initial consultation until February 6, 2003, nearly seven weeks from diagnosis. Because of scheduling problems in his office, Dr. Chabot had arranged his intake interview for several days later, so I actually completed my two sessions with Patient #16 before Dr. Chabot had determined his eligibility.

In the note documenting my first meeting with Patient #16, I indicated that under the care of a local naturopathic physician, he had begun a whole foods type diet though he described his appetite as poor:

> He went back to — and with friends who are interested in alternative medi-
> cine and with a local naturopath began an aggressive nutritional program that
> involved diet emphasizing fruits, vegetable [sic], nuts, seeds, and whole grains,
> and low in animal protein. He also began juices, some herbs, and some other
> nutritional supplements. He said on this program he felt better and he felt his
> stamina and energy improved and his appetite improved somewhat, although
> he is still losing weight. He said his appetite is not great.

In my summary of the session, I recorded my belief that this patient's poor food intake might disqualify him from the study:

History of metastatic pancreatic cancer. Again, I am not sure he is going to be eligible for the trial because he seems to be having a great deal of trouble eating. His last blood work is from late December, December 21. That probably should be repeated. Dr. Chabot will make that determination.

In addition, during that two-hour session with Patient #16, I became concerned that he seemed more interested in the financial benefits of the trial, rather than in the treatment regimen. In the "Assessment" at the end of my note, I commented on his apparent lack of determination to proceed with our therapy, a legitimate reason for exclusion:

> I am concerned over the fact that he seemed uncommitted to the program. He was not really sure whether he could do the program. We talked about it. Again, these issues will be discussed with Dr. Chabot.

That day, February 7, 2003, I e-mailed Dr. Chabot again, relaying my concern that Patient #16 seemed unmotivated to pursue our regimen:

> I saw [Patient #16]. Seems somewhat unfocused, he didn't have any of the information about when or where he was to meet with you on Monday.

The following Monday, Michelle Gabay, Dr. Chabot's assistant, called to inform me that the patient had been seen at Columbia but neither admitted nor rejected. Instead, Dr. Chabot had decided to withhold his decision until the Columbia Pathology Department reviewed the December 20, 2002 biopsy slides. Regardless, I was to proceed as if the patient had been formally admitted.

After his return home, I spoke with Patient #16 on February 12, 2003, a conversation I documented in my chart. When he told me he had not been contacted by Columbia regarding his status, I decided to e-mail Dr. Chabot:

> Was [Patient #16] accepted into the trial? We weren't sure yet (remember, we had reservations about his ability to focus and follow through)

Dr. Chabot in turn informed me by e-mail that "path is pending." I wasn't happy with the response, so hoping for a more specific answer I called Dr. Chabot, who told me he had no idea when the final Columbia report would be ready.

In the patient chart, I summarized these various conversations:

[Patient #16] still has not heard about the clinical trial and whether he is accepted or not. I spoke to Dr. Chabot who said the pathology needs to be reviewed and is not in yet so there is no decision.

In a note dated February 21, 2003, written after another phone call from the patient, I reported that neither of us had heard from Dr. Chabot. At that point, 63 days, exactly 9 weeks, had elapsed from the biopsy, so Patient #16 no longer qualified anyway by the eight-week rule. Nonetheless, I still heard no word from Dr. Chabot about the situation.

Twelve days later, on March 5, 2003, I described another phone conversation with Patient #16, who told me Dr. Chabot's office had yet to contact him. To my surprise, he also admitted he had not begun his treatment until the previous day, nearly a month since I had first met with him:

Unfortunately [Patient #16] did not start his program until yesterday. It is a month since I saw him. He does not have a good explanation. He is waiting to hear from Columbia about being on the clinical trial. I told him to start regardless because a valuable month has been lost.

In response to this new information, I e-mailed Dr. Chabot:

I spoke with [Patient #16] tonight. I had given him his protocol February 7, nearly a month ago. To my astonishment, he had not started any part of the protocol until yesterday, when he began the liver flush—despite the fact that I strongly and sternly advised him to start the program the day he got back to—regardless of whether he was on the clinical trial or not. . . .

He said he delayed because he hadn't heard from Columbia, but I had told him when I met him not to wait because of the aggressive nature of the disease. He agreed I had told him this. . . .

What do we do with a patient like this? I left a message for you to call, maybe we should discuss it over the phone at your convenience. It's another patient who isn't doing what he is supposed to do, in any way.

That same day, Ms. Gabay informed me that Patient #16 had been admitted.

Subsequently, on March 10, 2003 Ms. Gabay called me again, describing her own phone conversation with Patient #16 in which he claimed full compliance with the prescribed regimen since the day he arrived home a month earlier.

So, I e-mailed Dr. Chabot yet again:

> I spoke with Michelle about [Patient #16]. . . . He had done virtually nothing of the program after four weeks, except perhaps some of the foods. . . .

> I think he needs to be disqualified because not only was he not willing to do it, but apparently he misled Michelle. . . .

> As you know so well, it's just frustrating for us to face patients who don't do the therapy and yet will be counted as treatment failures.

A month later, on April 11, 2003, my assistant spoke at length with the patient's ex-wife who confirmed that Patient #16 had never followed the treatment plan, and had now deteriorated into a terminal state.

I recorded these latest developments in the chart:

> His ex-wife called and left a message with the staff. She stated that he is "at home and very terminal." She said that the patient wanted to be sure I knew that he believes that if he had started earlier he would have gotten more benefit.

> In retrospect, he lost valuable time when he decided for reasons which still remain unclear, not to start his therapy in a timely appropriate way.

To bring this story to an extraordinary conclusion, in 2005, more than two years after Patient #16 died, we learned that he had been sent to us as fully consented though he had never signed the required form.

I believe that this case, perhaps more than any other, illustrates the extraordinary lapses we repeatedly witnessed in the handling of patient entry. To this day, I do not know why Dr. Chabot insisted I treat the patient as if he had been an appropriate admission though he never signed the required consent document.

Even if we disregard the legitimate reasons for exclusion such as poor appetite, the lack of commitment to the therapy, the lack of social support, the apparent psychological disability and the missing signed consent, by the time Dr. Chabot's assistant Ms. Gabay told me Patient #16 had been admitted on March 5, 2003, 75 days had passed since the December 20, 2002 biopsy, more than 10 weeks. The eight-week window between diagnosis and entry had long passed, and meanwhile, as he waited for Chabot's decision, Patient #16 pursued no part of the therapy except perhaps for some of the diet. As a final footnote to this story, we learned much later that Dr. Chabot would claim that he had never approved Patient #16 in the first place.

Patient #23: Dr. Isaacs first met with Patient #23 on December 23, 2003, before her intake interview with Dr. Chabot. In the first sentence of her note from that day, Dr. Isaacs reported the patient's history of hypertension and clinical depression:

> HPI 52 yo WF w/ hx [history] of HTN, clinical depression. . . .

Parenthetically, Dr. Isaacs also described the patient's poor appetite:

> She "eats well but is not hungry"

Then on page 2 of her note, under the section titled "Med" (for Past Medical History), Dr. Isaacs wrote:

> Clinical depression—since 1999—has been more stable in last 6 months

The patient's local doctor had actually prescribed two drugs for the depression, Wellbutrin and Celexa. On page 3, in her summary of the case, Dr. Isaacs listed as one of the patient's problems "Clinical depression on 2 medications" and in the last section titled "Plan," she documented:

> As per pt request will proceed w/ [with] explanation of clinical trial protocol.
> Final assessment of eligibility as per Dr. Chabot.

This last sentence emphasized once again Dr. Chabot's complete authority over patient admission at that point. In this case, he subsequently approved this patient, despite the long history of psychiatric illness.

Unfortunately, shortly after returning home the patient's oncologist badgered her to quit the trial and begin chemotherapy. After a brief attempt at complying with the prescribed nutritional regimen, Patient #23 withdrew from the study to pursue conventional treatment, as per her doctor's advice.

To this day I do not understand the rationale of admitting a patient on high doses of two powerful anti-depressants into this clinical trial—though Dr. Chabot defended his decision in his April 22, 2006 letter to me:

> If you revisit the study protocol documents, please note the exclusion criteria
> refers to patients who have psychiatric conditions that preclude the ability to

obtain informed consent. Upon reviewing each of the two charts in question, I believe that both individuals were appropriate to the study, given the extent of their psychiatric conditions.

The written protocol, as we have seen, actually stated that trial candidates, to be eligible, must have:

> No serious medical or psychiatric illness preventing informed consent or intensive treatment (e.g., serious infection).

Dr. Antman and I included this phrase not for my benefit, but for the protection of those patients whose mental disability might hamper compliance with the prescribed therapy. What possible good can result from entering someone like patient #14, who for five weeks did no therapy whatsoever, or patient #16 who never took a single supplement? Who gains from this?

A patient lacking family or social support. The written protocol required supportive live-in family members for candidates to be eligible:

> 3.3 Since the Enzyme-Nutritional Therapy will be administered by the patients at home, they and their families must be willing to undertake the required work.

> 3.5 Non pregnant, non lactating
> Able to eat solid food, three meals per day . . .
> Supportive live-in spouse or other family member

Patient #15: On September 22, 1999 Dr. Isaacs first met with this patient, whom Dr. Chabot had approved for entry some four weeks after her initial contact with Columbia. Unfortunately, while she awaited Chabot's decision about her status, she had deteriorated dramatically. By the time of her initial consultation with Dr. Isaacs, Patient #15 reported a poor appetite as well as a recent 20-pound weight loss. Since the slow pace of Dr. Chabot's assessment had left her frustrated and discouraged, Dr. Isaacs and I did not argue against her admission.

On page 2 of her note from that day Dr. Isaacs described a list of somewhat formidable social problems. Nonetheless, Patient #15 also reported, as Dr. Isaacs documented, "Family is supportive," and that she had an active church life.

When Patient #15, after returning home, seemed unable to follow the treatment plan adequately, Dr. Isaacs questioned her about the social network she had described during her meeting in our office. After a phone conversation on October 20, 1999, Dr. Isaacs reported in the chart that Patient #15 admitted a lack of any help at home, and in fact, as sick as she was, she was herself caring for various family members including her adult son.

> She has no help—she is doing all this herself. She is tired, has a hard time getting help. But in further discussions, she is making meals for her grown son who lives with her even though he neither expects nor demands this.

> She is sleeping through enzyme doses—perhaps doing ½ the doses.

> I explained that doing what sounds like perhaps ½ of the program will not work. She needs to ask people to do small specific tasks for her. . . . I encouraged her to make a plan to get help.

As the patient worsened, Dr. Isaacs eventually helped arrange for hospice care. On November 15, 1999, Dr. Isaacs documented a phone conversation with a visiting nurse, who described a family missing in action:

> She apparently spends the whole day alone at home, there is no one in the family to help with medications or food.

In a note faxed to us describing a recent home visit, the nurse further elaborated the situation:

> Pt confused, @ home alone, pt drifting off to sleep during conversation. . . . PT describing very scared, being home alone.

The following day, November 16, 1999, Dr. Isaacs, as recorded in the chart, discussed the situation with the hospice doctor:

> Spoke w/ [with] hospice director. . . . He attempted to see the patient today, but no one responded to knocking. Apparently a social worker was able to see the patient later, she said she was asleep. They feel she needs their inpatient unit.

In a fax to Dr. Chabot dated November 17, 1999, Dr. Isaacs documented the lack of social support in this patient's case:

> Unfortunately, from the beginning she never did her program fully. . . . Her social support was not as she had indicated before she came in; in fact, she

had no assistance whatsoever and was sleeping through most of her doses of supplements. It also turned out she did **not** have a local physician [note: as required by the protocol] to help with her care contrary to what we believed. . . .

The patient is not cooperating with the hospice nurses, or anyone else according to her son.

Even if Patient #15 misrepresented her social and family situation to gain entry into the trial, once we learned the truth, she should have been disqualified—though we would have continued treating her for free off trial. Regardless, Dr. Chabot insisted that Patient #15 be counted as a properly entered, properly treated "Gonzalez patient."

Patients with no evidence of signed informed consent. In my Zerhouni monograph, I devoted an entire chapter to those patients admitted by Dr. Chabot who never signed the required consent forms. In my discussion of this issue for Dr. McNeilly, I added considerably more detail.

I started off by stating, as I had for Zerhouni, that to my knowledge all clinical trials, particularly those funded by the government, require each eligible patient who agrees to participate sign a consent form acknowledging in writing their decision. As carefully outlined on the official NCI website, such documents must, by explicit regulation, describe the purpose of the project, possible risks of treatment, potential benefits, options, and responsibilities. And, they must be signed:

Sec. 50. 27 Documentation of Informed Consent

(a) . . . informed consent shall be documented by the use of a written consent form approved by the IRB and signed and dated by the subject or the subject's legally authorized representative at the time of the consent. A copy shall be given to the person signing the form.[34]

The written protocol of our trial, in sections 3 and 4, clearly stated that each provisionally approved candidate must sign a consent form as part of the entry process.

3.8. Informed Consent. Each patient must be completely aware of the nature of his/her disease process and must willingly give consent for the chosen regimen. The patient must understand the alternatives, potential benefits, side-effects, risks, and discomforts.

4.4 Registration: To register the patient, fax or deliver the completed Eligibility Criteria Form and signed Informed Consent to the Cancer Center Protocol Office, located on MHB 6N-435. . . .

4.5 Required Forms:
Eligibility Criteria Form
Informed Consent

In accordance with the above written regulations, the Columbia team working with Dr. Isaacs and myself devised a lengthy document for this specific purpose. Though for the first 20 months of the study Dr. Isaacs and I could veto patient entry, from the beginning Dr. Antman insisted that only Dr. Chabot would supervise consent. The signed forms would then be kept in the appropriate files at Columbia, not in our charts. We were told that no patient would be officially considered as admitted—as the written protocol instructed—or even be sent to us for treatment as part of the trial unless all the completed documents were in hand at Dr. Chabot's office.

Though these rules seemed simple enough, in mid-2002, at a time Dr. Isaacs and I had been excluded from patient intake, we first became suspicious that all was not well with the consent routine at Columbia. As had been the case since the trial's inception, Dr. Chabot's office staff supervised the gathering of relevant patient records so that he could then begin his assessment. If Dr. Chabot subsequently approved a candidate for entry, his assistant would fax the documents to us so we could then arrange our own visits and begin the treatment process.

On July 17, 2002, Dr. Isaacs first met a new patient, a woman Dr. Chabot had already interviewed and qualified though his office had failed to mail or fax any of the medical records to us as documented in Dr. Isaacs' note:

CC [Chief Complaint]: pancreatic cancer

Source: pt—records currently not available

Dr. Isaacs conducted her initial consultation as instructed by Dr. Chabot, using the patient as the sole source of information since we lacked copies of the actual medical file—an odd circumstance for a government sponsored clinical trial. The following day, July 18, 2002, Dr. Isaacs, still without the records, completed her second session with the patient, who then returned home to start treatment. Unfortunately, she promptly experienced a series of strokes, deteriorated very rapidly, could not comply with the prescribed regimen, and entered a hospice program. She eventually died on September 26, 2002, 2 months and 9 days after her first visit with Dr. Isaacs.

Some time after her death, Dr. Chabot's assistant Michelle Gabay called our office to inform us, quite to our surprise, that the patient had never signed the consent form and had now been excluded from the trial. Apparently, during her initial meeting at Columbia, the patient asked if she could take the form home to "think about it," before signing and mailing the document back to Dr. Chabot. For reasons we do not understand, Dr. Chabot we were told agreed to this arrangement without notifying us, and then sent the patient to our office as if she had been properly consented—in violation of the written protocol requirements. Dr. Chabot's subsequent decision to disqualify the patient did not make right his handling of consent in this case.

At the time we assumed this episode, as strange as might be, represented an isolated incident, so we didn't make much of it. However, not long afterwards, we were to learn of the other two patients, #9 and #16 by our identifiers, who had been sent to us for treatment with no evidence of signed consent.

The story of these two began with an e-mail to us from Dr. Chabot's office assistant, Ms. DeRosa, dated April 21, 2003, in which she inquired if we had copies of the consent forms for Patient #9 and Patient #16:

> Also, do you keep consent forms on file for the nutritional arm. If you do I need
> a copy of the last page of the consent form for: [Patient #16 and Patient #9].

We found her request odd, since Dr. Chabot, who had supervised the consent process from the trial's beginning, had not sent copies of the signed forms of any study subjects to our office. In response to Ms. DeRosa's question, Dr. Isaacs called her by phone, explaining that we had seen none of these documents. When we didn't hear from her again about the issue we assumed the problem had been solved.

Some time later, in the summer of 2003, for the first time the Columbia administrators required that I sign a subcontract agreement with the University beginning each fiscal year, defining my specific responsibilities for the clinical trial. After reading the document, Dr. Isaacs and I realized that we were now required to keep copies of the signed consent forms in our own patient charts, in addition to the originals which would remain in Dr. Chabot's files. For us to comply with this new rule, we would need to get copies from Dr. Chabot's office.

On July 8, 2003, Dr. Isaacs e-mailed Michelle Gabay, offering to copy the forms herself at the time of the next regularly scheduled group meeting to be held at Columbia:

> Also, I will need to get copies of the consent form for every patient. The sub-contract that Nick had to sign specifies that he will keep consent forms for each patient on file. We tried to get them to modify it to say that you all were maintaining those records, but it didn't fly. I will be happy to come over early the day of the meeting and do it if you want.

Ms. DeRosa at Dr. Chabot's office subsequently responded:

> Dear Linda:
>
> Copies of the consent forms? All of them? When do you need them by?

Dr. Isaacs e-mailed back shortly afterwards:

> Can I get the copies on Thursday? We are coming over for a meeting that starts at 5, I can come up earlier if need be.

Ms. DeRosa did not reply, and as it turned out Dr. Chabot's staff was unprepared to copy the forms, or allow Dr. Isaacs to do so, the day of the July meeting. Subsequently, when we still did not receive the forms despite repeated conversations about the issue, on September 1, 2003 Dr. Isaacs again e-mailed Ms. DeRosa:

> I just wanted to see if we could set up time for me to come up and copy the consent forms.

Ms. DeRosa answered:

> Hi Linda:
>
> Just returned from a brief vacation. Anytime this next week would be fine. Alternatively, I can see if I have time to copy them this weekend.

During the ensuing two weeks, we contacted Ms. DeRosa repeatedly, hoping to arrange a mutually suitable time for Dr. Isaacs to go to Chabot's office and copy the forms. Finally, the date was set for September 15, 2003, but the day before, on September 14, 2003, Ms. DeRosa e-mailed Dr. Isaacs:

> We've been having difficulty with the e-mails coming through Columbia's pine network in a timely fashion so I just got this e-mail . . . Thought you were not coming. Ok today or tomorrow is fine. Got Chabot's area to allow you to use the photocopier here on my floor so we do not need to carry the charts far.

For a variety of reasons the scheduled rendezvous didn't happen, and it was not until October 2003 that Dr. Chabot's staff met with Dr. Isaacs at the Columbia Cancer Center for the purpose of copying the forms. However, while reviewing the files Dr. Isaacs noticed that the signed consents were missing from the charts of two patients, #9 and #16, considered as properly admitted into the study, but no one at Columbia seemed to know what had happened.

Some time later we were assured that the documents might be in a second set of charts kept in the surgery clinic, but this proved not to be the case. By July 2004, nine months after Dr. Isaacs' visit to Columbia, Dr. Chabot's staff still had not located the missing forms. Then on July 20, 2004, in preparation for another regularly scheduled meeting of the trial personnel at Columbia, Dr. Isaacs again e-mailed Michelle Gabay:

> Michelle:
>
> I just wanted to list the loose ends that we have in preparation for Thursday's meeting: . . .
>
> Consent form for [Patient #12, Patient #9, and Patient #16].
>
> Path report for [Patient #7] (did she ever send in her slides?)

The following day, July 21, 2004, Ms. Gabay responded:

> I sent your email to cara.

The missing documents were unavailable the day of the conference, but twenty-nine days later, on August 19, 2004, Ms. DeRosa e-mailed our office:

> Linda/Michelle:
>
> As noted previously, there are no consents in the charts for [Patient #9 and Patient #16] seen on 2–7–03 and 2–10–03. There is, however, a note by JC

[John Chabot] in the chart that the [Patient #16] was given the consent form at the time of the office visit. . . .

If you have additional questions, please do not hesitate to contact me.

So according to Ms. DeRosa's e-mail, the written record indicated that Dr. Chabot had given Patient #16 the form and not that he had been consented. Regardless, we were determined to learn the fate of the missing documents because of the new contract requirements. When we heard nothing more from Dr. Chabot's office about the issue, in December 2004 we decided to contact Dr. Victor Grann, one of the Columbia physicians supervising the study. At a recent staff meeting of trial personnel, Dr. Isaacs had discussed a number of errors on the Columbia data sheet with him, including a discrepancy between our records and Chabot's in terms of the total number of patients entered.

After the session, on December 13, 2004 Dr. Isaacs e-mailed Dr. Grann:

Victor:

Just as a followup to our conversation:

I would love to get our records in synch so that we all have the same number of people in our arm of the study.

I would also love to review the actual data entry, as there have been a number of little glitches (like only 2 people being alive instead of 3).

And finally, I have been trying to get copies of the consent forms for [Patient #9 and Patient #16] for about a year now. Cara refers me to Michelle and Michelle to Cara. I keep planning to ask at these meetings, but we run out of time. Perhaps these two patients were eliminated because there was no consent form, and that explains the discrepancy in our numbers. But I would like to know. According to a subcontract we have with Columbia, we are obligated to have copies of the consent forms.

Thanks for your help.

Linda

In a brief note to our office dated December 14, 2004, Dr. Grann wrote simply:

I emailed Cara.

Victor

So Dr. Grann had handled the problem by e-mailing Ms. DeRosa, who sixteen days later, on December 30, 2004, finally replied:

Linda/Victor:

The two patient's [sic] she mentions below without consent forms have been reported previously to the Cancer Center at the time of their registration. We also discussed this problem at our last meeting.

As we read this latest e-mail, we had no idea what Ms. DeRosa meant when she wrote that the patients have been "reported previously to the Cancer Center at the time of their registration," nor did we know what meeting she was talking about. We thought perhaps she was referring to some internal Columbia proceeding, since the elusive forms had not been discussed at any of the regularly scheduled group sessions we attended at Columbia.

Three days later, on January 2, 2004, Dr. Isaacs e-mailed both Ms. DeRosa and Dr. Grann:

Thanks for your response, but I wasn't present at the meeting you were at where these issues were discussed, and I still don't know what the answers are to the questions I asked.

Linda

When after a month we heard nothing in response, on February 4, 2005 I contacted Dr. Chabot directly. In my e-mail correspondence I queried him about the missing consent documents, as well as the ongoing disparity between our data sheet and his in terms of the total number of patients entered into the study:

John:

We have been trying for some time now to figure out why there is a discrepancy in our records regarding how many patients are on the study, and which patients are not on the study. Linda spoke with Victor briefly about this at the last meeting and e-mailed him in followup. He forwarded it to Cara, who sent us an answer we did not understand, referring to a meeting we did not attend. We received no response to our request for clarification. See below if you wish to review the correspondence. [note: I included the correspondence as a thread following my e-mail]

Any chance of getting this sorted out before the next meeting? We are also concerned that [patient] who is very much alive, had been listed as being dead. . . .

We have been trying to get copies of the consent forms for [Patient #9 and Patient #16] for quite some time now, and both Michelle and Cara say that the other person has them. Some intervention here would be appreciated since by the contract requirements, we are expected to keep copies in our charts. The subcontract with Columbia we signed says that we must keep them for all patients on the study. . . .

Nick

Four days later, on February 8, 2005, Dr. Chabot replied, without specifically answering my question about the consent forms:

Last week Michelle went through all the charts to confirm data accuracy. It is loaded loaded [sic] into the system now. I will get any new graphs to you when available.

JC

At that point, we decided to contact Michelle Gabay:

Michelle:

We got the e-mail below from Dr. Chabot and are very glad to hear you went through everything—that must have been quite an endeavor.

We are hoping that you can tell us why there is a mismatch between the number of patients we have listed and the number you have. Please see the attached spreadsheet, which is up to date as of February 1 . . .

Also, we would still like those wretched consent forms on [Patient #9 and Patient #16].

Thanks for everything

Nick and Linda

Ms. Gabay replied the following day acknowledging receipt of some documents we had sent her, but said nothing about the consent forms. When we heard nothing further about the missing documents, on March 8, 2005, nearly four weeks after Ms. Gabay's last note to us, Dr. Isaacs e-mailed her:

Michelle:

Did we hear that the study is accruing . . .?

Also, we still need the consent forms for [Patient #9 and Patient #16]. I noticed that the number of patients on the trial now matches between your records and ours. . . .

Linda

As more weeks passed with no explanation forthcoming from Dr. Chabot's office, I began to wonder if these two patients, who never followed the prescribed regimen, had ever signed the required forms. Subsequently, at the June 29, 2005 group meeting, we briefly discussed the problem, but Dr. Chabot still had no idea what might have happened. Nonetheless, it was our understanding these two patients were still being counted as "Gonzalez failures" in the tabulation of the interim data, despite the absent consent and the significant non-compliance. To me, their inclusion as properly vetted and properly treated made no sense.

When I heard nothing for nearly a month after the June 2005 session, on July 26, 2005 and in some frustration I again e-mailed Dr. Chabot:

John:

How are you? I hope you are surviving this miserable weather okay.

We just have a few odds and ends we'd like to wrap up.

The terms of the subcontract require that we have a copy of the consent form that the patient signs. Linda went to Cara's office and copied most of them nearly 2 years ago, but there were two that were not available when she came—[Patient #9 and Patient #16]. She has intermittently tried to get these from either Cara or Michelle ever since. Each said to check with the other, or would say that the consent form must be in a chart that was in another location, or something. Given that both of these patients did not follow through with their protocols, we would like to know if they even signed the consent forms. So we would appreciate either receiving a copy of these consent forms or getting an answer as to whether these patients are data points on the trial. . . .

Nick Gonzalez

The following day, Dr. Chabot responded:

I will F/U with Cara and Jane Lyons on these issues. Thx for the heads-up.

jc

Despite the assurances, we still received no explanation for the missing forms.

Dr. Smith of the NCI sent the minutes of the June 20, 2005 meeting to us on Sunday, September 11, 2005, the day before the scheduled September 12 session, which Dr. Isaacs and I did not attend. In response to what I perceived as the many errors in the record, I e-mailed the various trial personnel and again raised the issue of the missing forms:

> There are a number of very serious errors in the minutes. Under point 2, you have a question about how many patients are in the enzyme arm. So do we. For quite some time now, we have been trying to get copies of the consent forms of two of the patients on the enzyme arm . . . most recently in an e-mail to Dr. Chabot dated July 27, 2005. We still have not received these, and so we will now bring up the same question we brought up to him at that time. If the patients have consent forms, we want a copy, as the subcontract we were required to sign requires that we keep them. If the patients do not have consent forms, we would like to know if they are included in the clinical trial.

Our questions went unanswered. Frankly, by this point I wondered if Dr. Chabot hoped I would forget about the issue and go on to some other problem, but on October 19, 2005, I e-mailed him once more, hoping for some meaningful response:

> We are still waiting for an answer about the consent forms for [Patient #16 and Patient #9]. Do they exist, or don't they? If they exist, we would like a copy as is required by the subcontract we signed. If they don't exist, we would like to know if the patients are included as data points in the study. We continue to request them because, although your office was entrusted with the job of getting consent forms, as a part of the subcontracts we were required to sign, I am obligated to maintain copies of these consent forms. Linda started trying to get these consent forms in the summer of 2003. She finally came over and photocopied the bulk of them in October of 2003, but has been trying ever since to obtain copies of [Patient #16 and Patient #9] 's forms. We have repeatedly requested copies, or an indication of their status, since we were instructed to treat these patients as if they had met the criteria, including filling out consent forms.

Finally, in an e-mail dated October 26, 2005, Dr. Chabot confirmed in both cases the documents were missing:

The consent forms have not been identified. Both patients were accrued at times when Michelle was away and a research nurse from the cancer center was covering this clinical trial. The IRB was notified of this problem, in writing quite a long time ago and I have no further instructions. . . .

I didn't understand why Dr. Chabot had failed to inform us of this sequence of events months earlier. I was also somewhat surprised to learn that a substitute nurse had been assigned any part of the intake process, particularly informed consent, which we had been repeatedly told only Dr. Chabot would directly supervise. And I still could not tell from his note if he considered the two patients properly qualified treatment failures (I later learned, or at least I thought I learned, that he did).

My many written complaints about the error-filled June 2005 minutes would not be addressed until the March 20, 2006 group meeting, after Congressman Burton and Senator Harkin had questioned the management of the clinical trial in their respective letters to Dr. Zerhouni. According to the official notes, during that session Dr. Chabot provided a new explanation for the mysterious missing consent forms.

1. Number of subjects in the enzyme arm and missing consent forms:

The Columbia staff investigated this issue. Two consent forms from subjects entered in the enzyme arm are missing. Their follow up into this issue revealed that there are notes in both subjects' medical charts indicating that they were consented and in at least one of these cases, it is recalled that the patient requested to take the form with them and planned to return it. It appears that both these patients "walked off" with their forms. The IRB was informed of this and as both charts note that subjects were consented, the IRB left it up to the investigators to decide about inclusion of this data. The investigators conducted the statistical analyses both with and without these two subjects and there is no effect on the statistical conclusions.

I was taken aback to learn Chabot now claimed his chart notes confirmed that each of the two patients in question had been "consented" though the actual forms were missing. Never once prior to the minutes of the March 20, 2006 meeting had he or anyone else in his office implied that these two patients had been "consented" despite the absent documents.

In her e-mail to Dr. Isaacs dated August 19, 2004, some nineteen months earlier, Dr. Chabot's assistant Cara DeRosa reported finding a notation about the issue, apparently written by Dr. Chabot, only for Patient #16 after her search through the two charts. According to Ms. DeRosa, Chabot had indicated that the form had been *given* to Patient #16, not that he had been "consented."

I repeat for emphasis the relevant portion of that e-mail:

> Linda/Michelle:
>
> As noted previously, there are not consents in the charts for [Patient #9 and Patient #16] seen on 2–7–03 and 2–10–03. There is, however, a note by JC [John Chabot] in the chart that the [Patient #16] was given the consent form at the time of the office visit.

Presumably, if the chart of Patient #16 confirmed he had been "consented," Ms. DeRosa would have mentioned this finding to us. Furthermore she said nothing in her e-mail about any written comment in the file of Patient #9 concerning consent; if such a notation existed for this particular patient, it made no sense she wouldn't have told us.

Some six months after Ms. DeRosa's response to us, Dr. Chabot reported in a February 8, 2005 e-mail that a staff member "went through all the charts to confirm data accuracy," so by his own statement we know that charts were carefully reviewed yet again. If during this search his staff discovered each patient had been "consented" I did not understand why we weren't informed of this at the time.

In my Zerhouni manuscript, I discussed my surprise that the Columbia IRB did not, according to what Dr. Chabot himself said, seem unduly concerned about his serious oversight in sending three patients to us for treatment on a federally funded clinical trial without evidence of the required signed informed consent. Since I wasn't privy to any internal IRB conversations or memos, I don't know what its members may have discussed with Dr. Chabot, or what he might have said about the issue with them in the first place. Who knows what really happened?

I would also like to make several additional points about the above exchange of e-mails that span approximately two and a half years. These communications I hope prove that repeatedly and relentlessly Dr. Isaacs and I sought to learn the fate of the forms once we realized they were missing in mid-2003, and that repeatedly Dr. Chabot and his staff failed to explain what had actually happened.

Despite no evidence of signed consent for Patients #9 and #16, as far as we could tell Dr. Chabot counted both as properly entered for most of the study's duration, justifying their inclusion at the March 2006 group meeting as documented in the minutes. But when we received his final data sheet sent to us along with his April 22, 2006 letter defending his management of the trial, we realized he had expunged these two from the list of approved nutrition patients.

Summary of Patients Admitted Who Did Not Fulfill

Protocol Requirements at Time of Entry

(As Appearing in My McNeilly Manuscript)

Patients entered more than eight weeks after biopsy confirmation of diagnosis: Patients #14 and #34.

Patients who could not eat adequately at the time of entry as required for the protocol: Patients #2, #3, #4, #5, #6, #7, #8, #9, #12, #22, and #32.

Patients entered with psychiatric illness: Patients #16 and #23.

A patient lacking family or social support: Patient #15

Patients lacking evidence of signed consent: A patient entered in 2002 whom Dr. Chabot later disqualified, and consequently without, as far as we know, an identifying number. Note that although the required consent documents were missing from the charts of both Patient #9 and Patient #16, in my McNeilly manuscript I included #9 within the category of those **"who could not eat adequately"** and #16 as one **"entered with psychiatric illness."**

Chapter 30

Who Really Was in Charge of Patient Entry

In chapters 4–7 of my McNeilly monograph, I analyzed in great detail the evidence that Dr. Chabot, for the greater part of the study, solely evaluated the eligibility of trial candidates. I devoted considerable space to this issue since according to Dr. McNeilly, by claiming that Dr. Isaacs and I participated in the entry process throughout, Chabot now insisted that even if patients had been inappropriately admitted, I had no one to blame but myself.

In my counter-argument, I relied heavily on the official study documents, particularly the written protocol and the consent form. Between the project's beginnings in the fall of 1997 with its proposed randomized design and its reincarnation as a matched cohort in 2000, each of these had undergone at least five major revisions. The various drafts of both the protocol and consent form included clearly written sections defining the roles assigned to both Dr. Chabot and myself in the evaluation and approval of trial candidates. From this evidence, I easily demonstrated that for the greater part of the trial, Dr. Chabot exclusively managed all aspects of patient intake.

I began the fourth chapter of my McNeilly monograph by relating in some detail my initial discussions with Dr. Antman about the proposed project in the fall of 1997, long before Dr. Chabot's participation and long before the NCI came on board. Since at the time Procter & Gamble had agreed to provide full funding, we proceeded as if the project would be industry-supported.

As I previously discussed, during these conversations Dr. Antman insisted the study be randomized in design, though she readily agreed that both Dr. Isaacs and I should be fully involved with her office in the screening of all trial candidates. If Dr. Antman, Dr. Isaacs, and I approved a particular patient for entry, he or she would then be randomized by computer either to chemotherapy or to our nutritional regimen.

The first version of the written protocol, dated September 30, 1997, described our proposed role in Section 4.0:

4.0 **Patient Entry**

4.1 Evaluation by the study chair

4.2 Evaluation by Dr. Gonzalez or staff trained by him: All prospective patients must undergo extensive interviewing to determine their willingness to follow, and their suitability for, the Enzyme-Nutritional Therapy. This treatment is a complex dietary program that involves major changes in lifestyle and it is not suitable for all patients. Dr. Gonzalez has trained staff members to conduct such interviews, and it is suggested that someone from his staff be involved in the selection process.

Dr. Antman informed me the "study chair" referenced above would either be herself or perhaps Dr. John Chabot, whom we had not met at the time but whom she identified as a Columbia surgeon specializing in pancreatic cancer. Regardless, certainly Dr. Isaacs and I would help assess all trial candidates.

Furthermore, the September 1997 draft of the consent form, intended to be read and signed by those patients provisionally approved for the trial, indicated I would be involved in the admission process. Specifically, the section toward the end entitled "Questions" stated:

If you have any questions, we will do our best to answer them.

The physician in charge of this research at the Columbia Presbyterian Medical Center is Dr. Karen Antman. Her telephone number is (212) 305–8602. If you need more information about this study before you can decide whether to participate or at any other time, you may wish to contact her, or you could contact Dr. Gonzalez at (212) 213–3337.

If you have additional questions in the future, you can reach Dr. Antman at (212) 305–8602 and Dr. Gonzalez at (212) 213–3337.

If you have any questions on your rights as a research subject you can call the Institutional Review Board at (212) 305–5883 for information.

I have discussed this study with Dr. Antman, Dr. Gonzalez, or their associates, to my satisfaction. I understand that my participation is voluntary and that I can withdraw from the study at any time without prejudice. I have read the above and agree to enter this research study.

After Dr. Chabot officially joined the project as part of the Columbia team, Dr. Antman, perhaps with his assistance, rewrote the protocol in preparation for its submission to the Columbia IRB for final approval. This second draft, dated December 16, 1997, had been modified considerably, though Section 4.0, "Patient Entry," still indicated I would assist with the entry process:

4.0 **Patient Entry**

4.1 Evaluation by the study chair

4.2 **Evaluation by Dr. Gonzalez:** All prospective patients must undergo extensive interviewing to determine their willingness to follow, and their suitability for Enzyme-Nutritional Therapy, a complex dietary program that involves major changes in lifestyle and it is not suitable for all patients.

Note that Dr. Antman told us that the "study chair" at this point referred to Dr. Chabot, with whom we would share intake responsibilities.

The consent form, including the "Questions" section, had also been extensively rewritten, though I was identified again as part of the team.

If you have any questions, we will do our best to answer them.

The physician in charge of this research at the Columbia Presbyterian Medical Center is Dr. Karen Antman. Her telephone number is (212) 305–8602. If you need more information about this study before you can decide whether to participate or at any other time, you may wish to contact her, or you could contact Dr. Gonzalez at (212) 213–3337. . . .

If you have any questions on your rights as a research subject you can call the Institutional Review Board at (212) 305–5883 for information.

In early 1998, with the project still in its formative stages, Dr. Antman and her Columbia colleagues, again without my input, extensively revised the protocol document. To my surprise, she had removed my name from Section 4.0:

4.0 **Patient Entry**

4.1 Evaluation by the study chair

4.2 All prospective patients must undergo extensive interviewing to deter-mine their willingness to follow, and their suitability for Enzyme-Nutri-tional Therapy, a complex dietary program that involves major changes in lifestyle and it is not suitable for all patients.

The rewritten consent form reflected as well my apparent downgraded status. The "Questions" section, describing Dr. Chabot as the "physician in charge," instructed any prospective patient with questions about the trial or the two treatments to contact his office, not ours:

> If you have any questions, we will do our best to answer them. The physician in charge of this research at the Columbia Presbyterian Medical Center is Dr. John Chabot. His telephone number is (212) 305–8295. If you need more in-formation about this study before you can decide whether to participate or at any other time, you may wish to contact him.

> If you have any questions on your rights as a research subject you can call the Institutional Review Board at (212) 305–5883 for information.

Since both the protocol and consent form had changed so drastically, I called Dr. Antman, asking her to clarify my involvement with patient approval. She assured me that once the study was up and running, Dr. Isaacs and I would still participate, but our authority would be less formal in nature, not to be included as an official right in the written protocol. Her explanation made no sense to me: since this document represented the rule book for the trial, I argued our veto privilege, if real, should be explicitly defined in writing and not left to a verbal promise. She would not budge on the issue, before finally admitting the Columbia team thought it prudent to relegate us to a strictly secondary role in terms of evaluating trial candidates. In addition, she described new rules in place governing the initial processing of all patients once the project did open to accrual: Dr. Isaacs and I would be required to refer all those diagnosed with pancreatic cancer who contacted our office with an interest in joining the study immediately to Dr. Chabot. From that point, without our input he alone would supervise the gathering of pertinent patient records and the preliminary assessment.

For those whom he believed met all the entry requirements, one of his staff would conduct a phone interview to help evaluate eligibility further, as well as explain the nature of the clinical study and the two treatments under investigation. For those interested in joining the trial, Dr. Chabot or one of his assistants alone would answer questions about the project, even those questions pertaining to our therapy specifically, about which the Columbia team knew little. Should any patient undergoing review at Columbia contact our office wishing to talk to Dr. Isaacs or myself about our therapy or the trial, we were to redirect those patients back to Dr. Chabot without comment.

If and when Dr. Chabot finally approved a patient, we could then review the records ourselves and conduct our own interview by phone. After all this, if we objected to the admission of a candidate and if Dr. Chabot agreed that he or she for whatever reason did not qualify based on the explicit written entry criteria, he would then reject the patient. If our consensus favored approval, he would meet with the patient in his office for the intensive face-to-face discussion. At this time, he would reassess eligibility once more, and if all the criteria had been met, only then would he proceed with informed consent. Once qualified and consented, the patient would be randomized either to chemotherapy or to our nutritional regimen.

I asked Dr. Antman how we should handle patients contacting our office seeking information about the trial who did not meet the entry requirements, such as those who had already undergone the Whipple procedure or had received chemotherapy, clear reasons for exclusion. She suggested that I should refer even those patients to Dr. Chabot for his review without offering an opinion. However, we could continue to treat in our private practice, without directing them to Columbia, those patients diagnosed with pancreatic cancer who expressed no interest in the trial.

Up to this point in early 1998 and through the first versions of the protocol and consent documents, the project was still in its formative phases with its randomized design, we were not yet accruing patients, and the National Cancer Institute had not yet offered to fund the trial. In late spring 1998, after the NCI formally agreed to provide support, Dr. Antman and her staff revised the official documents to reflect the new government sponsorship. Both the "Patient Entry" section of the protocol and the "Questions" at the end of the consent form remained largely identical to the previous draft, confirming Dr. Chabot's increased authority.

In late 1998, the trial with its randomized design finally opened to patient accrual and as word spread in the media and on the Internet, patients expressing an interest in the project began calling our office. We dutifully referred all of these to Dr. Chabot, but many would get back to us some days, even some weeks later, complaining that they had called or faxed Columbia as we had instructed them to do, but no one had responded. We began to suspect that Chabot's office was simply overwhelmed, so to help smooth the process, in early 1999 Dr. Isaacs and I created a simple two-page document culled from the consent form, which we intended to distribute either by fax or by regular mail to potential study candidates who contacted us requesting information about the trial. The final version, dated February 10, 1999, read in part:

Dear Prospective Patient:

Thank you for your recent request for information regarding the study titled: "Evaluation of intensive pancreatic proteolytic enzyme therapy with ancillary nutritional support in the treatment of inoperable pancreatic adenocarcinoma." The study will be conducted in patients with adenocarcinoma of the pancreas. The study is funded by the National Cancer Institute and is being run under the direction of the Department of Oncology and Department of Surgical Oncology at Columbia Presbyterian Medical Center. It compares one type of therapy, intensive pancreatic proteolytic enzyme therapy (with ancillary nutritional support) with another type of therapy, gemcitabine, a chemotherapeutic agent. . . .

Because it is not known at the present time which treatment approach is best overall, the treatment program selected for you will be chosen by a method called randomization. This means that there is an equal chance that you will be assigned to receive either one of the two treatment programs. This letter is designed to give you a brief overview of the two therapies and of this study, to help you decide if you wish to pursue this option.

If you are interested in participating in this study, you will first be screened to be sure you meet certain eligibility criteria. This screening process will begin with a review of your medical history, pathology reports, and CT scans or MRI to determine the extent of your disease. The screening process also includes a telephone interview, at which time your history will be reviewed and your willingness to undertake either of these two therapies will be assessed. The pancreatic proteolytic enzyme therapy in particular requires a high degree of motivation and commitment.

You will then receive either the Enzyme-Nutritional Therapy or gemcitabine, the most recently approved chemotherapy drug for treatment of adenocarcinoma of the pancreas. . . .

If you participate in the clinical trial, you may be assigned to the nutritional therapy. Although all patients in the study will be evaluated at Columbia, patients in the nutritional group will be treated directly by either Dr. Nicholas Gonzalez or Dr. Linda Isaacs, through their office. . . .

The letter then included a five-paragraph description of our treatment, followed by a single paragraph summarizing gemcitabine and its administration as an intravenous drug. The document then ended as follows:

If you wish to proceed, please call Michelle Gabay at 212–305–9468 to begin the evaluation process. Thank you for your interest.

Note that we identified Dr. Chabot's team as in charge of entry into the trial, nowhere instructing patients to contact us for any reason at any time during their initial evaluation at Columbia.

In addition to this document, we wrote up a summary of the trial, its design and purpose, for use on our website. However, before distributing the printed information sheet or posting the online version, we submitted drafts of both to Dr. Antman for her review. She approved each, without any expressed reservation.

Despite these modest efforts to expedite the admissions process, the handling of study candidates by Chabot's office—based on feedback from frustrated patients—seemed to become only less efficient. Then, after only three suitable candidates sought entry into the trial in its randomized format during the first year of accrual—two of whom quit when assigned to chemotherapy—the NCI and NCCAM finally agreed to change to a matched cohort, so the patients, and not the computer, could choose their therapy. At this point Dr. Antman and staff rewrote the study documents in November 1999 to incorporate the new study design. Both the "Patient Entry" section of the protocol and the "Questions" portion of the consent form remained unchanged from the previous version, each identifying Dr. Chabot as the physician in charge of patient admission, with no mention of either Dr. Isaacs or myself. (Note that at the same time, we also revised our two-page information sheet and website summary to reflect the changes).

Despite the new format, few patients sought entry and by early summer of 2000, we had assessed a grand total of 10 candidates, only four of whom ultimately agreed to sign up. During this period we had dutifully followed Dr. Antman's instructions that we refer all patients diagnosed with pancreatic cancer who contacted our office with an interest in the trial to Dr. Chabot, whether we believed they met the written entry criteria or not. Unfortunately, we continued receiving phone calls from many trial candidates, complaining, sometimes angrily, about the intake process at Columbia. Repeatedly we heard that after the initial call or fax to Chabot, days and at times weeks had passed with no response. Out of frustration, these people had contacted us hoping we might intervene on their behalf. Few seemed aware of what the admission procedure actually involved or even what records they should send to Columbia, since no one from Chabot's office had called back to tell them. This to us was not a good sign.

Though at this point we could still veto patient entry, our role changed significantly beginning in July 2000. Those of us involved with the trial—the Columbia team, the NCI and NIH personnel, Dr. Isaacs and myself—planned to convene on July 24, 2000 at Dr. Chabot's office for one of our regularly scheduled group meetings. Some weeks before the session, Dr. Antman informed me that Dr. Isaacs and I could no longer distribute the two-page summary we had been faxing or mailing to prospective candidates who called or wrote our office seeking information about the project. Dr. Antman also insisted we must immediately remove any mention of the clinical trial from our website. She explained that the Columbia IRB had instructed her that any document created in our office related to the clinical trial and intended for public consumption through any venue, including the Internet, required their approval first. If we wished to submit the printed material we distributed or our posted website summary for review, Dr. Antman warned that the IRB could put the study on hold, perhaps for many months, while they critiqued the information. None of this made any sense to me, since Dr. Isaacs and I had created these simple documents by lifting whole paragraphs right out of the consent form which had already passed IRB scrutiny. Nonetheless, Dr. Antman insisted that if we wished to send out the sheet or include a description on our website, we had to submit the material for IRB consideration. Since so much time had already been lost during the disastrous one year of randomization, we agreed simply to stop distributing and posting the forms rather than push for official IRB blessing. Dr. Antman did, when pressed, suggest that we could substitute a short paragraph on our website, with Dr. Chabot's phone number, instructing patients interested in the NCI clinical trial to contact Columbia. But we could not describe or comment on the study itself.

Dr. Antman also warned us that both the Columbia IRB and the NCI supervisors felt uncomfortable with our continued involvement with the selection of trial candidates. The general consensus seemed to be that our participation might somehow allow the dreaded but unspecified "bias" to creep into the study and undermine its legitimacy. Though neither the IRB nor the NCI had come to a decision about this issue, she wasn't sure if Dr. Isaacs and I would retain our veto over patient entry much longer. Sensing the writing on the wall, Dr. Isaacs and I suspected we would eventually be removed from any managerial role, with Dr. Chabot given complete control over patient intake.

Six days before the planned July 2000 meeting, I received a revealing e-mail from Dr. Jeff White, the NCI supervisor of the trial, requesting information about our role in the entry process. In view of Dr. Antman's earlier comments, his note confirmed to us that our involvement with this aspect of the trial seemed to be a big concern in Washington:

> I have been asked to brief Bob Wittes and Steve Straus [from NCCAM] on some details about the Columbia study of your therapy, I thought I would e-mail the questions rather than call so as not to interrupt your work day too much and give you more time to respond. Our meeting is Monday the 24th, so I would appreciate if you could get me the answers by this Friday. . . .
>
> 1. Are all potential patients for the [sic] screened at Columbia or does your office identify and screen any?
>
> 2. Once a patient is identified and screened at Columbia and he/she selects the nutritional arm do you perform your initial and follow-up evaluations in your office or in the clinic at Columbia? If the evaluations are done in your office, are any of the Columbia investigators present during these evaluations?
>
> 3. Does anyone in your office participate in the consent process for protocol patients or have all patients that you [sic] for the protocol already signed the consent form?

I responded the same day:

> Dear Jeff:
>
> In answer to your questions:
>
> 1. All patients for the clinical trial are required to be screened at Columbia first, then screened by our office. So, each patient will be interviewed twice, and their records reviewed twice, to assess eligibility.
>
> We have "veto" power for a patient we feel doesn't meet the protocol criteria, but all patients must be screened and interviewed at Columbia. Slides on all patients are also going to be reviewed at Columbia.
>
> If a patient who might be eligible for the trial calls our office first, our staff has been trained to refer them directly to Michelle Gabay at Dr. Chabot's office. On rare occasions, a potentially eligible patient has faxed us extensive information before speaking to any of our staff. In that case, we review the records, then have our staff refer them to Columbia. But again, no patient enters the trial without approval and review at Dr. Chabot's office.
>
> 2. Once the patient is identified and screened, they are physically seen by Dr. Chabot at Columbia first, and then by either myself or Dr. Linda Isaacs in our office here. No one from Columbia Presbyterian has been present for the meetings in our office.
>
> 3. The consent process for the clinical trial is done exclusively at Columbia. We do not participate in this process. We do not discuss the clinical trial with prospective patients until after they have spoken with Michelle Gabay.

The group meeting went forward as planned. Unfortunately, the NCI did not begin distributing written minutes of these sessions until well over a year later, in September 2001. Consequently, I do not have in my possession any official notes summarizing the topics discussed in July 2000, or at the subsequent September 2000 conference, nor do I know if such notes even exist. I believe it was in July 2000 that Dr. Richard Kaplan of the NCI, whom I had not previously met, accompanied the rest of the Washington team to New York. Dr. Kaplan informed Dr. Isaacs and myself the NCI had decided that to protect the project from "bias," we could no longer participate with the intake process in any way—our veto power had, in essence, been revoked. Dr. Chabot would now assume cozmplete decision-making responsibility over the entry of all study candidates into each arm.

I want to remark that I cannot be sure whether Dr. Kaplan came to New York in July 2000 or in September 2000, since we have no official record of these events, but he did attend one of the two sessions and made his directives clear. I do remember Dr. Kaplan telling us sternly that henceforth we were to refer all patients with a diagnosis of pancreatic cancer who contacted our office in any way, whether by phone, fax, or letter, immediately to Dr. Chabot without comment or discussion. When I questioned him if he literally meant *all* patients, he expanded his point by saying that indeed we were to refer *all patients* who contacted our office with a diagnosis of pancreatic cancer to Dr. Chabot, including those who obviously did not qualify for the study, and to our astonishment, those with no interest in joining but who sought our treatment as private patients. Dr. Chabot, with no input from us whatsoever, would undertake the entire intake assessment for each of these patients, including the gathering of medical records and all interviews.

If, for whatever reason, someone whom we had routed to Columbia subsequently contacted our office while Dr. Chabot's evaluation was in progress and before he had come to a decision, even if to complain about a lack of responsiveness, our staff should offer no opinion but only insist they call Columbia. Only after Dr. Chabot officially approved a candidate for our arm of the study would he then notify us, so we could set up appointments to begin the treatment process. Subsequently, Dr. Chabot, in his face-to-face meeting with the patient, would complete informed consent, again with no input from us. And of course, we were forbidden from distributing any printed information about the project from our office, even if the documents only reproduced sections from the protocol or consent form. However, the one paragraph on our website directing patients interested in the clinical trial to Columbia could remain up.

For those patients who approached Columbia directly seeking our therapy as study participants without first contacting our office, Dr. Chabot was under no obligation to tell us anything until he had completed his review. If he admitted such a patient, only then would we be informed, and as for those patients approved for the chemotherapy arm, we would be told nothing, before or after their entry.

At our discretion, as part of our private practice we could treat, off study, any of those patients Dr. Chabot deemed ineligible, or those whom he may have qualified but who wanted no part of the study. By these new rules, we could not begin treating anyone with the diagnosis of pancreatic cancer who wished to consult with us as a private patient without first referring them to Columbia.

The assembled staff emphasized almost in chorus that Dr. Chabot's decisions henceforth would be final and binding, with no appeal possible at Columbia, at the NCI or at the NIH. If he admitted a patient into the nutrition arm, we were to treat the patient without question—and if we didn't like the rules, we could quit the study.

We found the requirements to say the least odd, and potentially damaging to the integrity of the trial since now a single individual, Dr. Chabot, had been granted unilateral authority over patient selection with no oversight. Nonetheless, the Columbia team along with the NCI and NIH personnel seemed convinced that Dr. Chabot alone could be trusted to manage patient intake, including informed consent, efficiently, effectively, and of course, without the dreaded bias, all for the greater good of the study. The reasoning left us somewhat baffled. By that point, on multiple occasions the Columbia evaluation process had proven itself to be less than ideal, and at times seemingly indifferent to those desperate patients awaiting an answer about their status. With this history in mind, Dr. Isaacs and I both argued for a continued role in selecting patients at least for the nutrition arm, pointing out that we just wanted another check on the procedure, no more. Our words fell on deaf ears, and now the entire clinical trial, our many years of research and work, would be at the mercy of Dr. Chabot's judgments about patient eligibility.

Unfortunately, after July 2000 Dr. Chabot's handling of trial candidates remained from our perspective inefficient. We continued receiving calls from frustrated patients awaiting some word from Dr. Chabot about their status, but according to the new rules, we could do nothing but instruct these people facing death to call Columbia. If we engaged in any discussion we had been warned we would be guilty of a protocol violation that might provoke closing the trial. So dutifully, thinking always of the greater good of the project, from that point onward my staff routed trial candidates who might contact our office during their intake processing back to Dr. Chabot without comment or discussion. We wondered how many of these callers, often incredulous that we could not discuss our own therapy or the study with them, had simply disappeared in annoyance to pursue some other treatment.

The situation deteriorated so significantly in the weeks after the July 2000 meeting that Dr. Isaacs and I looked for ways to ease the stress not only on study candidates, but also on our staff left dealing with the high volume of calls from often annoyed patients. We thought at the very least we should be allowed to send out a simple one or two page information sheet about the trial to those with a diagnosis of pancreatic cancer who called our office, letting them know what records they needed to send to Dr. Chabot so they might expedite the intake process.

After the September 2000 group meeting, we e-mailed Dr. Chabot about our suggestion:

> Something I forgot to bring up at the meeting:

> We frequently get calls from people who have pancreatic cancer but do not want to call Michelle or be a part of the trial because they are afraid that the screening process will be too slow, or who send in info according to the directions on our website [for non-trial patients] without even calling us first. . . .

> We have handled these folks in the past by gathering info such as blood work, path reports and CT scans, then forwarding it to Michelle, while minimizing our discussions with them here until after she has spoken with them. Is that acceptable? A lot of these folks have had their diagnosing doctors tell them that "time is of the essence," so they can be fairly persistent with the staff here.

> It would be very helpful to have something written we could send to these people. That way, they could go ahead and fax some info to Michelle instead of to us. I know that this material would have to have IRB approval. But it might be worth going through the process. I would be happy to draft something, using the informed consent paperwork as a guideline.

During a subsequent phone conversation, Dr. Chabot informed me, as had Dr. Antman before, that IRB blessing even for such a simple document could take weeks, even months, during which time the study might be put on hold. Since the last thing this trial needed was another long delay, once again we gave up the idea.

In the weeks that followed, when the situation in Dr. Chabot's office didn't improve, I felt I had to take some action for the sake of the patients contacting our office, frustrated as they waited to hear back from Columbia. I finally called Dr. Chabot on January 22, 2001, asking if we could at least inform those who clearly did not meet the entry criteria—such as those previously undergoing a Whipple procedure or who had received chemotherapy—that they would not be eligible. We thought such a simple and reasonable approach might save these people from undue distress as they waited, perhaps weeks, to hear Dr. Chabot tell them what we already knew, that they didn't qualify for this study. With their status immediately known, they would then be free to pursue some other treatment.

Dr. Chabot seemed only annoyed by my suggestion, as if in some way I sought to edge my way back into a managerial role, when I only hoped for a solution to a vexing problem, his delay in responding to patients. When I mentioned that in some cases we knew the person was not suitable, he seemed perturbed that I had in my possession any information on any prospective candidate.

That night, I e-mailed him, hoping to clarify the issue:

John:

Maybe we weren't clear to you. These patients sent us this information on their own and call us on their own, often because they are desperately waiting to hear from your office. We would be happier if they didn't—but they do call us, if a patient is clearly not eligible, and they've contacted you, and they still call us, how should we handle it?

After thinking about the situation some more, about an hour later I e-mailed Dr. Chabot a second time:

John—

Just a postscript to my earlier e-mail. All patients with pancreatic cancer who call our office on their own, independently, are referred to you—the problem we're running into is that when they don't hear from your office promptly, these patients who are coming to you from us start calling us, and it puts us in a difficult situation if we have a patient who clearly isn't eligible and we know it. Can't we tell them while they're waiting to hear from you? These people get anxious because if they're not eligible they want to look somewhere else, though of course there isn't much else to look into.

Linda and I feel a brief meeting with you and Karen might be useful to hash these kinds of things out—how does that sound?

When we spoke by phone later that day, Dr. Chabot repeated what he had said previously. All patients with the diagnosis of pancreatic cancer who called our office for whatever reason, whether seeking entry into the study or not, whether eligible or not, needed to be referred to his office without comment or discussion, regardless of our opinion about their suitability, and no matter how many times such patients might call us, or how inefficient we might perceive his intake process. We were not to engage with them in any way until he had reached a final decision about their status.

The following day I spoke again to Dr. Chabot, hoping to find some way to make the evaluation procedure less painful for study candidates, but to no avail. After our conversation, I decided to summarize our various discussions in an e-mail:

> John—
>
> Thanks for the clarification. In future, no matter how desperate, etc. we'll just insist they have to wait from [sic] you. We're not trying to be difficult, we just didn't know what to do with some of these folks. They call us sometimes insisting we give them input.

So clearly, as the study documents show, after July 2000 Dr. Chabot and only Dr. Chabot managed all aspects of patient entry.

Chapter 31

Instances in Which Dr. Isaacs and/or Dr. Gonzalez Argued Against Entry of Patients Approved by Dr. Chabot

As Dr. McNeilly requested, I provided him with ample documentation confirming Dr. Chabot admitted multiple patients into the nutrition arm who did not meet the entry requirements and that for the last five years of the study only he determined patient eligibility. But Dr. McNeilly had also requested I send him evidence responding to Dr. Chabot's third claim, that Dr. Isaacs and I had never objected to the entry of any patient into the nutrition arm of the study.

In answer to this last issue, I concentrated on the group of patients admitted after July 2000, when Dr. Chabot assumed unilateral authority over intake. Prior to that time, while we still retained veto privileges, we did object whenever Dr. Chabot provisionally approved a candidate we believed did not meet the specific written eligibility criteria. In such cases, Dr. Chabot accepted our opinions as valid, subsequently rejecting each of those we thought unsuited.

If we consider only those entered after July 2000, our records indicate that in the case of seven subjects Chabot qualified for treatment with us we questioned his decision for very specific reasons. Despite the evidence and our protests, Dr. Chabot nonetheless excluded none of this group.

In the section that follows I have extracted, with some editing, my answer to Chabot's charge as it appeared in my McNeilly manuscript. For the seven patients whose admission we did challenge, I reference the relevant written evidence, culled from both the charts and our multiple e-mail exchanges with Dr. Chabot and his office. Though I have discussed these patients earlier in other contexts, here I emphasize this specific point, that either Dr. Isaacs or I questioned the entry of each.

Our Objection to Entry of a Patient Entered More Than Eight Weeks After Biopsy Confirmation of Diagnosis

Patient #34: Dr. Isaacs and I first learned of this patient during the third week in August 2001. After contacting Columbia, she sent her medical records to Dr. Chabot for an initial assessment, but when she did not hear back from his office after several weeks she faxed the records to us on August 24, 2001. As I studied the file, I realized her biopsy dated from June 28, 2001, 57 days earlier, so that she had already missed the eight-week window required between diagnosis and entry. And at that point, Dr. Chabot had yet to evaluate her case, a process that would take additional time.

The day I received the records, I e-mailed Dr. Chabot expressing my opinion about her eligibility:

> Right before she left [for vacation], Michele [Gabay] called and let us know about the status on a few patients, since they have a tendency to contact us right after she leaves. Later the same day, we got an 80 page fax from [Patient #34] who, Michelle told us, hadn't sent in repeat labs. The patient said in her material that she had sent in 80 pages of material to your office, but never heard back. Perhaps the fax never went through to your office, and she apparently did not call to confirm that her fax was received. . . .
>
> Her biopsy was June 28, which I believe puts her outside the time limit for the trial.
>
> Anyway, she's waiting to hear about her status.

Dr. Chabot did not reply to my e-mail. Subsequently, though the patient clearly failed to qualify because of the eight-week rule, Dr. Chabot did not reject her immediately from the study as he should have. Instead he arranged to meet with the patient at Columbia two weeks later on September 6, 2001 for his intake evaluation, some 70 days from her biopsy. Then, to our surprise, Dr. Chabot approved her for entry, instructing us to begin the treatment process.

Our Objection to Entry of A Patient Admitted Despite a History of Psychiatric Illness

Patient #6: I first met with Patient #6 on September 5, 2002, before he had consulted with Dr. Chabot or been approved for the study. At that time he reported difficulty eating associated with a recent 12-pound weight loss over a six-week period, as well as a history of bipolar illness. In my chart note, I wrote that this patient's psychiatric history "may preclude him from entry into the clinical trial," and later in the "Assessment" section, the summation of the case, I questioned his suitability:

> History of metastatic pancreatic cancer. . . . I am not sure that he is completely eligible. The bipolar illness may preclude him. He is going to see Dr. Chabot next week.

In an e-mail to Dr. Chabot sent the same day of my initial consultation with Patient #6, I discussed the patient's long history of bipolar episodes. I advised Dr. Chabot, who had not yet evaluated Patient #6, that during my initial session he had downplayed these problems—which his wife more candidly discussed:

> I spoke to Michelle about [Patient #6], whom I saw for the first time today. . . . It turns out as we talked and I probed he has a long history of bipolar illness, with according to his wife obvious manic episodes, which he then downplayed. His wife says he tends to deny the seriousness of his illness. He is on Welbutrin [sic] now but not lithium. Again, in our experience, and as you know this program requires such focus, patients with psychiatric problems just don't do it. Certainly, he seemed nice enough, and was very grateful but the last thing we need is another non complier. I didn't discourage him because ultimately I know it's your decision, but I wanted you to be informed.

Nonetheless, Dr. Chabot approved the patient for treatment with us despite the poor appetite and psychiatric diagnosis.

As I reported in an October 28, 2002 note, although Patient #6 initially tried to follow the prescribed regimen, he declined rapidly. Here, I also again documented my reservations about the patient's admission into the study:

> [Patient #6] is having trouble with nausea, and he is not able to get his pills down. I think he is just too sick. I do not think he should have been entered into the trial.

Two days later, October 30, 2002, Patient #6's wife described her husband's dire situation, a conversation described in my note from that day:

> [Patient #6] is not doing well. He spent the day in bed. When I talked to him, he is overdosing himself on pain medication. He barely could talk. I spoke to his wife. He was slurring his words. He is on OxyContin. He was not sure of the dose. He is on some other pain medication; he was not sure of that. . . . He is not able to do this part of the program now, so we are headed for this downward spiral where the patient cannot do it.

Another two days later, on November 1, 2002, I documented a further phone discussion with the patient's wife:

> I spoke with Mrs. [Patient #6]. . . . a local internist wants to hospitalize [Patient #6]. He is not able to eat. It sounds like he is obstructing. She wanted reassurance, and I said he has to go into the hospital

Then five days later, on November 6, 2002, I e-mailed Dr. Chabot, once again expressing my concern that Patient #6 had been approved for the study:

> [Patient #6] is not doing well. He could never be stabilized in terms of his pain, nerve block didn't work, very quickly ended up with ascites. . . . He's not able to eat, hasn't been able to eat.
>
> This is part of our frustration which we expressed to you in our meeting, when patients just can't do the therapy properly. Some of these patients are just so sick, beyond what we would ever attempt to treat in our private practice. A patient like this would as you know would [sic] not have been entered on the Gemzar study because he could never be stabilized once he went back to —. Is it out of the realm of possibility to have at least a one week lead-in written into the protocol . . .?

So once again, I communicated to Dr. Chabot my belief he had qualified yet another patient too ill to follow through with the treatment.

Our Objection to Entry of Patients Who Could Not Eat Adequately at the Time of Entry As Required for the Protocol

Patient #8: Earlier, in Chapter 12, again in Chapter 19—my discussion of Dr. Chabot's April 22, 2006 letter to me—and in Chapter 26, I described this patient's history in some detail, though for different reasons and in different contexts. Here, I emphasize those records that show how strongly I questioned his admission into the trial.

In my intake note dated January 16, 2001, dictated before Dr. Chabot had consulted with Patient #8, I reported the patient's poor appetite:

> The patient reports that his surgeon, Dr. M— also told him that chemotherapy would not be particularly helpful and actually suggested he think of alternatives. One of the biggest problems is that the patient's appetite has been "terrible." A week ago one of his doctors (and he's not sure which one) started him on Megace 2-tsp day. With this his appetite has improved although it's still down. He reports a 20–25 lb. weight loss.

In the "Assessment" section at the end of that note I wrote:

> The patient was tentatively approved for the clinical trial but he doesn't meet the criteria at this point. . . . He has no appetite and he's on Megace for appetite. An inability to eat precludes his entrance into the trial. I discussed this with Dr. Chabot.

In the "Plan" section I again documented my doubts about the patient's eligibility:

> I am willing to start the patient on a program but I'm going to have to discuss with the various investigators whether he's appropriate for the clinical trial.

In an e-mail to Dr. Chabot dated January 16, 2002, the day of my first session with the patient, I restated my belief that he should not be entered:

> Since then he's lost 25 pounds, admitted he wasn't eating, couldn't eat and had no appetite until his Local MD put him on Megace a week ago. He is eating some now, but we have never had any success with a patient staying on the program who had to be put on Megace because of appetite. . . . I know from my experience he's already missed his window and I doubt he will stay on the program ten days.

After meeting with Patient #8 the following day, Dr. Chabot called me, reporting that he intended to order blood work before making a final determination about eligibility. As previously described, when the tests came back within the acceptable range, despite my objections Dr. Chabot approved Patient #8 for entry.

In a note dated April 15, 2002 dictated after a phone conversation with the patient's wife I expressed my concern that another patient had been admitted who could not comply with the treatment:

> [Patient #8] is not doing well. He had to be hospitalized over the weekend . . .

> The problem is he hasn't been able to eat since he started the program and he just wasn't really a suitable candidate for the protocol. That's the problem; he never was able to do it.

That same day I also e-mailed Dr. Chabot:

> Not unexpectedly, [Patient #8], though well meaning, has not been able to follow the diet virtually from day 1, and has been living on milk shakes. I am amazed he has lasted nearly four months since diagnosis with his stage IV disease and doing half the protocol. You may remember that he was on Megace when seen in your office because he couldn't eat, and hasn't been able to eat. . . .

> We are concerned that another two patients haven't been able to do it. . . . Maybe we should have a meeting to discuss all this?

Patient #8, who never could follow the therapy adequately, eventually passed away on April 19, 2002. For years after this patient first consulted with me, Dr. Chabot never disputed in any note, e-mail, or phone conversation my facts about the case, or my belief that this patient should not have been admitted. It wasn't until his April 22, 2006 letter to me, written after Congressman Burton and Senator Harkin had questioned the study's management with Dr. Zerhouni, that Dr. Chabot finally insisted this patient's entry was completely appropriate.

Patient #9: I first met with Patient #9 in my office on February 5, 2003, before his intake session with Dr. Chabot. In my chart discussion I expressed my belief that this patient, who appeared far too ill to comply with the treatment, should not be approved:

> Currently, he does not seem to be doing well. Frankly, I think he is too sick to enter into the clinical trial. He has developed chronic, dull lower back pain

that is resolved with Darvocet. His appetite is down. He lost about 20 pounds in the last six weeks. . . . His appetite is very poor and it sounds like he is starting to deteriorate.

In the "Assessment" section at the end of the note, I repeated my reservations about the patient's eligibility:

Widely metastatic pancreatic cancer. He [sic] last blood work is already a month old. I suspect it is much worse than it was. Liver function tests were elevated at the time. In the last week, there has been significant deterioration in his clinical status. I do not believe he is going to be strong enough to do the program. I think it is too late. I think he is probably not going to last very long. I will e-mail Dr. Chabot at Columbia and let him know about my feelings on this patient.

That afternoon I e-mailed Dr. Chabot:

I saw [Patient #9] today for his first session, you will be seeing him Friday. . . . However, he looked like a patient who is about to crash very soon. From my experience, I know he isn't going to make it. Over the past week, he and his wife both said there has been a significant deterioration, he is having trouble eating, he is getting pale, he gets short of breath going up stairs (his lungs sounded clear on exam so I suspect it's anemia). His window of opportunity has passed.

The following day, February 6, 2003, Patient #9 returned to my office to review the prescribed program. Though Dr. Chabot had not yet met with nor approved Patient #9, I proceeded with the session as I had been instructed to do. In the patient chart I restated my opinion that this patient did not qualify, though I offered to treat him off protocol and for free:

My feeling is that he is too sick and I suspect his liver functions tests will have worsened since they were done a month ago. He is going to discuss these issues with Dr. Chabot. He wants to do the program regardless of whether he is on the clinical trial or not and I agreed of course to do that.

Despite my strong objections, Dr. Chabot accepted the patient for treatment with us.

On February 18, 2003, just 12 days after our second visit, in a phone conversation with me Patient #9 admitted he could not eat, as I duly reported:

[Patient #9] complains he cannot eat. I thought he was far too sick to do the program. He is trying to get the pills down but it is difficult.

I e-mailed Dr. Chabot two days later, on February 20, 2003, reiterating my view that Patient #9 should have been excluded from the trial.

> I am concerned about [Patient #9]. He called after five days on the supplements to tell me he has no appetite and "can't eat." This was my concern when I first worked him up. I think patients like this are so desperate to get on the clinical trial they mislead you about their eating. We've had three patients recently who couldn't do it. . . .

In a note dated March 10, 2003, written after another phone conversation with Patient #9, I documented once again my belief that he should never have been admitted:

> I called [Patient #9] to see how he is doing. He is not doing well. I do not think he should have ever been entered into this clinical trial. He cannot eat. His local doctor put him on Megace because he cannot eat. His pain is poorly controlled with morphine and Darvocet.

In an e-mail to Dr. Chabot dated April 29, 2003, I once more questioned his approval of this patient:

> I had started to get suspicious about [Patient #9] from —. I hadn't heard from him for weeks. I called several times leaving messages, but no call back. Today his wife called saying he had died two weeks ago, not doing his program.
>
> As it turns out, for the record, within days of returning to — after his meetings with us his oncologist locally started him on Megace because he "couldn't eat." This was my concern about entering him into the study because he had lost some 20–25 pounds in the weeks before coming to New York and he and his wife said to us he couldn't eat well.

Dr. Chabot never responded, nor did he ever counter my charge that the patient did not meet the eligibility requirements. Regardless, in his data chart from April 2006 Dr. Chabot continued to count this subject as properly admitted and as fully treated, though Patient #9 never followed the prescribed regimen for any length of time.

Patient #12: Dr. Isaacs first met with Patient #12 on January 13, 2004, before his scheduled session with Dr. Chabot. As Dr. Isaacs' note from that day indicated, Patient #12, appearing quite emaciated, avoided responding to specific questions about his appetite, a warning sign to us he might be downplaying the situation hoping to gain entry into the study:

> Currently, he feels "not too bad." He did not clearly answer questions re food intake, but his wife and daughter reported he "eats something every meal." He is 15 lbs below his usual weight, but has stabilized since Amaryl was D/C'd [discontinued]. . . . On Phenergan for nausea

Dr. Isaacs recorded a height of 5′ 8 ½″, a weight of 130 lbs., and described his status as follows:

> Alert, cachectic male, NAD [No Acute Distress].

The same day of the initial visit with Patient #12, Dr. Isaacs e-mailed Dr. Chabot, documenting her reservations about the patient's suitability:

> I saw [Patient #12], the patient from —, today. Given his cachexia, it is difficult for me to believe that he will be able to do the program. From our experience, he's just too sick and coming too late.
>
> I would appreciate hearing about the results of his bloodwork and your final assessment of his eligibility.

I also e-mailed Dr. Chabot myself, arguing against this patient's acceptance into the trial, suggesting that perhaps he had overstated his appetite during the intake interview at Columbia. Regardless of what the patient claimed about his eating, the obvious cachexia should have been evidence enough for exclusion:

> I know Linda had e mailed you regarding the patient she saw today, and I think she underplayed it. He's not eating, and we think he wasn't straightforward with you in order to get into the protocol. . . . We've seen this several times, where we think that the patient is being less than candid in order to gain acceptance into the nutritional arm.

Dr. Chabot responded on January 19, 2004, six days later, with one word, "Noted," at least acknowledging receipt of my e-mail. Despite our objections, Dr. Chabot approved the patient and instructed us to begin the treatment process.

In a note from January 18, 2004, Dr. Isaacs reported that five days after his consultation in our office and only one day after beginning his supplement program, Patient #12 already reported difficulty complying with the treatment. A day later, he was hospitalized because of severe dehydration, thereafter never pursuing the prescribed regimen. Nonetheless, on his data chart from April 2006 Dr. Chabot included Patient #12 as properly admitted and fully treated, though he never attempted to follow the therapy beyond one or two days.

Patient #22: Dr. Isaacs first met with Patient #22 on April 2, 2003, before his intake appointment with Dr. Chabot. During his initial conversation with Dr. Isaacs, he described ongoing diarrhea and told two different stories about his food intake, one of a "good" appetite, while at the same time reporting a recent 30-pound weight loss. In the "Assessment" section, Dr. Isaacs included, as one of the patient's problems, "Early satiety, diarrhea, pain, wt loss. . . ."

The "Plan" section immediately following summarized Patient #22's problems that argued against admission:

> Pt has questions re likelihood of success on program + advisability of pursuing other RX [treatment] in addition to this which I answered—reason for doing trial is to be able to answer this sort of question. I told him frankly that I had some doubts whether he would be able to do this secondary to early satiety and poor po [oral] intake for which LMD [local doctor] prescribed appetite stimulant. He will return tomorrow for protocol. I will verify approval for trial w/ Columbia. He also wanted to know which aspects of program are most important—I responded that they all are.

After the consultation with the patient, Dr. Isaacs e-mailed Dr. Chabot, expressing her hesitation about his eligibility:

> Did [Patient #22] meet with your approval? He is on an "appetite stimulant" presumably Megace—he left his list at home. He will let me know what it is tomorrow. He has lost 40 pounds in 3 months, so from what we put together eating is a major problem. He also had questions that typically go along with poor compliance—"what are the most important things to do" and "how do I know if I'm responding" being some of them. He also asked about chemotherapy.

The following day, April 3, 2003, Dr. Isaacs met again with Patient #22 for the scheduled second session as if he had been approved. After interviewing the patient at Columbia later that afternoon, Dr. Chabot finally responded to Dr. Isaacs's e-mail of the previous day:

I thought he was very intelligent, highly motivated and despite my challenge very committed. We are awaiting path confirmation. jc

As we expected, Dr. Chabot subsequently approved Patient #22 for the trial, despite the poor appetite and 40-pound weight loss. Thereafter, the patient rapidly declined before passing away on June 28, 2003.

In this case, we have solid evidence of a subject Dr. Chabot qualified for the nutrition arm who couldn't eat, who admitted to significant weight loss, and who in fact required an "appetite stimulant." We have documentation that Dr. Isaacs, in an e-mail sent the day she first met with the patient, notified Dr. Chabot of her concerns including his lack of commitment to the proposed treatment regimen. Dr. Chabot chose not to address the eating problems in his response to Dr. Isaacs, only lauding the patient for his intelligence before entering him into the trial.

Our Objection to A Patient Admitted Despite Multiple Reasons for Exclusion

Patient #16: I have previously discussed this patient at length both in Chapter 12 and in Chapter 26. Here, I include his case history again, as I did in my McNeilly manuscript, as an example of yet another patient whose admission by Dr. Chabot we questioned.

I believe this patient actually failed to satisfy at least six separate entry criteria as previously documented. These include: first, his poor appetite; second, his lack of motivation to follow the program, evident during the initial session with me; third, his lack of social support; fourth, his psychological disability that became apparent during his first visits; fifth, the fact that Dr. Chabot did not approve him until well beyond the eight-week window from diagnosis; and finally, Dr. Chabot's failure to obtain the required written consent before sending this patient to us for treatment.

Patient #16 underwent exploratory surgery and biopsy proving pancreatic cancer on December 20, 2002, although I did not see him in my office for his initial consultation visit until February 6, 2003, nearly seven weeks after his diagnosis. Dr. Chabot had arranged his intake interview several days later because of scheduling problems in his office, so I actually completed my two sessions with Patient #16 before Dr. Chabot had even determined the patient's eligibility.

In my note after our first meeting, I documented that under the care of a local naturopathic physician where he lived at the time, Patient #16 had begun a whole foods type diet, though he reported a very poor appetite:

> He went back to — and with friends who are interested in alternative medicine and with a local naturopath began an aggressive nutritional program that involved diet emphasizing fruits, vegetable [sic], nuts, seeds, and whole grains, and low in animal protein. He also began juices, some herbs, and some other nutritional supplements. He said on this program he felt better and he felt his stamina and energy improved and his appetite improved somewhat, although he is still losing weight. He said his appetite is not great.

In the "Assessment" of the note, I summarized the situation:

> History of metastatic pancreatic cancer. Again, I am not sure he is going to be eligible for the trial because he seems to be having a great deal of trouble eating. His last blood work is from late December, December 21. That probably should be repeated. Dr. Chabot will make that determination.

In addition, during that two-hour session with Patient #16, I became concerned that he seemed motivated by the financial benefits of the trial, rather than any interest in following the nutritional regimen. In a chart note I commented on his lack of commitment, a legitimate reason for exclusion from the study:

> I am concerned over the fact that he seemed uncommitted to the program. He was not really sure whether he could do the program. We talked about it. Again, these issues will be discussed with Dr. Chabot.

That day, February 7, 2003, I e-mailed Dr. Chabot, relaying my reservations:

> I saw [Patient #16]. Seems somewhat unfocused; he didn't have any of the information about when or where he was to meet with you on Monday.

The following Monday, Dr. Chabot met with the patient as planned. After the session, Michelle Gabay, Dr. Chabot's assistant, called to inform me that Patient #16 had neither been admitted nor rejected. Instead, Dr. Chabot had decided to withhold his decision about his eligibility until the Columbia Pathology Department reviewed the December 20, 2002 biopsy slides. Regardless, I was to proceed as if the patient had been entered.

After Patient #16 returned home, I spoke with him by phone on February 13, 2003, as documented in the chart. When I learned he had not been informed about his status, I decided to e-mail Dr. Chabot:

> Was [Patient #16] accepted into the trial? We weren't sure yet (remember, we had reservations about the ability to focus and follow through)

Dr. Chabot responded with a curt "path is pending." I wasn't happy with the brief answer, so I called Dr. Chabot hoping he might be more specific, but he only told me he had no idea when the final Columbia report would be available.

My chart note from that day summarized the various conversations:

> [Patient #16] still has not heard about the clinical trial and whether he is accepted or not. I spoke to Dr. Chabot who said the pathology needs to be reviewed and is not in yet so there is no decision.

During another phone discussion on February 21, 2003, Patient #16 told me that he still had heard nothing from Dr. Chabot. At that point, 63 days, exactly 9 weeks had elapsed since the biopsy confirmation of disease, so Patient #16 no longer qualified because of the eight-week rule. Nonetheless, I still heard no word from Dr. Chabot about the situation.

In another phone conversation 12 days later on March 5, 2003, Patient #16 reported that Dr. Chabot's office had yet to contact him. To my surprise, he also admitted that he had not begun his treatment until the previous day, nearly a month since I had met with him

I recorded the latest developments in the patient's chart:

> Unfortunately [Patient #16] did not start his program until yesterday. It is a month since I saw him. He does not have a good explanation. He is waiting to hear from Columbia about being on the clinical trial. I told him to start regardless because a valuable month has been lost.

After my conversation with Patient #16, I also e-mailed Dr. Chabot:

> I spoke with [Patient #16] tonight. I had given him his protocol February 7, nearly a month ago. To my astonishment, he had not started any part of the protocol until yesterday, when he began the liver flush—despite the fact that I strongly and sternly advised him to start the program the day he got back to — regardless of whether he was on the clinical trial or not. . . .

He said he delayed because he hadn't heard from Columbia, but I had told him when I met him not to wait because of the aggressive nature of the disease. He agreed I had told him this. . . .

What do we do with a patient like this? I left a message for you to call, maybe we should discuss it over the phone at your convenience. It's another patient who isn't doing what he is supposed to do, in any way.

Then on March 10, 2003, Ms. Gabay called me, telling me she herself had spoken with Patient #16, who for some reason insisted he had been fully compliant with the prescribed regimen since the day he arrived home.

In response, I e-mailed Dr. Chabot yet again:

I spoke with Michelle about [Patient #16]. . . . He had done virtually nothing of the program after four weeks, except perhaps some of the foods. . . .

I think he needs to be disqualified because not only was he not willing to do it, but apparently he misled Michelle. . . .

As you know so well, it's just frustrating for us to face patients who don't do the therapy and yet will be counted as treatment failures.

Subsequently, on April 11, 2003 the patient's former wife spoke with my assistant, confirming that Patient #16, never having followed the treatment plan, had now deteriorated into a terminal state. I summarized the conversation in a chart note:

His ex-wife called and left a message with the staff. She stated that he is "at home and very terminal." She said that the patient wanted to be sure I knew that he believes that if he had started earlier he would have gotten more benefit.

In retrospect, he lost valuable time when he decided for reasons which still remain unclear, not to start his therapy in a timely appropriate way.

To bring this story to an extraordinary conclusion, in 2005, more than two years after Patient #16 died, we learned that he had been sent to us as fully consented though he had never signed the required form.

As the above notes demonstrated, I repeatedly questioned Dr. Chabot about this patient's eligibility for the trial, without much of a response. After the project came to a close, Dr. Chabot apparently claimed that he never officially approved this patient, even though we were instructed to begin the treatment process as if he had been formally admitted. It was our understanding from a telephone conversation with Ms. Gabay that Dr. Chabot had qualified Patient #16 on March 5, 2003. During the 2 ½ years we tried to learn what happened to this patient's consent form, neither Dr. Chabot nor any of his staff ever told us he had been excluded from the trial. Furthermore, if Patient #16 had not been entered, why did Dr. Chabot's assistant, Cara DeRosa, e-mail us on April 21, 2003 asking if we had a copy of his signed consent?

Summary of Cases in Which Dr. Isaacs and/or Dr. Gonzalez Argued Against Entry of Patients Approved by Dr. Chabot

As I have now documented, after we were excluded from the entry process in July 2000, Dr. Isaacs and I objected to the entry of seven patients approved by Dr. Chabot and sent to us for treatment.

These include:

Patient #34, admitted into the study ten weeks after biopsy despite our objection.

Patient #6, #8, #9, #12, #22, admitted over our objections despite evidence of poor appetite, significant weight loss, and in one case, that of Patient #12, cachexia.

Patient #16, admitted over our objections despite evidence of poor appetite, a lack of motivation to follow the program, absent social support, apparent psychological disability, approval for entry well beyond the eight-week window from diagnosis, and lack of signed informed consent.

The records of these seven cases also confirmed that by July 2000, Dr. Isaacs and I had been completely removed from the intake process. After that point, even when we presented evidence that an approved trial candidate failed to meet one or more entry criteria, our concerns were disregarded.

So if Dr. Chabot admitted patients whom we believed did not legitimately qualify, why then did we agree to treat them as part of the study? As I have already stated, when the NCI revoked our veto privilege in July 2000, we were sternly instructed that once Dr. Chabot reached a decision about a particular patient's eligibility, the decision stood regardless of our opinion. We had no right to object, nor was any oversight or appeal process in place. We had only two choices; either accept Dr. Chabot's judgments, or quit the study—and we weren't about to walk away after years spent fighting for a test of our treatment. As a more productive option we decided to stay involved, continue pointing out managerial mishaps as they occurred, and hopefully guide the clinical trial under Dr. Chabot's supervision toward a fair and equitable end.

In summary, we believe the documentation we gathered for Dr. McNeilly unquestionably showed that Dr. Chabot admitted multiple patients into the nutrition arm of the study who did not satisfy the entry criteria; that for the greater part of the trial he alone supervised the intake process; and that on multiple occasions we did object to his approval of inappropriate patients.

Chapter 32

Inefficient Screening of Study Candidates at Columbia

O ver a period of three months, as I organized my response for Dr. McNeilly I reviewed many thousands of pages of documents created during the nine years of the clinical trial's history, dating back to my first meetings with Dr. Antman and Dr. Wynder in the fall of 1997. As part of this effort, I studied the records of all patients Dr. Chabot had qualified for the nutrition arm including those who, though approved, ultimately decided against proceeding any further. As I read through these many charts, I carefully tracked those instances in which Dr. Chabot's processing of study candidates appeared to have been problematic. Though Dr. McNeilly had not specifically asked me about such cases, I found so many that I decided to address this issue in some detail in the monograph prepared for him.

From the time he first came on board in 1998 until the study's close in 2006, Dr. Chabot supervised all aspects of the *initial* evaluation of prospective study candidates, even during the period prior to July 2000 when we exercised veto power over entry. By the third protocol draft completed in late 1998 and before we had accrued any patients, Dr. Chabot's carefully defined responsibilities included gathering and reviewing of pertinent medical records for those patients seeking admission, then conducting preliminary intake interviews by phone to help assess eligibility further. At that point we could evaluate those patients Chabot had provisionally accepted, with the authority to reject those that we felt did not meet the entry criteria. For those we agreed did qualify, Dr. Chabot would then arrange for his face-to-face interview in New York for his final evaluation. If the patient passed this last test and agreed to proceed, Dr. Chabot would then complete informed consent, obtaining, as a necessary step, the signed copy of the required documents. As I previously discussed, after the NCI rescinded our veto in July 2000, Dr. Chabot exercised complete control over every aspect of patient entry and approval with no appeal allowed. If he accepted a patient, the patient was accepted.

Though the study formally opened to accrual in early 1999, as we have seen the randomized format very efficiently discouraged patient interest. It was not until some eight months later, on August 9, 1999, that Dr. Chabot's assistant Michelle Gabay sent over the records of the first trial candidate, whom I will call Candidate #1, for our review. Dr. Chabot believed, based on his assessment of the case and his staff's phone interview with the patient, that he seemed suitable. Furthermore, despite the randomized design, this patient had agreed to join the study, so after months of waiting, we thought we might finally have our first appropriate subject. However, when Dr. Isaacs and I studied the file we immediately realized that several of his blood results were outside the required range, so we didn't understand why Dr. Chabot had tentatively approved him.

That same afternoon I received this patient's file, I faxed a long note to Dr. Chabot expressing my doubts about his eligibility, with pertinent points extracted below:

> Our concern was that his albumin and bilirubin are outside the criteria for acceptance of the study. Although in a week his bilirubin dropped from 3.8 to 3.3, the inclusion criteria require a bilirubin no higher than 1.5 outside the Upper Normal Limit. His albumin has stayed at 2.5, and the criteria require an albumin greater than 3.2. . . .
>
> I wasn't sure what we do, since two major blood parameters are outside the criteria. . . .
>
> Linda did interview Mr. [Candidate #1], and in terms of attitude, etc., he's fine. Let me know what you think.

I want to point out that for someone diagnosed with pancreatic cancer, these two factors, bilirubin and albumin, are not esoteric inconsequential tests, but critical reflections of overall status. As it turned out, in this case Dr. Chabot agreed with our opinion, ultimately rejecting the patient from further consideration.

The next patient we evaluated, Candidate #2, took a circuitous journey before being finally randomized to the nutrition arm. Only days after her diagnosis of inoperable pancreatic cancer on August 12, 1999, she learned of our approach from a patient with the disease whom we had successfully treated some ten years earlier. With no knowledge of the clinical trial, she sent copies of her records directly to our office along with a long note dated August 24, 1999, expressing her wish to begin our treatment.

From our reading of her file, Candidate #2 seemed eligible for the clinical trial, so on August 27, 1999, Dr. Isaacs called her, discussed the study briefly, and referred her to Dr. Chabot. Since her finances were tight, she was grateful to learn of the study and for the chance to receive our treatment for free. So, that same day of her conversation with Dr. Isaacs, she called Dr. Chabot's office to begin the formal entry process. In addition, Dr. Isaacs faxed a note to Dr. Chabot, summarizing Candidate #2's medical history.

We didn't hear any more about Candidate #2 until September 13, 1999, 17 days later, when Michelle Gabay called our office, informing us that some repeat blood tests had come back within the acceptable range. From Dr. Chabot's perspective, Candidate #2 now seemed appropriate for admission, as she seemed to us as well. We faxed a note to Ms. Gabay, advising her that we approved this patient's entry and didn't need to interview her again since Dr. Isaacs had already spoken with her at length.

Two days later, on September 15, 1999, Candidate #2—who would become Patient #15 by our clinical trial identifiers—called our office, concerned that 19 days since her first contact with Columbia, she still had not been informed about her status. We could not understand why Chabot's office hadn't contacted her since we all agreed she was eligible. Regardless, from the patient's perspective, with her diagnosis of rapidly progressive and terminal disease she knew she couldn't wait any longer even if it meant seeing either Dr. Isaacs or myself as a private patient.

My assistant summarized the conversation in writing:

> She decided to forgo the clinical trial. They still are not giving her an answer and she can't wait any longer. She asked them to fax over recent blood reports today. Wants to come in ASAP.

I called Dr. Chabot's office repeatedly inquiring about her status, but heard nothing back until September 17, 1999, when Ms. Gabay informed us that Candidate #2 had been conditionally approved and randomized for Enzyme-Nutritional Therapy. I say the candidate had been "conditionally approved," because she still needed to meet with Dr. Chabot in person before she could be fully qualified.

Once aware of Dr. Chabot's decision, Candidate #2 arranged her trip to New York and finally met with Dr. Isaacs on September 22, 1999, nearly four weeks after she had first contacted our office. Today, Dr. Isaacs and I still do not understand Dr. Chabot's delay in accepting her for treatment, since we had faxed her records to his office, with an accompanying explanatory note, the day we received them, on August 27, 1999. In our minds he could have made his preliminary decision within a few days.

Unfortunately, by the time of Candidate #2's visit with Dr. Isaacs she had deteriorated significantly since her initial contact with us. As she patiently waited for to hear from Dr. Chabot, her appetite had plummeted precipitously, she had lost 20 pounds, and we believed she no longer qualified for the trial.

During her initial sessions in our office, Dr. Isaacs also discovered Candidate #2 had somewhat misrepresented her social situation, which proved far less rosy than she had first suggested. Despite the legitimate reasons for excluding her from the trial and though we still possessed veto power, Dr. Isaacs and I chose not to argue against Candidate #2's admission. We thought, frankly, such action on our part would be cruel in view of what she had endured to that point, particularly with her stressed finances. After all, she had contacted our office soon after her diagnosis hoping to begin our treatment quickly as a private patient, not because of any interest in the clinical trial of which she at the time knew nothing. As Dr. Antman and Dr. Chabot had instructed us to do in such cases, Dr. Isaacs discussed the study with her, urging that she consider entry into the study, and referred her to Columbia. Her decision to follow our well-intentioned suggestions ultimately cost her four weeks of valuable treatment time while Dr. Chabot processed her case. By the time she finally met with Dr. Isaacs, she was frightened, angry, and frustrated by the four weeks lost as she waited to learn of her status.

So, despite her weakened condition, without any hesitation we began treating her as a trial patient, even though we believed her window of opportunity for possible response to our therapy had passed. Unfortunately, Candidate #2, unable to follow the regimen for any length of time, ultimately died in November 1999, only two months after her meetings with Dr. Isaacs in New York.

Dr. Isaacs and I hoped that in the future, Dr. Chabot would manage the intake of trial candidates more expeditiously. We reasoned that since Candidate #2 was one of the first applicants seeking entry into the study, perhaps his office just needed some time to refine their intake procedures. Unfortunately, Dr. Chabot's handling of Candidate #2 would prove typical, rather than exceptional.

At one of the group meetings in early fall of 1999, Dr. Antman and Dr. Chabot reported on the progress of the project. At this time we learned that in the one year since the trial officially opened to accrual, some 260 patients diagnosed with pancreatic cancer had contacted the Columbia offices inquiring about the study, but all but two—those discussed above—declined to proceed once informed they could be randomized to chemotherapy. As we had predicted, all these patients with an interest in the project wanted only our therapy.

With this data before us, we argued once again for a change to a case-control or matched cohort design, allowing patients to choose their treatment. Based on the continuing level of interest in the trial we suspected this approach would more easily attract the patients needed to fill the nutrition arm. I thought we most likely could create the control-chemotherapy group from those seeking conventional approaches at Columbia with no interest in our alternative nutritional regimen. Dr. Chabot had already informed us the Columbia oncology team treated some 75 patients with newly diagnosed pancreatic cancer annually, a large group from which to choose. On the other hand, if we did not modify the design, it was clear to us the study would never enroll sufficient numbers to succeed.

For the first time, Dr. Antman, Dr. Chabot, and the NCCAM and NCI supervisors agreed with us. Shortly after the meeting, Dr. Antman and her team rewrote the protocol, redefining the study as a matched cohort, before petitioning the IRB at Columbia to allow the change. Concurrently, the NCI personnel submitted the revised plan to their respective oversight committees. As the new protocol made its way through the various regulatory channels, the trial remained open in its randomized form, pending official permission to switch over.

On November 8, 1999, we learned of the next patient seeking entry into the study, Candidate #3, whose medical records Dr. Chabot's assistant Michelle Gabay faxed over to us with a note stating that the "Pt is ready for her phone interview." From our review of the file, Candidate #3, diagnosed a month earlier during the first week in October, appeared to be quite ill. Oddly, the packet from Ms. Gabay included a fully signed consent form, witnessed by relatives and dated November 8, 1999, the same day we received her records even though she had not yet been seen by Dr. Chabot. We wondered why his office would have sent her the form and why she would have signed it, since Dr. Chabot supposedly reviewed informed consent only during his in-person New York interview. When our calls to Chabot for clarification went unanswered, one of my staff contacted the patient, who lived some distance from New York, to find out what might be going on. To our surprise we learned that she had been hospitalized for some time.

On November 9, 1999, Dr. Isaacs faxed a note to Ms. Gabay:

> We tried to set up phone interview with her today but got a call from her MD that she was in the hospital because of trouble breathing from her pulmonary mets. One of the staff here called her and she sounded nervous and unclear about why she was in the hospital. . . . We left it that she should contact us when she is out of the hospital.

Ms. Gabay then phoned our office and spoke with Dr. Isaacs, as our notes from that day confirmed:

> Michelle called back—she had never advised her to call here.

Ms. Gabay's response left us completely baffled, so we decided to await instructions from Columbia before taking any further action, but we heard nothing more. Ten days later, on November 19, 1999, now five weeks since the first contact with Columbia, the patient's elderly mother called our office, expressing her frustration with Chabot's lack of response.

My staff member who took the call documented the conversation:

> [Candidate #3] has pancreatic cancer and is interested in the clinical trial. [Candidate #3's mother] called Michelle Gabay when [Candidate #3] was first diagnosed—that was 5 weeks ago. [Candidate #3's mother] has tried unsuccessfully to get an answer about [Candidate #3]'s acceptance in the trial. I

think she was told to call us, or perhaps she decided on her own to call us to
try to find out what is going on.

I told her I would relay the information to the doctors and she should call us
back on Monday and also try to reach Michelle on Monday. I also apologized
for the delay in getting an answer.

She wasn't hostile or desperate, she realized that time is running out. (Personally I think a 5 week delay is inexcusable)

As the note indicated, the handling of the situation at Columbia upset even my
assistant. In any event, the patient had so deteriorated she could not possibly
travel to New York to continue the evaluation process or begin treatment, so
any question about her eligibility became moot. Dr. Chabot never explained
the long delay between the first contact with his office and his lack of response,
nor did I ever learn why this patient had signed the consent form before she
had been formally approved.

Dr. Chabot's slow pace of handling these three candidates did not inspire our
confidence in the intake procedures at Columbia. He should have immediately
rejected the first patient, whose abnormal blood results were well outside the
required range. The second applicant waited nearly four weeks for an answer
about her status during which time her condition rapidly deteriorated, before
Chabot finally approved her. The third candidate, far too sick for admission,
apparently had not heard from Columbia after five weeks.

We responded to Dr. Chabot within hours of receiving and reviewing the records
of each of these patients, so I didn't understand the slow pace of his assessment.
We began to be concerned that the handling of patient intake at Columbia,
if continued unchanged, might easily undermine the entire study. Four and
five week delays between first contact and a final decision about eligibility, for
those diagnosed with a deadly disease like advanced pancreatic cancer, could
mean the difference between treatment success and treatment failure.

In late November 1999, I received a copy of the revised protocol, now defining
the study as a matched cohort. However, the document still required approval
by the Columbia IRB as well as the NCI before we could actually implement
the new format, a process that can take months. We were told that in the
interim, the trial would remain open but with its earlier randomized design.
By that point, after a year a grand total of three patients had been formally

approved, two of whom promptly quit after being assigned to chemotherapy. We hoped once the new structure was in place, more suitable patients would actually agree to participate, and that with more experience, Dr. Chabot might evaluate study candidates more efficiently.

According to our records, no other patients sought entry during the waning months of 1999. As I recall in early 2000 the study closed to accrual while the revised protocol made its way through the various bureaucratic channels. Finally, in late spring 2000 both the Columbia IRB and the NCI granted us permission to reopen with the matched cohort format so that patients, at last, could choose which of the two treatment options they wished to pursue. Though Dr. Chabot remained in charge of the initial phases of patient assessment, Dr. Isaacs and I could still veto entry of those preliminarily approved by Dr. Chabot if we demonstrated that they failed to meet the explicit written eligibility criteria.

During the second week of June 2000, Michelle Gabay sent for our review the incomplete records of Candidate #4, the first patient seeking admission into the trial in its new incarnation. Though he seemed appropriate by his history, the packet sent us from Columbia lacked a copy of the biopsy report, the ultimate proof of diagnosis and perhaps the single most important piece of information we needed to determine his suitability. We couldn't understand why the records had been forwarded to our office for our consideration with this vital document missing.

We spoke with Dr. Chabot's staff repeatedly, trying to learn why this patient had passed the initial evaluation. Apparently, Dr. Chabot had given his approval without the biopsy report, which the patient's doctors had inadvertently failed to send. Subsequently, Dr. Isaacs obtained a copy of the document from the patient's local physician, faxed it to Dr. Chabot, interviewed the patient herself, and found him, after all this confusion, acceptable. Candidate #4 promptly set up his New York visits with Dr. Chabot for his required interview and with Dr. Isaacs to begin treatment. However, during the third week of June he cancelled his appointments and we never heard from him again.

On June 16, 2000 Ms. Gabay sent the next set of records, those of Candidate #5, whom Dr. Chabot had tentatively accepted into the study. The files of this patient, diagnosed not only with pancreatic cancer but also with uncontrolled diabetes, described a poor appetite that alone should have disqualified him, associated with a recent 20-pound weight loss. Nonetheless, since Dr. Chabot had already given him a preliminary green light, three days later, on June 19, 2000, Dr. Isaacs conducted her phone interview with Candidate #5 who as it turned out, smoked—a habit that required exclusion. As the written protocol clearly stated, active smokers were ineligible and former smokers needed to be cigarette-free for at least a year to qualify. Based on the entry criteria, Dr. Chabot should have rejected this trial candidate outright and not even have sent his records to us. Once again we wondered if anyone at Columbia had actually read the records or adequately interviewed the patient, as they were supposed to do.

After her conversation with Candidate #5, Dr. Isaacs faxed a brief note to Michelle Gabay expressing our position:

> I interviewed him today. Very nice man. Unfortunately, he is not suitable—he is not eating well at all, his diabetes is out of control, and he is smoking. Who delivers the news? Please advise.

We did not hear from Ms. Gabay, nor apparently did the patient, whose daughter called us on June 20, 2000 wondering about her father's status. My staff informed her that he was not eligible for the trial.

On June 26, 2000, Dr. Chabot's office faxed over the next batch of records, those of Candidate #6, conditionally approved at Columbia and awaiting our decision about his status. The handwritten note from Dr. Chabot's assistant accompanying the documents read simply:

> re: [Candidate #6]
> ?ok for protocol?

After reviewing the file the day it arrived in our office, we found the patient most assuredly *not* "ok for protocol." The written entry criteria required a serum level of albumin, a marker of liver function and general nutrition, of at least 3.2. In this case, the most recently available reading of 2.6 from May 17, 2000, nearly six weeks earlier, fell far below the acceptable minimum.

That day, June 26, 2000, Dr. Isaacs faxed Ms. Gabay:

> Mr. [Candidate #6]'s albumin was 2.6 on 5/17/2000, which is out of range. The other bloodwork that was sent dates from 4/99 and from 10/98, so that the normal albumins on those dates don't make me feel better about the ab- normal value from 5/2000. I cannot get an overall feel of his story from the

material that was sent, so I don't know if this abnormal albumin from May represents short term or long-term problems with eating. However, given that they were motivated to check various tumor markers last December, it would make me wonder if he has been sick for quite a while. If the low albumin was during some acute situation that may have improved, it would be worthwhile to recheck it.

In response, Dr. Chabot informed the patient we required more recent blood tests before determining his eligibility. When a new albumin level came back within the normal range, Dr. Isaacs then interviewed the patient by phone. During this conversation, the patient reported an extremely poor food intake and an extraordinary 72-pound weight loss during the previous two months—approximately nine pounds a week. In the hopes of jumpstarting his eating, he had recently started hydrazine sulfate, an appetite stimulant not approved in the U.S. but available via the alternative underground. To make matters worse, for his unrelenting pain his local doctors had prescribed large doses of Duragesic and Roxanol, both strong narcotics that suppress appetite.

We could not comprehend Dr. Chabot granting provisional approval to someone with a catastrophic 72-pound weight loss in an eight-week period and who required an appetite stimulant. In our opinion, Candidate #6 appeared to be in the final stages of terminal disease, someone we would never even attempt to treat in our private practice.

On June 28, 2000, Dr. Isaacs faxed a curt note to Dr. Chabot's office relaying our opinion about the situation:

Interview done. Not acceptable.

He will be calling you tomorrow.

At this point, with our veto authority still intact, Dr. Chabot did reject this completely inappropriate patient. But Dr. Isaacs and I were again troubled that Chabot had provisionally accepted yet another trial candidate who was so obviously ineligible.

On June 26, 2000, Ms, Gabay faxed over information regarding another patient, Candidate #7, diagnosed with stage IV pancreatic cancer with extensive metastatic disease in both the lungs and liver. Though she was obviously very ill, on initial review Dr. Isaacs and I thought this patient might actually be acceptable. However, although Dr. Chabot had given his preliminary approval, we noticed that the records sent us lacked liver function tests, which the protocol required fall within a certain range. After several discussions back and forth with Dr. Chabot, we finally received the blood work, which did meet the entry criteria.

On March 12, 2001, Candidate #8, the man who would become Patient #38, called our office, explaining to my staff that he had been diagnosed with pancreatic adenocarcinoma two weeks earlier. After investigating various treatment options, both conventional and alternative, he had decided our regimen sounded most promising. During this first conversation, he seemed unaware of the clinical trial, so as the NCI required, my assistant explained the situation and referred him to Dr. Chabot. We heard nothing again about the case until Candidate #8 sent us an urgent fax on April 5, 2001, 24 days after his original call to us, and more than 6 weeks since his biopsy diagnosis. As his note explained, he had contacted Dr. Chabot's office as per our instructions but weeks later still had heard nothing back concerning his status. With his life in the balance, he had grown frantic as the days passed with no response from Columbia:

Dear Dr. Gonzalez:

I am urgently in need of your assistance.

I am a —year-old male living in — diagnosed with pancreatic adenoductal carcinoma on Feb. 27. I researched the treatment options available and decided that the proteolytic enzyme treatment you offer is the best option for me. I contacted your office and was told I had to apply for the clinical trial at Columbia Presbyterian Medical Center.

I contacted Dr. John Chabot's office on March 12 regarding the trial, providing initial information on my case. Since then, I've encountered one delay after another in getting approval for the clinical trial—even though I believe I meet all the eligibility requirements.

Attached is a summary of my contacts with Dr. Chabot's office for the clinical trial.

I want to stress that the program co-coordinator, Michelle Gabay, and her assistant Suzanne, have always been extremely positive and courteous.

I was originally told by Michelle that scheduling an appointment would "only take few days" [sic] once I was approved. However, the "paper work" obstacles have dragged on for almost three weeks now—putting me in the agonizing position of having to [put] my treatment program on hold.

I need to know where I stand regarding the clinical trial. <u>I would prefer to see you directly, and as quickly as possible.</u> I am prepared to come to New York, at any time.

Dr. Gonzalez—can you please help me with this?

Along with his note to us, Candidate #8 included a copy of a fax he had sent to Dr. Chabot ten days earlier, on March 26, 2001, pleading for some response. At the time Candidate #8 assumed, since he had not heard from Columbia, that Dr. Chabot had rejected him because of his specific tissue diagnosis which in fact did not disqualify him for the study.

Dear Dr. Chabot:

I am most anxious to participate in the clinical trials using the pancreatic proteolytic enzyme therapy. I have researched Dr. Gonzalez' treatments and results and am convinced this is the right treatment program for me right now. In fact I have been utilizing elements of his program while waiting for the past two weeks to see if I qualify.

I believe I qualify in all essential respects for the trial. <u>Please do not exclude me from the program because my diagnosis is adenoductal carcinoma.</u>

<u>Since I must go through the clinical trial screening program in order to see Dr. Gonzalez, you are my only hope for getting this treatment—which I desperately need.</u>

When Dr. Chabot failed to respond after ten days, Candidate #8 then faxed us his April 5, 2001 letter.

We did call Dr. Chabot's office on Candidate #8's behalf, hoping to expedite a decision about his status. Though we left repeated messages, Dr. Chabot never contacted us about the case directly, though eventually he approved Patient #38 for admission into the nutrition arm. Finally, on April 16, 2001, exactly five weeks after his initial contact with Columbia, Dr. Isaacs met with Candidate #8 to begin the treatment process.

Though Candidate #8 tried valiantly to comply with his nutritional regimen, he eventually died in May 2002, some 13 months after his first consultation with Dr. Isaacs. We believe Dr. Chabot's five-week delay before determining this patient's eligibility compromised his chances for a better response to our treatment.

I would also like to point out that in his fax to Columbia of March 26, 2001, Candidate #8 identified Dr. Chabot as solely responsible for patient screening and for all decisions about patient entry. He repeated what my staff had told him, that Dr. Isaacs and I could not consult with any patient diagnosed with pancreatic cancer, whether on trial or off, until Dr. Chabot completed his evaluation. I thought it strange to hear from Dr. McNeilly some six years later that Chabot would insist Dr. Isaacs and I participated in the intake process for the duration of the trial.

Even today, when I reread Candidate #8's faxes, I find myself troubled by the handling of this case at Columbia. Ironically, all the administrators from the various institutions seemed convinced that Dr. Isaacs and I, if not watched carefully, might somehow inappropriately undermine the trial and negatively influence its outcome. Yet not once did any of them appear even slightly concerned by Dr. Chabot's slow pace of evaluating trial candidates, an issue we had raised with them and a problem which created an obvious handicap against us. Over the course of the trial, patient after patient lost weeks of valuable time, perhaps setting the stage for treatment failure, before Chabot approved them for entry.

Chapter 33

The Changing Protocol and Consent Form

As part of my effort to prove to Dr. McNeilly that Dr. Chabot, for the greater part of the trial, alone supervised patient admission, I reviewed various versions of the official protocol and consent form for the study—I counted eight of each in our own records—beginning with the first, written way back in September 1997. Certainly these documents helped make my case, providing considerable information about the entry process and the specific investigator in charge. In addition, as I reread each of these drafts spanning a period of some three years, I became aware of a peculiar trend I had not previously observed—and came to believe the revisions over time reflected a changing, more negative attitude toward me and my treatment on the part of the Columbia team.

In the discussion that follows, I first review the history of the forms as they were first created, then track in detail the modifications illustrating my point. I have chosen to concentrate on six of the eight editions, omitting from consideration two early versions that incorporated only slight alterations.

In mid-1997, Dr. Karen Antman, at the time Director of the Columbia-Presbyterian Cancer Center (later changed to the Herbert Irving Comprehensive Cancer Center), first offered to help organize and supervise a large-scale controlled clinical trial evaluating my therapy. Despite the controversy already swirling around my approach, she took the initiative at Dr. Wynder's suggestion based on the preliminary results of the pilot study. Though the National Cancer Institute had not yet committed resources to the effort, Procter & Gamble, which had already invested more than $5 million in research support for my therapy, agreed to fund the study.

During that period, Dr. Antman, Dr. Wynder and I met multiple times to discuss the project and its design. Dr. Chabot did not attend these first sessions, but since Dr. Antman considered him an expert in the surgical management of pancreatic cancer, she eventually suggested that he should assume some supervisory responsibility. In those initial meetings, against our strong objections Dr. Antman also insisted we adopt a randomized format. However, she did agree that Dr. Isaacs and I could participate with Dr. Chabot in both the intake assessment of study candidates as well as the informed consent process.

Late that summer of 1997, Dr. Antman and I completed the first drafts of the protocol and consent documents, using as a guide the Columbia Cancer Center template for clinical trials. For any study, the protocol serves as a detailed rule-book and roadmap to govern a clinical trial and guide it along its often complicated pathway. The consent form, when signed, serves as critical proof a study candidate understands the risks and benefits of all treatments being evaluated.

In the sections that follow, I first describe significant changes in the official Protocol over the years, then do the same for the Consent Form, as each evolved from the first draft completed in September 1997, to the last in 2000. Keep in mind that though I had helped write the originals of these documents with Dr. Antman, the Columbia team under her direction compiled all subsequent versions.

The September 30, 1997 Protocol:
The First Version

On page 1 of this draft, entitled "Evaluation of Intensive Pancreatic Proteolytic Enzyme Therapy with Ancillary Nutritional Support in the Treatment of Inoperable Pancreatic Adenocarcinoma," Dr. Antman, Dr. Isaacs and myself were listed as the "Chief Investigators." The document described the design as randomized, with Procter & Gamble identified as the "Pharmaceutical sponsor," since the NCI was not yet involved.

Section 1.2, "Background on pancreatic proteolytic enzyme therapy" included a discussion of Dr. Beard, more recent scientific support for my approach, and a summary of my Kelley study conducted under Dr. Good, followed by a description of the treatment as applied today. I excerpt here the paragraphs that specifically referenced my prior research efforts:

1.2 **Background on pancreatic proteolytic enzyme therapy:** The planned therapy overall involves four components: pancreatic proteolytic enzymes, dietary modification, adjunctive nutritional supplements, and detoxification procedures. The pancreatic enzymes remain the main anti-cancer component of the program, while the other nutritional aspects function in a supportive, rather than anti-cancer, role.

A. Pancreatic Enzyme Therapy: The Scottish embryologist, Dr. John Beard, first proposed in papers dating to 1902 that the pancreatic proteolytic enzymes represent the body's main defense against cancer, and he suggested that such enzymes would be useful as a cancer treatment. Initially Dr. Beard's thesis attracted some attention and generated considerable controversy in orthodox research circles. During the first two decades of this century, a number of case reports appeared in the mainstream literature documenting tumor regression and even cure in a number of terminal cancer patients treated with only pancreatic enzymes. In 1911, Dr. Beard published a monograph entitled The Enzyme Therapy of Cancer [sic], which summarized his therapy and the supporting evidence.

After Dr. Beard's death in 1923 [sic], the enzyme therapy was largely forgotten. Periodically, alternative type therapists have rediscovered Dr. Beard's work, and used pancreatic proteolytic enzymes as a treatment for cancer.

Basic science support for this work, though certainly not extensive, does exist: in 1965, two articles appeared documenting a significant anti-cancer effect for the enzymes in a tumor prone animal model. Leighton King, a researcher at St. Joseph's Hospital in Arizona, reported complete prevention of tumors in a group of C3H mice carrying Bittner's milk factor virus who received oral pancreatin, compared to 100% tumor occurrence in the control group. In a second article, King proposed an immune enhancement effect for orally ingested pancreatin: in an experimental group of Swiss mice, he described a 260% increase in antibody production with the addition of 2% pancreatin to the diet.

The actual mechanism of action for the enzyme effect has not been described. The proteolytic enzymes may have a direct anti-cancer capability, as well as indirect activity mediated via immune enhancement or differentiation pathways. Basic science and animal studies are currently being developed to coincide with the clinical trial.

The section that followed, 1.3, "Background on new treatment," similar in title to section 1.2, reported in some detail my early investigations of the enzyme approach, as well as the more recent pilot study data presented in chart form. Not surprisingly, and appropriately, my name appeared here throughout:

1.3 **Background on new treatment:** Dr. Nicholas Gonzalez, one of the investigators of this study, began researching the use of intensive oral pancreatic proteolytic enzyme therapy as a treatment for cancer in 1981 while a medical student. Later, as an immunology fellow, Dr. Gonzalez conducted an intensive retrospective review of 1306 patients who had been treated over a twenty year period by an unconventional practitioner who used enzyme therapy along with adjunctive dietary and nutritional support. This study included a review of pancreatic cancer patients in particular, some of whom survived in excess of five years.

Since 1987, Dr. Gonzalez has been applying proteolytic enzyme therapy to patients with advanced, poor prognosis cancer. The treatment also includes dietary modification, nutritional support in the form of supplements, and detoxification routines such as coffee enemas.

In his clinical experience with pancreatic adenocarcinoma, Dr. Gonzalez finds that a low fat, low animal protein diet, emphasizing whole grains, fresh fruits, vegetables, nuts and seeds enhances the effectiveness of the pancreatic enzyme treatment. Dr. Gonzalez sees the diet as supportive and adjunctive to the enzymes.

In collaboration with the NCI, Dr. Gonzalez developed a formal protocol to study 10 patients with pancreatic adenocarcinoma, which was ultimately funded by the Nestec (Nestle) Corporation.

The data chart for the pilot study, updated as of 1997, then followed.

Section 4.0, entitled "Patient Entry," clarified my role in the intake processing of study candidates:

4.0 **Patient Entry**

4.1 Evaluation by the study chair

4.2 Evaluation by Dr. Gonzalez or staff trained by him: All prospective patients must undergo extensive interviewing to determine their willingness to follow, and their suitability for, the Enzyme-Nutritional therapy. This treatment is a complex dietary program that involves major changes in lifestyle and it is not suitable for all patients. Dr. Gonzalez has trained staff members to conduct such interviews, and it is suggested that someone from his staff be involved in the selection process.

Dr. Antman informed me the "study chair" referenced above would either be herself or Dr. John Chabot. As Section 4.2 made clear, Dr. Antman intended I would be directly involved with evaluation of patient eligibility.

Shortly after we completed the first drafts of the protocol and consent form, Dr. Chabot officially joined the Columbia team, and it is our understanding that with his help Dr. Antman rewrote the subsequent versions. At that point the documents had not yet, as I remember, been submitted to the Columbia Institutional Review Board for approval.

The second protocol draft, dated December 16, 1997, had been considerably modified.

The December 16, 1997 Protocol: The Second Version

On page 1, Procter & Gamble was identified as the sponsor, the study was described as "Randomized," but now Dr. Chabot, along with Dr. Antman, Dr. Isaacs, and myself, were listed as the "Investigators." We all appeared to be of equal stature.

Section 1.2, "Background on pancreatic proteolytic enzyme therapy," had also been rewritten, but more for style than for content. It resembled the earlier draft, paragraph for paragraph, providing the same basic discussion of Dr. Beard, the laboratory evidence supporting enzyme treatment, and the therapy as used today. Dr. Antman and her team had, however, shortened section 1.3, "Background on new treatment," which now consisted of only two paragraphs:

Background on new treatment: Dr. Nicholas Gonzalez, who began researching the use of intensive oral pancreatic proteolytic enzyme therapy as a treatment for cancer in 1981, retrospectively reviewed 1306 patients [sic] **records?** treated over a twenty year period with enzyme therapy and adjunctive dietary and nutritional support. In this some pancreatic cancer patients survived more than five years. **Reference?**

In collaboration with the NCI, Dr. Gonzalez developed a formal protocol to study 10 patients with pancreatic adenocarcinoma, which was ultimately funded by the Nestec (Nestle) Corporation.

The data chart, as before, then followed.

Section 4.0, "Patient Entry," had also been rewritten, but still indicated I would assist with patient selection:

4.0 **Patient Entry**

4.1 Evaluation by the study chair

4.2 **Evaluation by Dr. Gonzalez:** All prospective patients must undergo extensive interviewing to determine their willingness to follow, and their suitability for Enzyme-Nutritional Therapy, a complex dietary program that involves major changes in lifestyle and it is not suitable for all patients.

Note that Dr. Antman informed us that the "study chair" now referred specifically to Dr. Chabot, with whom we would share patient intake responsibilities.

The March 20, 1998 Protocol:
The Third Version

In early 1998, Dr. Antman and her Columbia crew, again without my input, completely rewrote the protocol. On the first page of this new edition, dated March 20, 1998, my name appeared along with that of Dr. Isaacs, but this time within a new category, "Non-Columbia Collaborators." Dr. Antman, Dr. Chabot, and three other Columbia staff were identified as "Columbia Faculty."

The discussion of Dr. Beard, the supporting laboratory research, and the treatment as applied today appearing in section 1.2 remained largely intact. The two paragraphs describing the pilot study along with the data chart in section 1.3 also seemed identical to the prior December 1997 draft, with my name prominently displayed. But section 4.0 had been modified:

4.0 **Patient Entry**

4.1 Evaluation by the study chair

4.2 All prospective patients must undergo extensive interviewing to determine their willingness to follow, and their suitability for Enzyme-Nutritional Therapy, a complex dietary program that involves major changes in lifestyle and it is not suitable for all patients.

I was somewhat perplexed that my name had been deleted from this important section. In any event, as before the "study chair" referred to Dr. Chabot.

The November 11, 1998 Protocol:
The Fourth Version

The project took a new and somewhat unexpected course when in the spring of 1998 NCI Director Dr. Richard Klausner promised full federal support, both in terms of funding and personnel. By November of that year, the Columbia team had revised the protocol once again, this time to reflect the study's new status as an official NCI clinical trial. The design remained "randomized," both Dr. Isaacs and I were again listed on page 1 as "Non-Columbia Collaborators," and section 1.2 included the same discussion of Dr. Beard's early research, the laboratory evidence in support of enzyme therapy, and the treatment as applied today. The two paragraphs referring to the pilot study in Section 1.3, as well as the data chart, were identical to the prior edition, with my name still present. Similarly, the "Patient Entry" section 4.0 remained unchanged with my name absent, and the "study chair" (Dr. Chabot) apparently in charge of the intake process.

The November 14, 1999 Protocol:
The Fifth Version

After the wasted first year, when the various supervisors finally agreed to a non-randomized design, the study documents were rewritten for a fifth time. The revised November 14, 1999 protocol described the trial as a matched cohort effort, but otherwise remained much the same in content. As before, on page 1 the names of Dr. Chabot, Dr. Antman, and two other colleagues were grouped under "Columbia Faculty" with Dr. Isaacs and me described as "Non-Columbia Collaborators."

Section 1.2, "Background on pancreatic proteolytic enzyme therapy," once again discussed Dr. Beard's work, the more recent laboratory investigations, and briefly described the treatment as administered today. Section 1.3, with my name appearing twice, included the same paragraphs devoted to my research efforts, summarizing my Kelley investigation conducted under Dr. Good as well as the pilot study with the data in chart form.

Section 4.0 on page 7 entitled "PATIENT ENTRY" remained unchanged from the prior version. However, section 13.1 reflected the new format:

> 13.1 **Study Design:** We propose a nonexperimental [note: nonrandomized] study in which patients will be allowed to choose between two therapeutic modalities: proteolytic enzymes versus standard chemotherapy. Patients will be matched on an individual basis for known predictors of survival outcome.

Non-randomized clinical trials fall into certain distinct categories. For our project, we had agreed upon—or at least Dr. Isaacs and I thought we had agreed upon—a matched cohort approach, in which the two patient groups would be, as much as possible, equivalent by stage, clinical status, even by sex and age. This format, we believed, offered the fairest and most effective way to test our treatment. Though the above paragraph did not include the specific term "matched cohort," by requiring that Dr. Chabot create two similar groups in essence the Columbia team had defined our study in this way.

In early 2000, the Columbia staff again revised both the protocol and the consent form, though we did not receive copies of the documents, dated February 28, 2000, until mid-June. This proved to be the final version of the protocol, though the consent form would undergo slight modification in late 2000.

The February 28, 2000 Protocol:
The Sixth Version

The February 2000 protocol remained much the same in content as the previous draft. As before, on page 1 the names of Dr. Chabot, Dr. Antman, and two other colleagues appeared under "Columbia Faculty" with Dr. Isaacs and me described as "Non-Columbia Collaborators."

Section 1.2, "Background-Pancreatic Proteolytic Enzyme Therapy," discussed, without any changes, Dr. Beard's work, the more recent laboratory investigations, and briefly described the treatment as administered today. Section 1.3 consisted of the same paragraphs devoted to my research efforts, my Kelley investigation conducted under Dr. Good, and the pilot study with the data in chart form. However, for some reason my name now appeared six times, not twice as in the previous edition.

Section 4.0, "PATIENT ENTRY," had been considerably revised. Since these paragraphs would govern patient admission for the next six years, I include them here:

4.0 **PATIENT ENTRY**

Evaluation by the study chair (John Chabot, M.D.).

Patients electing to participate in <u>the nutritional therapy arm</u> must undergo extensive interviewing to determine their willingness to follow, and their suitability for Enzyme-Nutritional Therapy, a complex dietary program that involves major changes in lifestyle and it is not suitable for all patients.

Staging: evaluate all areas of disease.

Eligible patients who wish to participate must sign an informed consent.

Registration: To register the patient, fax or deliver the completed Eligibility Criteria Form, Cancer Center demographic form, and signed Informed Consent to the Cancer Center Protocol Office, located on. . . . Send hard copy for intra-hospital mail.

Required Forms:

Eligibility criteria form, Informed consent, Cancer Center demographic form

This time around, with our names again absent, Dr. Chabot was clearly identified as the "study chair," responsible for assessing trial candidates and conducting "extensive interviewing to determine their willingness to follow, and their suitability for Enzyme-Nutritional Therapy." Though Drs. Antman and Chabot still verbally assured us our veto rights over patient selection remained intact, nowhere did the protocol acknowledge such authority.

Section 16.1, "Study Design," had been considerably enlarged, this time around describing the non-randomized format in greater detail. As I read this section I thought that without our input, once again the rules had been significantly modified:

We propose an observational study in which eligible patients will select their preferred therapy: either proteolytic enzymes or standard chemotherapy. In the experimental arm, patients will receive intense proteolytic enzyme therapy with prescribed adjunctive dietary modification, supplementation with vitamins, minerals. . . .

Patients on the conventional arm will receive standard chemotherapy treatment for adenocarcinoma of the pancreas.

All eligible patients will undergo an intensive intake interview to determine their interest in following either the nutritional treatment or the chemotherapy protocol. Patients who are suitable candidates for either treatment will be entered into the arm of their choice.

Self-selection of patients into treatment arms may result in a biased estimate of the treatment effect because the arms may differ on important predictors of survival. Consequently we will record data on various known and suspected predictors of survival. Our primary analysis will be a survival analysis that adjusts for these differences by the propensity score method for bias reduction.

The word "observational" as used above—and not appearing in any earlier protocol document—refers in a general sense to any type of non-randomized clinical trial, of which, as we have seen, there are several, including matched cohort. Though the Columbia authors of the previous November 14, 1999 draft did not use the term "matched cohort," they described our study as such by including the phrase "Patients will be matched on an individual basis for known predictors of survival outcome." But now this very important instruction had been deleted, technically freeing Dr. Chabot from the requirement he create two similar groups. Furthermore, the worrisome term "propensity score" popped up for the first time. This convoluted statistical application allows researchers to run confusing data from unmatched groups through a series of mathematical filters, in the hope of generating "meaningful" data. I myself have long considered "propensity scores" as an elaborate mechanism for making flawed data seem valid and important.

Note that at that time, in mid-2000, the "standard chemotherapy" consisted of gemcitabine alone.

I will now review relevant changes as they appeared in the consent form over time, reflecting, perhaps more so than the protocol revisions, a growing negative feeling about the project at Columbia.

The September 30, 1997 Consent Form:
The First Version

I helped write this first draft, entitled simply "Consent," which accompanied the September 30, 1997 protocol. This document consisted of nine pages, beginning with a basic introduction to the consent process:

> You have been asked to participate in a clinical research study. To decide whether or not you should agree to be part of this research study, you should understand enough about its risks and benefits to make an informed judgment. This process is known as informed consent.

> This consent form gives detailed information about the research study which your physician will discuss with you. Once you understand the study, you will be asked to sign this form if you wish to participate.

The section entitled "Study purpose" outlined my past research, beginning with my medical school investigations of the enzyme treatment, before moving on to my 1993 presentation at the NCI. A lengthy description of the pilot study, at the time still in progress, and its preliminary data, then followed. Not surprisingly, my name appeared in five of the seven paragraphs:

> **Study purpose:** The purpose of this research study is to determine whether a new nutritional treatment for cancer, called Enzyme-Nutritional Therapy, is effective in treating pancreatic cancer (adenocarcinoma). You were selected as a possible participant in this study because you have been diagnosed with adenocarcinoma of the pancreas and have not previously received chemotherapy or radiation. Furthermore, you are able to eat normally and care for yourself, both requirements for entrance into the study.

> Background: Dr. Nicholas Gonzalez, one of the investigators of this study, began researching the use of intensive oral pancreatic enzyme therapy as a treatment for cancer in 1981. While a medical student, and later as an immunology fellow, Dr. Gonzalez evaluated 1306 patients who had been treated by an unconventional practitioner who over a twenty year period used enzyme therapy along with dietary and nutritional support. This study included a review of pancreatic cancer patients who survived in excess of five years while receiving this nutritional therapy.

> Since 1987, Dr. Gonzalez has been applying the proteolytic enzyme therapy to patients with advanced, poor prognosis cancer. The treatment also includes

391

dietary modification, nutritional support in the form of supplements, and detoxification routines such as coffee enemas.

In July of 1993, Dr. Gonzalez was invited to present a series of case reports from his own practice at the National Cancer Institute in Bethesda, Maryland. As a result of that session. [sic] it was suggested that Dr. Gonzalez conduct a pilot study of his treatment in ten patients suffering pancreatic adenocarcinoma using survival as the end point. In collaboration with the NCI, Dr. Gonzalez developed a formal protocol for the study, which was ultimately funded by the research division of the Nestec (Nestle) Corporation.

The study commenced in January, 1994. Eleven patients were eventually entered onto the study and all the patients entered into the trial had advanced or metastatic disease. All, when first seen by Dr. Gonzalez, had a history of significant symptoms consistent with progressing illness.

Despite the advanced state of the patients, the survival overall far exceeded what would be expected for pancreatic cancer. Nine of the eleven patients (including one who quit the study) lived longer than one year. Four patients have already survived 2.5 years, and a fifth, doing very well despite a history of pelvic involvement, will be at two years this December. At that time, three patients will have survived three years and five will have survived at least two years. This data certainly surpasses the results for gemcitabine, the drug recently approved for treatment of pancreatic adenocarcinoma. In the gemcitabine trials, no patient lived 18 months. [sic: one patient actually lived 19 months].

Dr. Gonzalez presented the results of this pilot study on August 4, 1997 at a joint NCI-NIH conference in Bethesda, Maryland. As a result of that conference, it was suggested that Dr. Gonzalez undertake a definitive controlled clinical trial to document more definitively the efficacy of the treatment with pancreatic cancer. Procter & Gamble has agreed to fund the study in its entirety.

I want to emphasize that though I wrote much of the above, Dr. Antman herself edited and approved each statement.

Dr. Wynder, who had agreed to help supervise the study, actually composed most of the section entitled "Potential Benefits of Study Treatments," which likewise referenced the pilot study data accurately, if somewhat enthusiastically:

Potential Benefits of Study Treatments

It is not possible to predict whether your cancer will respond to either the Enzyme-Nutrition, or gemcitabine, treatment. If your cancer does respond you may feel better and live longer. It is hoped that the results of this study will be useful in the development of future treatment for patients with pancreatic cancer.

Specifically, in the pilot study of Enzyme-Nutritional Therapy, patients with pancreatic cancer have lived—and a number of patients continue to live—far longer than would be expected with this serious illness. In addition, the quality of life of these patients has generally been greatly improved by the aggressive nutritional support.

Patients receiving gemcitabine have enjoyed a slight prolongation of life and a significant improvement in their quality of life.

Your participation in this study may be of great benefit to society at large, because you will be involved in helping document whether a non-toxic, nutritional therapy can be of benefit in the treatment of pancreatic cancer. Should the Enzyme-Nutritional Therapy prove to be beneficial to patients, this finding could open up a new avenue of scientific investigation.

The final paragraphs under "Questions" identified me as an integral part of the research team:

If you have any questions, we will do our best to answer them.

The physician in charge of this research at the Columbia Presbyterian Medical Center is Dr. Karen Antman. Her telephone number is (212) 305–8602. If you need more information about this study before you can decide whether to participate or at any other time, you may wish to contact her, or you could contact Dr. Gonzalez at (212) 213–3337.

If you have additional questions in the future, you can reach Dr. Antman at (212) 305–8602 and Dr. Gonzalez at (212) 213–3337.

If you have any questions on your rights as a research subject you can call the Institutional Review Board at (212) 305–5883 for information.

I have discussed this study with Dr. Antman, Dr. Gonzalez, or their associates, to my satisfaction. I understand that my participation is voluntary and that I can withdraw from the study at any time without prejudice. I have read the above and agree to enter this research study.

The December 16, 1997 Consent Form: The Second Version

This draft, now titled "Columbia Presbyterian Medical Center—Consent to Participate in a Research Study," like the accompanying protocol, had been drastically restructured. Though the brief introductory two paragraphs had not changed, in the section that followed, "Study purpose," Dr. Antman had deleted all reference to the pilot study, as well as to my name. I found these omissions very odd, since the preliminary pilot study data provided the entire rationale for this second clinical trial:

> **Study purpose:** The purpose of this research study is to determine whether Enzyme-Nutritional Therapy is effective in treating pancreatic adenocarcinoma. About 40 patients will participate in this study. You were selected as a possible participant in this study because you have been diagnosed with adenocarcinoma of the pancreas and have not previously received chemotherapy or radiation. . . .
>
> We want to compare how well patients respond to treatment with Enzyme-Nutritional Therapy or to a drug called. [sic] If treatment works in your case, it may shrink your tumor or cause it to disappear. . . .

The section "Potential Benefits of Study Treatments" had likewise been significantly edited down and now lacked any mention of the pilot study or Dr. Wynder's enthusiastic words about new avenues in cancer research:

> ### Potential Benefits of Study Treatments
>
> It is not possible to predict whether your cancer will respond to either the Enzyme-Nutrition, or the gemcitabine, treatment. If your cancer does respond you may feel better and live longer. The results of this study may be useful in the development of future treatment for patients with pancreatic cancer.

The "Questions" section at the end, though shorter, still referred to me as part of the supervisory team:

> If you have any questions, we will do our best to answer them.

The physician in charge of this research at the Columbia Presbyterian Medical Center is Dr. Karen Antman. Her telephone number is (212) 305–8602. If you need more information about this study before you can decide whether to participate or at any other time, you may wish to contact her, or you could contact Dr. Gonzalez at (212) 213–3337. . . .

If you have any questions on your rights as a research subject you can call the Institutional Review Board at (212) 305–5883 for information.

After reading the revised documents, I spoke with Dr. Antman at length, voicing my concern that the consent form now excluded all mention of the pilot study. Why ignore, I asked, the very research that had encouraged Procter & Gamble, as well as Columbia itself, to support a second investigation? Why leave out the very data that might encourage patients to join our current clinical trial? She listened, and said she would rethink her decision to remove the relevant passages. She also advised me that Dr. Chabot would assume the role of Principal Investigator, while I would now be considered a "Collaborator," not an "Investigator."

The March 20, 1998 Consent Form:
The Third Version

The rewritten form accompanying the March 20, 1998 protocol draft reflected not only my apparent downgraded status, but in my mind a changed attitude on the part of Columbia toward my treatment. Though Dr. Antman had added back some information about the pilot study under "Study purpose" on page 1, the tone was distinctly negative with my name omitted:

Study purpose: The purpose of this research study is to determine whether enzyme-nutritional therapy is as effective as a drug called gemcitabine for treating pancreatic adenocarcinoma. We also want to find out what kind of side effects these treatments cause and how often they occur.

Many Americans who develop advanced cancer for which standard treatments have little to offer turn to alternative or complimentary [sic] therapies. Enzyme-nutritional therapy is such a study [sic] which has been reported, in a pilot study of 11 patients, to produce a median survival of 18 months. This survival could have been a result of selection of healthier patients (those able to eat normally). The only way to determine if enzyme nutritional therapy benefits patients with advanced pancreatic cancer is to compare it to standard therapy, gemcitabine.

As a first point, I didn't understand why Dr. Antman classified my treatment among "alternative or complementary therapies," terms I do not use and which I believe carry a pejorative connotation.

I also thought unreasonable the statement that the very impressive pilot study survival data might have reflected no more than "the selection of healthier patients." Here Dr. Antman seemed to be implying that Dr. Isaacs and I had chosen, apparently deliberately, patients who might have lived just as long without any treatment, so the seemingly positive results really didn't mean much. After I read these comments, I spoke with Dr. Antman, challenging the plausibility of her reasoning. First of all, I repeated what I have said so many times since, eight of the 11 entered into the pilot study had been diagnosed with stage IV disease, and all were headed for quick demise. Such patients usually die within 3–6 months, and no subgroup of "healthier" stage IV patients, no lucky few destined for prolonged survival of two, three, and more years has ever been identified to my knowledge in any scientific paper or textbook anywhere at any time.

For example, in the 1997 published report of the main Gemzar clinical trial, of a total of 126 subjects receiving two different chemotherapy regimens, including 72% at stage IV, the gemcitabine-treated group survived an average of 5.6 months. Only 18% lived a year despite aggressive therapy, and not one patient in either arm lasted beyond 19 months. If a subpopulation destined for long-term survival despite advanced disease truly existed, as Dr. Antman claimed, one wonders how they managed to make their way into my 11 patient pilot study but eluded the large-scale Gemzar clinical trial, with more than ten times as many subjects entered? Where were they? Though we did require patients be able to eat because of the dietary-nutritional nature of our therapy, we treated very sick patients, as the actual medical records easily confirmed. Despite my arguments, Dr. Antman refused to change the wording.

In any event, the section "Potential Benefits of Study Treatments" remained unchanged:

Potential Benefits of Study Treatments: It is not possible to predict whether your cancer will respond to either the Enzyme-Nutrition, or the gemcitabine, treatment. If your cancer does respond you may feel better and live longer. The results of this study may be useful in the development of future treatment for patients with pancreatic cancer.

On page 5 under "Questions," Dr. Antman identified Dr. Chabot as the "physician in charge," and now instructed all study candidates to direct any of their questions about the project or the two treatments to his office, with no mention of Dr. Isaacs or me:

> If you have any questions, we will do our best to answer them. The physician in charge of this research at the Columbia Presbyterian Medical Center is Dr. John Chabot. His telephone number is (212) 305–8295. If you need more information about this study before you can decide whether to participate or at any other time, you may wish to contact him.

> If you have any questions on your rights as a research subject you can call the Institutional Review Board at (212) 305–5883 for information.

The November 11, 1998 Consent Form:
The Fourth Version

Along with the protocol, in the fall of 1998 Dr. Antman (with presumably Dr. Chabot) once again rewrote the consent document, which was dated November 2, 1998. The "Study Purpose," with the same negative inferences about the pilot project, once again excluded any mention of me. In the lengthy description of the two treatments, identified respectively as "Standard Arm Chemotherapy" and "Experimental Arm Enzyme-Nutritional Therapy," my name oddly was missing. In the section "Potential Benefits of Study Treatments," still the same brief paragraph, the pilot study, its data, and I were again not mentioned, and in fact the authors failed to reference me anywhere in the consent document.

The rewritten "Questions" at the end of the form defined Dr. Chabot's authority in greater detail than had the third draft of March 1998. It appeared that as my role diminished, that of Dr. Chabot had only expanded:

> You are deciding whether or not to take part in this study. If you sign, it means that you have decided to volunteer after reading and understanding all the information on this form.

> Dr. Chabot and his staff will be instructing you on the techniques necessary for all treatments related to this protocol as they pertain to you. If you have any additional questions, please do not hesitate to ask, and we will do our best to

answer them. Dr. John Chabot, the physician in charge of this research at the Columbia Presbyterian Medical Center, may be reached at (212) 305–9468 prior to and during your participation in this study should you have any questions about this study. In addition, if you have any questions on your rights as a research subject, you can call the Institutional Review Board at (212) 305–5883 for information.

Eventually, I believe in late 1998 or very early 1999, the Columbia IRB and the NCI approved the rewritten protocol and consent form, so the trial, still randomized in design, opened to accrual—with, as we predicted, disastrous results.

We received the fifth version of the protocol in late November 1998. Though we assume the Columbia team rewrote the consent form at the same time, they did not send us a copy so I have no idea how it might have been revised. However, Dr. Antman did fax us the sixth edition dated February 28, 2000:

The February 28, 2000 Consent Form:
The Sixth Version

This document ran seven pages, with some significant modifications from the prior drafts, though the opening paragraph addressed directly to the patient remained the same:

> You are being asked to participate in a clinical research study. To decide whether or not you should agree to be part of this research study, you should understand enough about its risks and benefits to make an informed judgment.
>
> This consent form gives detailed information about the research study which your physician will discuss with you. Once you understand the study, you will be asked to sign this form if you wish to participate.

Under "Study Purpose," the writers, presumably Dr. Antman and Dr. Chabot, described the pilot data in terms more negative and ominous than in any previous version of the consent form:

> **Study Purpose.** The purpose of this research study is to determine whether enzyme-nutritional therapy is as effective as a drug called gemcitabine for treating pancreatic adenocarcinoma. We also want to find out what kind of side effects these treatments cause and how often they occur.

Many Americans who develop advanced cancer for which standard treatments have little to offer turn to alternative or complimentary [sic] therapies. Enzyme-nutritional therapy is such a study [sic] which has been reported, in a pilot study of 11 patients, to produce a median survival of 18 months. This survival could have been a result of selection of healthier patients (those able to eat normally). The only way to determine if enzyme nutritional therapy benefits patients with advanced pancreatic cancer is to compare it to standard therapy, gemcitabine. The rationale of those advocating this alternative medicine approach will be explained to you by the physicians and staff involved in this part of the study. However, there is no current conventional medical support for the therapies and assumptions underlying the use of nutritional therapy. The Columbia University College of Physicians and Surgeons does not support its use except as part of a properly conducted clinical trial such as this one.

Unfortunately, despite the facts and despite my complaints, Dr. Antman and the Columbia team continued claiming the positive pilot study data might only be an artifact, resulting from my careful selection of a group of stage IV patients, previously unidentified in the scientific literature, who would have lived longer regardless of treatment. I also disagreed with the fourth sentence, "The only way to determine if enzyme nutritional therapy benefits patients with advanced pancreatic cancer is to compare it to standard therapy, gemcitabine." Such a controlled clinical trial as described represented *one way* to assess the value of a treatment, but it was hardly the only way.

In the past the Food and Drug Administration has approved conventional cancer treatments based solely on pilot study or anecdotal data. For example, in 1992 the FDA gave its blessing to interleukin II for treatment of kidney cancer based on essentially anecdotal results, data in my opinion far less impressive than what we had observed in our own pilot study. Especially for a disease as deadly as advanced pancreatic adenocarcinoma, with the well-documented life expectancy so dismal, pilot study data such as ours can indicate real benefit from treatment. The significantly improved survival we had reported in the spring of 1999, before the consent draft had been finalized, indicated some effect from therapy—despite Dr. Antman's suggestion that the extraordinary results might reflect only selection of stage IV patients who would have lived longer anyway.

In the fifth sentence of the paragraph, "The rationale of those advocating this alternative medicine approach will be explained to you by the physicians and staff involved in this part of the study," I assumed here the writers meant the Columbia team under Dr. Chabot, who at this point seemed to be in charge of everything, though he knew little about our treatment.

The two sentences that followed troubled me far more, of course. The statement "However, there is no current conventional medical support for the therapies and assumptions underlying the use of nutritional therapy" reduced to nothing Beard's impressive—and very conventional in nature—body of research.[5;9] It also ignored the more recent efforts of scientists such as Leighton King from the 1960s, whose animal research confirmed a significant anti-cancer, immune enhancing effect for pancreatic proteolytic enzymes.[71] Furthermore, by implication the writers suggested that our very carefully designed, carefully supervised pilot study signified little.

Even the more controversial aspects of our regimen such as the coffee enemas have been recommended for a variety of conditions in the peer-reviewed medical literature.[2-4] So I was disappointed that Drs. Antman and Chabot would include such a sweeping, dismissive statement about our treatment without first consulting me or reviewing my extensive documentation supporting most of what we do.

I found the final sentence of the paragraph equally peculiar: "The Columbia University College of Physicians and Surgeons does not support its use except as part of a properly conducted clinical trial such as this one." First of all, I thought the tone unnecessary. No one to my knowledge, including no one in my office and certainly neither Dr. Isaacs nor myself, has ever even vaguely intimated that the Columbia University College of Physicians and Surgeons had authorized, supported, recommended, embraced, etc., my treatment approach in any way at any time. During the many years of the study, when asked about my relationship to that medical center, we always responded with the truth, that the Institution served as the site for our NCI-supervised, NIH-funded clinical trial and nothing more. I also did not understand how this very guarded declaration in the consent document would encourage any patient to join the study—on the contrary, I thought it would have quite the opposite effect. I wondered if Dr. Antman and Dr. Chabot now wished to distance themselves and Columbia from us, as far as possible.

The section "Patient Selection of Treatment" at the bottom of page 1 informed candidates the choice of therapy would be theirs, whether our nutritional regimen or chemotherapy:

> Your treating physicians will discuss both treatments that are available to you. Based on this information, you will decide which treatment program you would like to participate in (chemotherapy or enzyme-nutritional therapy).

The descriptions of the two interventions that followed resembled the statements in the prior draft, and, the "Potential Benefits of Study Treatments" remained unchanged, with no reference to the pilot study, its data, or my name:

> **Potential Benefits of Study Treatments.** It is not possible to predict whether your cancer will respond to either the Enzyme-Nutritional Therapy, or gemcitabine treatment. If your cancer does respond you may feel better and live longer. The results of this study may be useful in the development of future treatment for patients with pancreatic cancer.

Under "Questions" beginning at the bottom of page 5, the authors again defined Dr. Chabot's role:

> You are deciding whether or not to take part in this study. If you sign, it means that you have decided to volunteer after reading and understanding all the information on this form.

> Dr. Chabot and his staff will be instructing you on the techniques necessary for all treatments related to this protocol as they pertain to you. If you have any additional questions, please do not hesitate to ask, and we will do our best to answer them. Dr. John Chabot, the physician in charge of this research at the Columbia Presbyterian Medical Center, may be reached at (212) 305–9468 prior to and during your participation in this study should you have any questions about this study. In addition, if you have any questions on your rights as a research subject, you can call the Institutional Review Board at (212) 305–5883 for information.

The first sentence of the second paragraph above indicated that "Dr. Chabot and his staff" would be educating all prospective study candidates about the two therapies being compared, the Gemzar based chemotherapy and our "Enzyme-Nutritional Therapy." Though Drs. Antman and Chabot assured Dr. Isaacs and myself that our role in the admitting process had not changed, my name and that of Dr. Isaacs appeared nowhere in the entire seven-page consent document.

The Late 2000 Consent Form:
The Seventh Version

Though the February 28, 2000 draft of the protocol would be its last incarnation—as far as we know—in late 2000 the Columbia team sent us a slightly modified consent form with a new paragraph entitled "Side Effect of Enzyme-Nutritional Therapy," warning of the alleged dangers of coffee enemas:

> Patients occasionally develop hemorrhoids from the coffee enemas. Should this happen your doctor may prescribe a medication to help reduce the hemorrhoids and may discontinue the enemas. **In addition, there have been reported deaths associated with coffee enemas. In each of these cases the doses were far in excess of those used in this study. Therefore, it is very important that you adhere to the prescribed frequency and dosage for this study.**

During my five-year evaluation of Dr. Kelley's therapy in the early 1980s, I had reviewed the medical literature searching for cases of so-called "deaths associated with coffee enemas," which even at that time had created some stir in the media. After considerable effort, I located only three, though for two the data appeared to be at best borderline.[72;73] Below I have extracted the relevant section from *One Man Alone,* which documents my original Kelley investigation completed in 1986 and includes my analysis of the fatalities that had to that point been attributed to the enemas. I am unaware of any more recent cases, and though these reports date back some 25 years and more, the vocal critics of alternative cancer treatments, including critics of my work, still reference these three examples to "prove" the dangers of coffee enemas:

> Obviously, the orthodox medical world finds little of value in Dr. Kelley's methods. However, many physicians target one specific aspect of the program, the coffee enemas, for particular ridicule and criticism, and several articles appearing in the medical literature in recent years have specifically questioned their safety. A widely discussed report in the October 30, 1980 issue of the *Journal of the American Medical Association* helped fuel this concern.
>
> In their paper entitled "Deaths Related to Coffee Enemas," two pathologists from the Seattle Medical Examiner's Office, Drs. Eisele and Reay, describe two fatalities they directly attribute to the use of coffee enemas. Neither of the

victims, I should add, had ever consulted Dr. Kelley, but followed nutritional programs designed by other unconventional therapists.

The first patient discussed, a 46-year-old woman, had not been diagnosed with cancer, but instead had a long history of numerous, chronic digestive problems. In the days prior to her death, she developed acute gastrointestinal distress associated with frequent vomiting, and began, of her own accord, using coffee enemas at the rate of three or four an hour. Subsequently, after more than 30 enemas, she developed an electrolyte (blood salt) imbalance, lapsed into coma and died.

Severe vomiting can itself cause life-threatening fluid and electrolyte loss. In this particular situation, the obvious overuse of coffee enemas may indeed have contributed to the disturbance and her death.

The second example presented, a woman with terminal breast cancer that had metastasized widely, seems far less clear cut. Though this patient did self-administer coffee enemas as prescribed by an alternative practitioner, a postmortem evaluation of her blood revealed "only a small amount of caffeine." Though the authors offer no solid evidence for an electrolyte imbalance, strangely they still try to make a case:

> Using 0.95 L [liter] of this liquid [coffee] three or four times an hour certainly could produce sodium and chloride depletion and fluid overload . . .

This supposed scenario could, of course, lead to death. The writers conclude:

> We are unable to evaluate the prevalence of coffee enemas and are unaware of any other deaths attributed to this treatment. When the second case was publicized by the news media, we received telephone calls and letters from numerous individuals and groups who were using or prescribing coffee enemas. With the current wave of popularity of naturopathic medicine, one would expect an increase in this therapy and consequent morbidity and mortality.[72]

In a "Letter to the Editor" appearing in the March 1984 issue of *Western Journal of Medicine*, two physicians from the University of California, San Diego, describe sepsis—blood-borne bacterial infection—in a 23-year-old woman, diagnosed with widely metastatic breast cancer, who had been self-administering coffee enemas. When chemotherapy failed to halt her disease, she sought an

403

"alternate therapy"—but not the Kelley program—in Mexico. She eventually developed liver failure due directly to her cancer, entered University Hospital in San Diego, and died. Cultures taken prior to her death confirmed bacterial infection in the blood, attributed to the coffee enemas.

"We believe," the authors write, "that our patient's polymicrobial septicemia from two unusual enteric [intestinal] pathogens was induced by enema therapy in the setting of severely compromised hepatic function and portal hypertension. This complication should be considered an additional potential risk of coffee enema therapy."[73]

I found this article informative, although severely ill, terminal cancer patients can develop sepsis after brushing their teeth.[74(pp44-46)]

To put all this in perspective, however valid these cases may or may not be, I have read that more than 10,000 Americans die yearly as a direct result of aspirin use. Furthermore, during my Kelley project I interviewed over 1000 of his patients, all of whom had incorporated daily coffee enemas into their lives, some for more than ten and 15 years. Not one reported a significant side effect; and nearly all told me they felt much better with the enemas.

I have now described the evolution of the written protocol and consent form for our trial, from first versions to the last. These documents illustrate, over a two year period, changes in my official title, my role in the study, the significance of my previous research, the prominence of my name, and the overall attitude of Columbia toward the project. Though some modifications seem minor and perfectly understandable, others appear to us far more significant and troubling.

I would now like to look at these five specific areas from a somewhat different perspective, by directly comparing the relevant sections from the first drafts of the study documents dated September 30, 1997, to the last, dated February 28, 2000. Here, for the sake of this discussion, I will consider the February 2000 Consent document to be the last, since it accompanied what we believe to have been the final version of the protocol.

In so doing, I hope to demonstrate that my diminished standing as apparent in the written protocol and particularly in the consent form, and the profound shift in attitude toward me and my therapy, indicated not inconsequential editorial revisions but perhaps a major transformation in the thinking of the Columbia team.

Comparison of the First and Sixth Versions of
The Protocol

My title. On page 1 of the September 30, 1997 protocol draft, Dr. Antman, Dr. Wynder, Dr. Isaacs and myself were listed as "Investigators," of apparently equal stature.

The February 28, 2000 version identified Dr. Antman, Dr. Chabot and two other Columbia staff as "Columbia Faculty." My name, along with that of Dr. Isaacs, appeared under the category "Non Columbia Collaborators." A third grouping, "Supervisory Board for the Study" listed Ernst Wynder, M.D. along with seven other scientists from various academic centers. In this case, the changes of course seemed perfectly reasonable.

My role. The September 30, 1997 protocol defined my responsibilities in section 4.0:

4.0 **Patient Entry**

4.1 Evaluation by the study chair

4.2 Evaluation by Dr. Gonzalez or staff trained by him: All prospective patients must undergo extensive interviewing to determine their willingness to follow, and their suitability for, the Enzyme-Nutritional Therapy. This treatment is a complex dietary program that involves major changes in lifestyle and it is not suitable for all patients. Dr. Gonzalez has trained staff members to conduct such interviews, and it is suggested that someone from his staff be involved in the selection process.

The equivalent section from the February 28, 2000 draft read:

4.0 **PATIENT ENTRY**
  Evaluation by the study chair (John Chabot, M.D.).
  Patients electing to participate in <u>the nutritional therapy arm</u> must undergo extensive interviewing to determine their willingness to follow, and their suitability for Enzyme-Nutritional Therapy, a complex dietary program that involves major changes in lifestyle and it is not suitable for all patients.
  Staging: evaluate all areas of disease.
  Eligible patients who wish to participate must sign an informed consent.

Registration: To register the patient, fax or deliver the completed Eligibility Criteria Form, Cancer Center demographic form, and signed Informed Consent to the Cancer Center Protocol Office, located on. . . . Send hard copy for intra-hospital mail.

Required Forms:

Eligibility criteria form, Informed consent, Cancer Center demographic form

Here we can see how my position, as defined in the official protocol, had changed over two years, from directly supervising the assessment of study candidates to contributing nothing to the process.

Significance of my research. Both the first and last versions of the protocol summarized the history of enzyme therapy, as well as its current application, within subchapters 1.2 and 1.3. Section 1.2 remained virtually identical over the years, consisting of four paragraphs summarizing Dr. Beard's early research and the more recent laboratory studies of Leighton King. My name did not appear in either draft. By February 28, 2000, the writers—presumably Dr. Antman and other Columbia staff—had condensed section 1.3 considerably.

The September 30, 1997 protocol read:

1.3 **Background on new treatment:** Dr. Nicholas Gonzalez, one of the investigators of this study, began researching the use of intensive oral pancreatic proteolytic enzyme therapy as a treatment for cancer in 1981 while a medical student. Later, as an immunology fellow, Dr. Gonzalez conducted an intensive retrospective review of 1306 patients who had been treated over a twenty year period by an unconventional practitioner who used enzyme therapy along with adjunctive dietary and nutritional support. This study included a review of pancreatic cancer patients in particular, some of whom survived in excess of five years while receiving this nutritional therapy.

Since 1987, Dr. Gonzalez has been applying proteolytic enzyme therapy to patients with advanced, poor prognosis cancer. The treatment also includes dietary modification, nutritional support in the form of supplements, and detoxification routines such as coffee enemas.

In his clinical experience with pancreatic adenocarcinoma, Dr. Gonzalez finds that a low fat, low animal protein diet, emphasizing whole grains, fresh fruits, vegetables, nuts and seeds enhances the effectiveness of the pancreatic enzyme treatment. Dr. Gonzalez sees the diet as supportive and adjunctive to the enzymes.

In July of 1993, Dr. Gonzalez was invited to present a series of case reports from his own practice at the National Cancer Institute in Bethesda, Maryland. As a result of that session, the then Associate Director of the NCI suggested Dr. Gonzalez conduct a pilot study of his treatment in ten patients suffering pancreatic adenocarcinoma, using survival as the end point. In collaboration with the NCI, Dr. Gonzalez developed a formal protocol to study **10 patients with pancreatic adenocarcinoma,** which was ultimately funded by the Nestec (Nestle) Corporation.

The data chart for the pilot study then followed.

For the final version dated February 28, 2000, section 1.3 had been significantly edited:

1.3 Background-New Treatment

Dr. Nicholas Gonzalez, who began researching the use of intensive oral pancreatic proteolytic enzyme therapy as a treatment for cancer in 1981, retrospectively reviewed records of 1306 patient [sic] treated over a twenty year period with enzyme therapy and adjunctive dietary and nutritional support. In this some pancreatic cancer patients survived more than five years. . . .

In collaboration with the NCI, Dr. Gonzalez developed a formal protocol to study 10 patients with pancreatic adenocarcinoma, which was ultimately funded by the Nestec (Nestle) Corporation.

The pilot study data was still included, and though Dr. Antman had deleted much out of section 1.3, my name still appeared.

Prominence of my name. In the September 30, 1997 protocol, my name appeared ten times, including my listing on page 1 as one of the "Investigators." The February 28, 2000 version mentioned me eight times—admittedly only a slight change.

Change in overall attitude of Columbia toward Dr. Isaacs, myself, and our therapy. The above comparison between the September 30, 1997 and the February 28, 2000 documents shows some alterations in my title, my role, the significance of my research and to some extent even the prominence of my name. Certainly, in terms of my title and the mention of my name, the changes are either appropriate or trivial. However, I thought the modifications regarding my role, along with the heavily reduced discussion of my research, indicated a more negative vision of me and my work on the part of the Columbia team.

Comparison of the First and Sixth Versions of The Consent Form

My title. Though the various consent form drafts discussed my research at length in several places, I was not assigned an official title as in the protocol.

My role. In the "Questions" section of the September 30, 1997 consent document I was described an integral part of the research team:

Questions

If you have any questions, we will do our best to answer them.

The physician in charge of this research at the Columbia Presbyterian Medical Center is Dr. Karen Antman. Her telephone number is (212) 305–8602. If you need more information about this study before you can decide whether to participate or at any other time, you may wish to contact her, or you could contact Dr. Gonzalez at (212) 213–3337.

If you have additional questions in the future, you can reach Dr. Antman at (212) 305–8602 and Dr. Gonzalez at (212) 213–3337.

If you have any questions on your rights as a research subject you can call the Institutional Review Board at (212) 305–5883 for information.

I have discussed this study with Dr. Antman, Dr. Gonzalez, or their associates, to my satisfaction. I understand that my participation is voluntary and that I can withdraw from the study at any time without prejudice. I have read the above and agree to enter this research study.

The equivalent paragraphs from February 28, 2000 read:

Questions

You are deciding whether or not to take part in this study. If you sign, it means that you have decided to volunteer after reading and understanding all the information on this form.

Dr. Chabot and his staff will be instructing you on the techniques necessary for all treatments related to this protocol as they pertain to you. If you have any additional questions, please do not hesitate to ask, and we will do our best to answer them. Dr. John Chabot, the physician in charge of this research at the Columbia Presbyterian Medical Center, may be reached at (212) 305–9468 prior to and during your participation in this study should you have any questions about this study. In addition, if you have any questions on your rights as a research subject, you can call the Institutional Review Board at (212) 305–5883 for information.

In the earlier version, Dr. Antman was identified as "The physician in charge of this research," and I was referred to by name three times as an important member of the intake team. Patients were instructed to direct their inquiries, whatever they might be, either to Dr. Antman or to myself. In the last draft, Dr. Chabot now reigned supreme, my name appeared nowhere, and patients were advised to call his office with any questions they might have about the study—even questions pertaining to my treatment.

Significance of my research. The initial September 30, 1997 consent form included a lengthy, objective, truthful report of my previous research efforts, highlighting the positive pilot study data:

> **Study purpose:** The purpose of this research study is to determine whether a new nutritional treatment for cancer, called Enzyme-Nutritional Therapy, is effective in treating pancreatic cancer (adenocarcinoma). You were selected as a possible participant in this study because you have been diagnosed with adenocarcinoma of the pancreas and have not previously received chemotherapy or radiation. Furthermore, you are able to eat normally and care for yourself, both requirements for entrance into the study.

> Background: Dr. Nicholas Gonzalez, one of the investigators of this study, began researching the use of intensive oral pancreatic enzyme therapy as a treatment for cancer in 1981. While a medical student, and later as an immunology fellow, Dr. Gonzalez evaluated 1306 patients who had been treated by an unconventional practitioner who over a twenty year period used enzyme therapy along with dietary and nutritional support. This study included a review of pancreatic cancer patients who survived in excess of five years while receiving this nutritional therapy.

> Since 1987, Dr. Gonzalez has been applying the proteolytic enzyme therapy to patients with advanced, poor prognosis cancer. The treatment also includes

dietary modification, nutritional support in the form of supplements, and detoxification routines such as coffee enemas.

In July of 1993, Dr. Gonzalez was invited to present a series of case reports from his own practice at the National Cancer Institute in Bethesda, Maryland. As a result of that session. [sic] it was suggested that Dr. Gonzalez conduct a pilot study of his treatment in ten patients suffering pancreatic adenocarcinoma using survival as the end point. In collaboration with the NCI, Dr. Gonzalez developed a formal protocol for the study, which was ultimately funded by the research division of the Nestec (Nestle) Corporation.

The study commenced in January, 1994. Eleven patients were eventually entered onto the study and all the patients entered into the trial had advanced or metastatic disease. All, when first seen by Dr. Gonzalez, had a history of significant symptoms consistent with progressing illness.

Despite the advanced state of the patients, the survival overall far exceeded what would be expected for pancreatic cancer. Nine of the eleven patients (including one who quit the study) lived longer than one year. Four patients have already survived 2.5 years, and a fifth, doing very well despite a history of pelvic involvement, will be at two years this December. At that time, three patients will have survived three years and five will have survived at least two years. This data certainly surpasses the results for gemcitabine, the drug recently approved for treatment of pancreatic adenocarcinoma. In the gemcitabine trials, no patient lived 18 months [sic: should be 19 months].

Dr. Gonzalez presented the results of this pilot study on August 4, 1997 at a joint NCI-NIH conference in Bethesda, Maryland. As a result of that conference, it was suggested that Dr. Gonzalez undertake a definitive controlled clinical trial to document more definitively the efficacy of the treatment with pancreatic cancer. Procter & Gamble has agreed to fund the study in its entirety.

As we have seen, in the later version from February 28, 2000, the authors portrayed the pilot study in far more negative terms, with my name now edited out and the tone ominous:

Study Purpose. The purpose of this research study is to determine whether enzyme-nutritional therapy is as effective as a drug called gemcitabine for treating pancreatic adenocarcinoma. We also want to find out what kind of side effects these treatments cause and how often they occur.

Many Americans who develop advanced cancer for which standard treatments have little to offer turn to alternative or complimentary [sic] therapies. Enzyme-nutritional therapy is such a study [sic] which has been reported, in a pilot study of 11 patients, to produce a median survival of 18 months. This survival could have been a result of selection of healthier patients (those who could eat normally). The only way to determine if enzyme nutritional therapy benefits patients with advanced pancreatic cancer is to compare it to standard therapy, gemcitabine. The rationale of those advocating this alternative medicine approach will be explained to you by the physicians and staff involved in this part of the study. However, there is no current conventional medical support for the therapies and assumptions underlying the use of nutritional therapy. The Columbia University College of Physicians and Surgeons does not support its use except as part of a properly conducted clinical trial such as this one.

The lengthy section "Potential Benefits of Study Treatments," initially written by Dr. Wynder and approved by Dr. Antman, underwent major revisions over the years. The September 30, 1997 version included a positive summary of my pilot study, an honest appraisal of the published Gemzar data, and a hopeful vision for the current project:

Potential Benefits of Study Treatments

It is not possible to predict whether your cancer will respond to either the Enzyme-Nutrition, or gemcitabine, treatment. If your cancer does respond you may feel better and live longer. It is hoped that the results of this study will be useful in the development of future treatment for patients with pancreatic cancer.

Specifically, in the pilot study of Enzyme-Nutritional Therapy, patients with pancreatic cancer have lived—and a number of patients continue to live—far longer than would be expected with this serious illness. In addition, the quality of life of these patients has generally been greatly improved by the aggressive nutritional support.

Patients receiving gemcitabine have enjoyed a slight prolongation of life and a significant improvement in their quality of life.

Your participation in this study may be of great benefit to society at large, because you will be involved in helping document whether a non-toxic, nutritional therapy can be of benefit in the treatment of pancreatic cancer. Should

411

the Enzyme-Nutritional Therapy prove to be beneficial to patients, this finding could open up a new avenue of scientific investigation.

In all subsequent drafts this section had been significantly reduced in length and neutered in tone. The final February 28, 2000 issue read:

> **Potential Benefits of Study Treatments.** It is not possible to predict whether your cancer will respond to either the Enzyme-Nutritional Therapy, or gemcitabine treatment. If your cancer does respond you may feel better and live longer. The results of this study may be useful in the development of future treatment for patients with pancreatic cancer.

Prominence of my name. The September 30, 1997 consent document referenced me by name 18 times, the February 28, 2000 edition, not once.

Change in overall attitude of Columbia toward Dr. Isaacs, myself, and our therapy. The two sections "Study Purpose" and "Potential Benefits of Study Treatments" excerpted above revealed in our opinion a significant alteration in attitude on the part of the Columbia team toward us and our treatment. The "Study Purpose" had evolved from a positive—and honest—portrayal of our prior research efforts to the strange warning:

> However, there is no current conventional medical support for the therapies and assumptions underlying the use of nutritional therapy. The Columbia University College of Physicians and Surgeons does not support its use except as part of a properly conducted clinical trial such as this one.

Dr. Antman did send us copies of each draft of the trial documents as they became available, and we did protest, as best we could, all the issues discussed above. But our concerns were either ignored or discounted. It seemed to us that with each new rewrite, Dr. Antman, perhaps Dr. Chabot, and Columbia as an institution sought, at least to some extent, to marginalize both Dr. Isaacs and myself, and make our prior research efforts appear less significant, our therapy less promising. I didn't understand how a negative tone in the official study documents would encourage potentially suitable candidates, all with their lives in the balance, to join the trial. After some prodding on my part, Dr. Antman explained that she faced a largely unsympathetic Columbia administration, particularly several new IRB members who felt they had inherited a trial of a disreputable treatment. Apparently, these individuals would have preferred their institution sever all relation to me, and this study.

Once again, Dr. Isaacs and I felt trapped between our wish to have our therapy appropriately tested and the need to compromise endlessly. Our powerful advocate, Dr. Wynder, had died the previous summer, so he could no longer argue the case on our behalf. But after our conversations with Dr. Antman in the fall of 1999, we believed that unless we asccepted the changes, even the implausible statements about the pilot study in the consent form, the whole project would most likely come to an end.

Nonetheless, I could not comprehend how we could all work together toward the same goal, a fair and honest assessment of my treatment, if the very institution serving as the project site perceived me as less than sympathetic and my treatment less than defensible. If any bias towards us and our therapy existed within Columbia or influenced Columbia policy, I feared it could ultimately undermine the study itself.

Despite our serious doubts about the future of the project, and though we thought about quitting, ultimately we chose not to walk away. As a matter of principle, I do not like abandoning anything midstream, and I knew my mentor Dr. Wynder would have insisted I stay on, whatever the costs, to keep fighting for a just study. So we continued participating and continued cooperating for the sake of the trial which we thought so important, for the benefit of cancer patients everywhere.

Chapter 34

Errors in Data Collection by Dr. Chabot and His Staff

As the project first took shape in 1998, Dr. Antman and I discussed at length the procedures that would be put in place for organizing and interpreting the final results. She emphasized the critical importance, for the trial's purpose to be fulfilled, of collecting reliable data on all entered patients that could then be used to calculate survival time and quality of life for each of the groups of the study. She proposed that the pertinent information on participants should be gathered and updated in an ongoing fashion as the project progressed, to allow for periodic assessments of the effects of the two treatments. At the trial's conclusion, Columbia's statisticians would then analyze the final numbers for presentation in article form.

As we have seen Dr. Antman initially agreed Dr. Isaacs and I could help evaluate study candidates, but from the outset she insisted the Columbia team under her direction would solely assume responsibility for collecting, maintaining, and interpreting all statistical information for each arm, while the trial was in progress and at its conclusion. When Dr. Chabot came on board in early 1998, Dr. Antman informed us he and his staff would henceforth directly supervise the gathering of data and its analysis, with the help of the Columbia statisticians, and with no input from us. Later, when the NCI and NCCAM joined the project, their respective personnel assigned to the study agreed that Dr. Chabot should remain in charge of this aspect of the trial.

Of course, we were to assist Dr. Chabot in his task by providing copies of all records, as they were created, of all patients assigned to the nutrition arm, whether reporting an office visit with us, a phone call with the patient, a lab test, or radiology study. We were also to pass on to Dr. Chabot copies of all additional information we might receive such as a letter from a consulting doctor. Dr. Chabot and his team would organize these documents in the respective patient files, enter the information on the Columbia computers, and periodically calculate the survival statistics for the two groups.

Once the trial began accruing patients, we cooperated fully with these requirements, sending to Dr. Chabot, on an ongoing basis, copies of every record generated on every study subject sent to us for treatment. In addition, though we understood that Dr. Chabot and his staff were ultimately in charge of the process, Dr. Isaacs and I created a flow sheet for our patients on our office computer, which we regularly updated. This chart included each patient's identifying number, date of biopsy, stage of disease at the time of diagnosis, date of first consultation in our office, status as of last contact, survival time, and any pertinent comments related to compliance or physical condition.

Beginning in March of 2003, Dr. Isaacs and I began handing out copies of this document to the Columbia, NCCAM, and NCI staff attending the regularly scheduled group meetings. Though we assumed Dr. Chabot also kept a similar chart for the two arms of the trial, to that point he had been distributing only a summary statement of survival for the nutrition and chemotherapy groups presented in graph form, but not a listing of each individual patient entered into the two arms with their stage and status identified.

More than a year later, at the July 29, 2004 group meeting, Dr. Chabot distributed a sheet containing more detailed information, this time listing every patient admitted into each arm, the date of entry into the study, the treatment each received, their status (alive or dead), and the date of death for those that had died. At the time Dr. Chabot described a total of 38 nutrition patients but only 12 in the chemotherapy group. Unfortunately, the chart did not include information about the staging distribution of patients, so we couldn't compare the two groups in this important regard—this data would not be made available to us until the pivotal December 13, 2004 session.

Dr. Isaacs and I could not independently verify the survival information for the chemotherapy patients, since we had been kept in total darkness regarding this group. But after the meeting, as we carefully reviewed the information on our own patients provided by Dr. Chabot, we identified nine errors, some minor, some major, which I list below (using Dr. Chabot's identifying numbers):

Patient #103: wrong date of death listed, actually died a year earlier than reported

Patient #107: wrong date of death listed

Patient #110: wrong date of death listed

Patient #118: wrong date of death listed

Patient #119: wrong date of death listed

Patient #120: wrong date given for two year survival

Patient #125: wrong date given for six month survival

Patient #129: wrong date of death listed, died a year earlier than reported

Patient #135: reported as entering the trial many months after she actually entered

Patient #139: wrong date of death listed, died a year earlier than reported

In response to the multiple errors, Dr. Isaacs and I created an erratum, which on August 2, 2004 we e-mailed to all the Columbia, NCCAM, and NCI supervisors who had attended the meeting. When Dr. Isaacs and I discussed the situation further after sending our corrections, we agreed Dr. Chabot's staff might require some oversight, to help insure the data on our patients would be properly recorded. So that afternoon I e-mailed Dr. Chabot, asking if either Dr. Isaacs or myself could go to his office to check the information entered into the Columbia computer system, with the intent of rectifying any additional errors:

We assume you got our earlier e-mail with the corrections for the "Data Chart" that was presented at the meeting.

We forgot to bring it up on Thursday, but another issue we wanted to discuss was when we might have the opportunity to proof the information that has been entered about our patients in whatever system is being used for analyzing the data. Linda was at a meeting with Cara some time back during which Cara was ready to characterize a patient's worsened liver functions as worsening liver metastases when in fact it was biliary obstruction. That, along with the corrections as above, and knowing the pressure Cara has been under recently, makes us want to double check things.

In a subsequent phone conversation, Dr. Chabot informed me we would not be allowed to review any records in his office, period.

During the December 13, 2004 group meeting, Dr. Chabot handed out his "updated" data sheet that now included staging information for the two groups. He had arranged the patients in two columns, one headed "Chemotherapy," the other "Enzyme therapy," with the total number entered into each arm appearing at the top of the respective column. To my surprise he listed only 36 nutrition patients, not the 38 that had been actually approved and admitted, and which we had carefully documented on our own chart we distributed that same day.

Further down on the page, he grouped the patients by stage, with 12 nutrition subjects or 35.3% described at stages II and III, and 22, or 64.7% at stage IV. None of this made any sense for several reasons. First of all, 12 earlier stage and 22 later stage patients added up to 34—a number at odds with the 36 "Enrolled" patients reported at the top of the same column. The numbers weren't even internally consistent within the chart, and certainly did not match up with the 38 that had actually been qualified. Furthermore, of the 38 nutrition subjects that to that date had been actually accepted into the study, Dr. Isaacs and I had identified, based on the medical records, 24% at stages II and III, 76% at stage IV, percentages far different from what Dr. Chabot reported.

Unfortunately, it was impossible for us to pinpoint the source of the discrepancy, since he had provided only the total numbers he had assigned to each stage without identifying the individual patients and their stage. When I questioned Dr. Chabot about the differences between our data and his regarding the numbers entered into our group and the staging distribution, he had no answers but said he would "look into it." Dr. Isaacs and I were concerned that within the same chart, in the space of several lines, Dr. Chabot had cited two different total numbers for those entered into the nutrition arm, first 36, then 34, neither correct by our tally. These errors, which Dr. Chabot could not explain, left me troubled.

Later that day, after we returned to our office from Columbia, Dr. Isaacs e-mailed Dr. Grann hoping he might intervene to correct the errors:

Victor:

Just as a followup to our conversation:

I would love to get our records in synch so that we all have the same number of people in our arm of the study.

I would also love to review the actual data entry, as there have been a number of little glitches (like only 2 people being alive instead of 3).

In that e-mail Dr. Isaacs also discussed our unsuccessful efforts to learn the status of the two missing consent forms.

Two weeks later, on December 30, 2004, Dr. Chabot's assistant Cara DeRosa contacted us after Dr. Grann had forwarded our earlier e-mail to her.

Linda/Victor:

The two patient's [sic] she [meaning Dr. Isaacs] mentions below without consent forms have been reported previously to the Cancer Center at the time of their registration. We also discussed this problem at our last meeting.

With regard to who is alive/deceased: I believe — and — are still alive. I just received a death notice on —.

Regards,

Cara

We had no idea what meeting Ms. DeRosa meant, since the informed consent issue had not been discussed at our previous group session. So three days later, on January 2, 2005, Dr. Isaacs replied:

Thanks for your response, but I wasn't present at the meeting you were at where these issues were discussed, and I still don't know what the answers are to the questions I asked.

Meanwhile, during this period I completed my lengthy letter to Dr. Killen written in response to his statements at the December 13, 2004 group meeting. I sent this out to the various study supervisors during the first week of January 2005, and as we awaited a reply we still received no clarification from either Dr. Grann or Ms. DeRosa regarding the discrepancies between the official Columbia data and ours, and the missing consent forms. Finally, on February 4, 2005, we wrote Dr. Chabot directly about these two specific issues:

John:

We have been trying for some time now to figure out why there is a discrepancy in our records regarding how many patients are on the study, and which patients are not on the study. Linda spoke with Victor briefly about this at the last meeting and e-mailed him in followup. He forwarded it to Cara, who sent us an answer we did not understand, referring to a meeting we did not attend. We received no response to our request for clarification. See below if you wish to review the correspondence.

Any chance of getting this sorted out before the next meeting? We are also concerned that [Patient #28] who is very much alive, had been listed as being dead. . . .

We have been trying to get copies of the consent forms for [Patient #16] and [Patient #9] for quite some time now, and both Michelle and Cara say that the other person has them. Some intervention here would be appreciated. . . .

Dr. Chabot responded as follows:

Last week, Michelle went through all the charts to confirm data accuracy. It is loaded loaded [sic] into the system now. I will get any new graphs to you when available

Nonetheless, the errors in data entry at Columbia would continue.

Chapter 35

A Second Look at Patients Misstaged On Dr. Chabot's April 22, 2006 Data Chart

D r. Chabot entered the final patient into the nutrition arm in April 2005, several months before the study closed to accrual. I did not receive the final listing of each trial subject admitted into the two arms until April 27, 2006, more than a year later. As I have discussed, Dr. Chabot sent the document along with a letter in which he strongly defended his management of the study and denied he had admitted any patient into the nutrition arm who failed to meet the entrance criteria.

On the data sheet, this time Dr. Chabot included every patient he had approved for the nutritional and chemotherapy arms, their stage when admitted, and their calculated survival at the time the study closed. Again, we had no way to judge the accuracy of the entries for the chemotherapy patients, since we had never seen their records and knew only what Dr. Chabot told us about them. As for the nutrition group, Dr. Chabot had tallied a total of 37 patients, not the 39 we had been counting since the last subject approved a year earlier, and one less than the 38 he had identified in his previous March 2005 chart. Once again, he had modified the numbers with no explanation. And of the 37 Dr. Chabot now included as admitted and treated, he reported 22 subjects, or 59%

of the group as stage IV, and 15, or 40.5% as earlier stages. His numbers didn't essentially differ from those provided in March 2005, when he reported 38 total nutrition patients with 23, or 60.53% at stage IV, and 15, or 39.47% at stages II and III, but his calculations differed from our tabulation of the staging distribution. But now, since on his April 2006 data chart Chabot had identified each patient with his version of their stage, I could finally determine why his numbers and ours differed so significantly.

We immediately noticed that he no longer included two stage IV subjects, Patients #9 and #16, for whom no evidence existed for the required signed consent forms. During the March 2006 group meeting Dr. Chabot had claimed, as the official minutes confirmed, that the Columbia IRB approved the inclusion of these two patients as valid entries despite the missing documents.

We also noticed that Dr. Chabot identified five patients, #3, #14, #26, #27, and #33, at a lesser stage than we believed appropriate according to their medical records. To add some context, by that late date we had criticized Dr. Chabot repeatedly for entering primarily early stage patients into the chemotherapy arm, and largely late stage IV subjects for treatment with us, arguing that such an imbalance alone invalidated any comparison between the two groups. By eliminating Patients #9 and #16—both diagnosed as stage IV—from the nutrition group and by reassigning five additional patients to a lesser stage, Dr. Chabot had, whether intentionally or not, helped neutralize the staging disparity between the two arms.

Earlier in Chapter 2, I mentioned these five patients Dr. Chabot assigned to a lesser stage than we believe appropriate. In the discussion that follows I enlarge on my earlier analysis somewhat, referencing the actual medical records that indicated a diagnosis of stage IV disease in these five patients. Note that these documents had been gathered by Dr. Chabot's own staff, so certainly he had access to this information himself, and as PI he was required to read them all.

Patient #26: Dr. Isaacs first met with this patient on November 20, 2000. In her note from that day, she clearly reported the diagnosis of extensive, stage IV metastatic cancer:

> Then had CT scan 10/20/00 [showing] multiple liver mets, largest was 2.0 X 1.5 cm. . . .

The actual CT report confirming stage IV disease read:

> Multiple low attenuation regions in the liver compatible with presumed areas of metastatic disease.

Patient #3: Dr. Isaacs first met with Patient #3 on November 26, 2002. In her note from that day she documented the findings of stage IV metastatic pancreatic cancer:

> Subsequently, she was referred to Vanderbilt University Med Center where she underwent laparoscopy on 11/21/02. She was found to have encasement of the hepatic artery and biopsy with one peritoneal biopsy + [positive] for adenocarcinoma. She was therefore deemed unresectable.

The operative report from her surgery read:

> In the peritoneum overlying the right subcostal margin, there was another nodule that appeared more suspicious to me. The liver had a couple of little small white plaque like lesions which I did not think were metastases, but I could not be sure. . . .

> I biopsied the liver twice. . . . The liver upper quadrant nodules were biopsied. The right upper quadrant nodule was biopsied.

The liver lesions proved to be benign, but the peritoneal lesion was consistent with metastatic adenocarcinoma, confirming stage IV disease.

Patient #27: Dr. Isaacs first met with Patient #27 on October 24, 2003. In her note from that day, she described extensive stage IV metastatic malignancy:

> CT of abd/pelvis [showed] small L pleural effusion; pulmonary emboli in RLL; irregular thickening of omentum; soft tissue fullness in pancreatic body. . . .

> CT scan guided needle biopsy of omental mass was done on 10/6/03, and was + [positive] for poorly differentiated carcinoma.

The official cytopathology report of the omental biopsy unequivocally described poorly differentiated carcinoma, confirming stage IV.

Patient #14: After meeting with Patient #14 on December 18, 2002, in her note from that day Dr. Isaacs recorded metastatic disease:

> On 11/8/02 she underwent FNA of peripancreatic lymph node [showing] adenocarcinoma. Based on metastatic disease, she was felt to be unresectable.

The report of a CT scan dated December 2, 2002 indicated:

1. Pancreatic head/neck cancer with extensive infiltration surrounding the celiac axis. SMA [Superior Mesenteric Artery] SMV [Superior Mesenteric Vein] and root of the small bowel mesentery rendering the lesion unresectable. . . .

2. Shotty mesentery and retroperitoneal lymphadenopathy.

Dr. Chabot, before rendering his decision about eligibility, requested the Pathology Department at Columbia review the slides of the lymph node biopsy to verify the diagnosis. The final Columbia report dated December 26, 2002 described "Poorly differentiated adenocarcinoma."

The 6th Edition of the DeVita text, *Cancer: Principles & Practice of Oncology*, current during the time of the trial, provided a chart defining each of the four stages of pancreatic cancer. Stage IV not only included those patients diagnosed with distant metastases into an organ like the liver or lung, but as in this case when:

> Tumor extends directly to any of the following: stomach, spleen, colon, or adjacent large vessels.[29(p1131)]

The positive lymph node biopsy, the CT findings of tumor invading into the "large vessels" of the abdomen, and the multiple additional enlarged lymph nodes proved stage IV disease in this patient.

Patient #33: I first met Patient #33 on December 6, 2001, at which time he reported that an initial CT scan showed no evidence of metastasis. However, after his biopsy diagnosis at a local hospital but prior to seeking entry into our trial, he had traveled to MD Anderson in Houston for a second opinion. There, he told me that a second CT scan of the abdomen had revealed multiple lesions in the liver consistent with stage IV disease.

In my note describing this first meeting with the patient I summarized the new information:

> Then on October 25, 2000, the patient underwent ERCP with biopsy of the lesion in the pancreatic head. Pathology diagnosis showed adenocarcinoma of the pancreas. . . .

> In late October, the patient went to MD Anderson. He spent several days there and was seen by the specialist in pancreatic cancer, Dr. Abruzzi [sic, should be Abbruzzese]. At MD Anderson (again, according to the patient) the CAT scans

were repeated confirming a tumor in the head of the pancreas. According to the patient, they thought that there was evidence of liver metastases.

For reasons that remain unclear to me, Dr. Chabot had not sent us—as was his responsibility—the MD Anderson records. Perhaps Dr. Chabot simply wasn't aware the patient had been to Houston, or of the testing completed there, so the records were never requested. Perhaps his staff did request the records, which MD Anderson then failed to send. Perhaps they were received, but then lost—who knows? In my initial conversation with Patient #33 I did learn easily enough of the MD Anderson visit, duly recording this information about the trip in my note from that day, copies of which my staff then sent on to Dr. Chabot. Even if Dr. Chabot, during his own intake interview, somehow failed to hear of the MD Anderson consultation and the testing done there, he had in his possession copies of my office files on this patient which as Principal Investigator he was supposed to read carefully.

Therefore, from my records alone Dr. Chabot should have been cognizant of the MD Anderson evaluation, the CT scan apparently done there, and the presumed findings of stage IV disease. He should also have requested, as was his duty, copies of the relevant records if the patient had failed to provide them to his office.

Once Dr. Isaacs and I realized Dr. Chabot had officially categorized this patient at a stage lower than IV, and that the MD Anderson files apparently had never been requested, or if requested, had never been received, or if received, had been lost, we ourselves did try to obtain the missing documents. By law, no hospital or doctor can legally release copies of medical records to anyone, including another physician, without an authorization signed by the patient, or, for those who are deceased, an authorization signed by the legally appointed executor of the estate. Unfortunately, by the time we began our efforts, the patient had died and we could never locate any surviving family members, so to this day the MD Anderson records remain missing. Consequently, this patient is best described at "indeterminate" stage, or "presumptively at stage IV." Certainly the patient should not be classified definitively at a lesser stage, as did Dr. Chabot on his data chart.

Some Final Comments About Dr. Chabot's Errors

Of course, an occasional mistake in data entry, with so many numbers to track, would hardly prove much. However, the above documentation illustrates a pattern of errors over the years of the trial requiring our vigilance for correction. Some of these admittedly may have been minor in nature, but some—like the downgraded staging of five patients in Dr. Chabot's final data sheet—represent significant deviations from the facts.

It's ironic that NCCAM and the NCI, the institutions ultimately responsible for overseeing this study, not only excluded Dr. Isaacs and myself from the evaluation of trial candidates, but also prohibited us from monitoring Dr. Chabot's handling of the data. Furthermore, in 2004, after we first became aware of the multiple inaccuracies in the notes he distributed to us, Dr. Chabot rejected outright our suggestion that one of us go to his office to check his computerized flow sheets for accuracy. He and his staff apparently did not need our help, they would do it all themselves. So the errors continued right up until the last data chart sent us in April 2006, in some ways the most inaccurate of all.

Chapter 36

My Growing Concerns About OHRP

After finishing the first draft of my McNeilly monograph in mid-August 2007, I immediately began work on a final rewrite. About a week later, Dr. McNeilly phoned my office while I was in the middle of a patient consultation. I took the call with the patient sitting in front of me, and to my surprise and without asking if I could talk freely, in an angry tone Dr. McNeilly demanded I explain why I hadn't sent the documentation, as he said, "you claim to have." He then announced that *my* delay in responding to his "simple" request had held up the entire investigation—as if the process had taken over a year because of me. Listening to him, for the first time I began to wonder if OHRP had really taken my complaints seriously.

I remained calm for the sake of the patient in my office who already must have been wondering who the caller might be. I reminded Dr. McNeilly that he had initially asked for "all documents" that might help counter Chabot's various claims, an enormous undertaking in and of itself. Due to its complexity, I explained, the project had taken some time, and since the mass of written evidence numbered many hundreds of pages, I had decided to write up a narrative to accompany the records and clarify their significance.

He responded in an even angrier tone, telling me he had never suggested anything be written, all he wanted were the "documents." His office, he made clear with great irritation, "could figure out what to do with the papers without your help." I responded that the copied records would not make much sense without an explanation, a roadmap so to speak, and I needed only a few more days to complete the final editing. I reminded him that when we had talked earlier in June he never once implied I faced an imminent deadline of any sort, in fact quite the opposite. I also repeated what he had told me in our previous phone conversation, when he assured me I had no target date to meet and should get the material to him when it was ready.

McNeilly retorted that he didn't care about editing or final drafts, he wanted the records before the weekend. I told him his demand would be impossible to meet since we still needed to copy the documents and arrange them in final order before sending them out. Collating these papers, which Dr. Isaacs and I would do between our patient responsibilities, might take several days. He only sternly repeated his demand that the documents be sent immediately, before getting off the phone.

After finishing my patient session, I discussed the situation with Dr. Isaacs and later over the phone with Beth Clay, the Washington consultant who many times had helped me maneuver through the various federal bureaucracies. Ms. Clay was disappointed in the turn of events and McNeilly's attitude, particularly since Dr. Borror at OHRP had already informed me that Columbia had been given some six months to answer my original charges.

I worked on the manuscript non-stop through the weekend, but hadn't quite finished the editing when McNeilly called early the following week, again while I was with a patient. He appeared to be even more irate this time around, demanding to know why he had not received the documents I had "promised to send." When I told him I hadn't promised to send anything before the weekend and needed only a couple more days to finish the project properly, he answered that there were no more "days," he wanted all the information shipped to him by Labor Day (the following weekend). Since I seemed to have little choice, I agreed to send the materials but warned I had not finished cleaning up the narrative for any remaining grammatical or spelling errors. When he became still more exasperated, I then challenged him, asking him why he had not told me weeks earlier of this impending deadline. As hard as I had been working on this in the context of a full load of patients, if necessary I could have stayed even later in the evenings and longer on weekends.

Suddenly, his manner changed abruptly. He told me, his voice still full of frustration but not anger, that he was leaving OHRP within two weeks and needed to get this project finished. To my complete surprise, he then said that "Columbia is pressing us to get back to them." I thought to myself, since when did Columbia, the object of this investigation, set the ground rules for OHRP?

When, trying to make conversation and diffuse the situation, I asked him if he was staying within the NIH or going into industry, he responded, "staying within the government." I had no idea what had transpired at OHRP, but whatever the reason for his upcoming departure, I suspected his superiors were urging him to finish this investigation quickly and he simply transferred the pressure onto me.

So on August 30, 2007 I did send a box of documents, including my not quite finished manuscript, to Dr. McNeilly, followed five days later by the corrected and edited final version of the narrative. This most recent episode with McNeilly, his manner on the phone while I was in the midst of consulting with patients, his statement about Columbia, his planned transfer out of OHRP—all left me feeling less than confident about the situation. From that time forward Dr. Isaacs and I prepared ourselves to expect that the ultimate government findings, whenever they might appear and whatever they might be, most likely would not reflect the full truth of this eight-year long clinical trial.

In the days following my last conversation with McNeilly, I went to the official OHRP website a number of times to study their online postings, referred to as "determination letters," summarizing previous investigations of alleged mismanagement. Most ORHP actions seemed prompted by fairly mild instances of human error, the result of misunderstanding or carelessness, not deliberate malfeasance. Often the penalties levied appeared to be equivalently tepid in nature, a rap on the knuckles, gentle warnings, in some more serious cases suggestions about retraining of staff in the methods of clinical trial management. I began to wonder, as I read all this, if OHRP had the moxie to tackle the many serious issues I had raised regarding my clinical trial.

Chapter 37

OHRP Doesn't Come Through

After sending off the newest batch of documents to Dr. McNeilly, Dr. Isaacs and I waited for OHRP to reach some sort of conclusion about the management of our study. Dr. Borror had long ago advised me that upon completing its investigation, her office would post the findings on the OHRP website under the category "Determination Letters." I checked the section at least once a week, but time passed with no word. By November 2007, some 17 months after my first contact with OHRP and three months since my last conversation with Dr. McNeilly, we still had heard nothing. I discussed my frustration over the slow pace with Beth Clay and Congressman Burton's aide Monica Knab who had been following the issue closely. Finally, in mid-November 2007, the Congressman, himself somewhat perplexed about the situation, wrote to Dr. Ivor Pritchard, the OHRP acting director, recounting some of my grievances, summarizing again the alleged mismanagement, and asking for an update on the status of the OHRP evaluation.

After enumerating four major areas of concern, the Congressman wrote:

> While I do not wish to compromise an ongoing investigation, I am extremely interested in the final resolution of this matter and would greatly appreciate an update on where your investigation stands.

As you may know, the Pancreatic Proteolytic Enzyme Therapy study was the first direct clinical comparison funded by NIH of a non-traditional cancer treatment protocol versus conventional chemotherapy. In the opinion of many, this study represented a groundbreaking effort to scientifically validate the success of complimentary [sic] and alternative forms of cancer treatment. As am [sic] sure you can appreciate, should the allegations of misconduct prove true, it would compromise the study results and represent a serious blow to other efforts to scientifically-support the so far anecdotal evidence of the power of alternative and complimentary [sic] forms of medicine. In addition, should the allegations prove true, it would reinforce in the minds of many America [sic] who believe in alternative therapies that our Federal health agencies are biased against non-traditional, non-pharmaceutical-based medicine.

I appreciate that the professional reputations and perhaps the livelihoods of Dr. Chabot and members of the NCI and NCCAM staff are at stake and that you owe it to them to conduct a thorough investigation. However, I hope that you appreciate that the longer your investigation drags out—particularly if the allegations prove true—the stronger the suspicion grows in the minds of some that NIH is attempting to suppress bad news that undermines a scientific result the agency politically agrees with.

In my opinion, there is an expectation among the scientific community and the general public that all NIH-funded studies are conducted with an open mind, scientific rigor and proper attention to all human research protections. I believe that we owe it to the American people, and especially the cancer community, to reinforce that expectation by removing the cloud of uncertainty hanging over the Pancreatic Proteolytic Enzyme Therapy study as soon as possible.

A month later, in a three-paragraph note dated December 13, 2007, Dr. Pritchard responded to Congressman Burton, essentially saying nothing of any substance. He summed up his position by stating what we all already knew:

As you are aware, OHRP has initiated an evaluation of the matter referenced in your letter. The evaluation is ongoing and may take some time to complete. OHRP will advise Dr. Gonzalez and you when the evaluation has been completed.

Finally, on March 10, 2008, 21 months after my initial conversation with Dr. Borror, OHRP posted its findings on their website in the form of a letter addressed to Steven Shea, M.D., Vice President & Dean's Office, Columbia

University Medical Center. Dated February 25, 2008, the report consisted of less than a full page of text, with the relevant paragraphs reading:

Thank you for your January 15, 2008 response to our letter of September 14, 2007 regarding the above-reference research. Based on the information submitted to us, we make the following determination regarding this research:

(1) Subject 113 was enrolled into the study more than 8 weeks after undergoing biopsy of his pancreatic tumor, which was inconsistent with the inclusion criteria stipulated in the institutional review board (IRB)-approved protocol. Department of Health and Human Services (HHS) regulations at 45 CFR 46.103(b)(4)(iii) require that the IRB review and approve all proposed changes in a research activity, during the period for which IRB approval has already been given, prior to initiation of such changes, except when necessary to eliminate apparent immediate hazards to the subjects. We determine that the enrollment of subject 113, who did not meet all eligibility criteria, represented a change in the research activity that was implemented without IRB approval.

(2) We note that Columbia University Medical Center (CUMC) found that for 40 of 62 subjects it appeared that informed consent was not documented with a signed written consent form prior to the initiation of research activities involving human subjects (e.g., receipt and analysis of identifiable private information and pathology tissue specimens, or completion of rating forms or patient diary entries), although it was documented prior to the subjects undergoing other research interventions dictated by the protocol. HHS regulations at 45 CFR 46.177(a) require that informed consent be documented by the use of a written consent form approved by the IRB and that is signed by the subject, or the subject's legally authorized representative, unless the IRB waives this requirement. We determined that the informed consent for the 40 of 62 subjects referenced by CUMC was not documented prior to the start of research activities, nor was the requirement for documentation waived by the CUMC IRB for subjects in this study.

Required Action: Please provide us with a corrective action plan that addresses the above determinations by March 21, 2008. If you need assistance in developing a corrective action plan, please feel free to contact us.

We appreciate the continued commitment of your institution to the protection of human research subjects. Please do not hesitate to contact me should you have any questions.

Paul J. Andreason, M.D., identified as "Compliance Oversight Coordinator" had signed the document.

As I read and reread the letter, I felt somewhat perplexed by its brevity, considering I had provided well over 600 pages of evidence to the OHRP including my two monographs accompanied by supporting documents. So, I thought to myself, less than a full page after all this?

True, some of the determination postings I had studied on the OHRP website were short, but few were as brief as this one, and many went on for pages. For example, one six-page letter dated February 27, 2008 appeared online around the time of the Columbia response. Addressed to an official at the University of Washington Office of Research in Seattle, the report discussed at length a *single* waived consent form not appropriately documented in the records. Did such an innocent sounding oversight warrant such in-depth analysis, but my hundreds of pages of evidence only a comparatively meager response?

At least in the first paragraph of its Columbia letter, OHRP substantiated my claim that Chabot admitted Subject 113 into the nutritional arm of the study beyond the eight-week cutoff from biopsy, a clear protocol violation. However, Dr. Andreason said nothing about the two other patients Chabot sent to us for treatment who failed the eight-week rule.

Furthermore, in the second long manuscript I prepared for Dr. McNeilly, I had discussed in some detail a total of 16 patients Chabot accepted into the nutrition arm who by the available evidence we believed did not qualify for the study. In addition to the three patients diagnosed more than eight weeks from biopsy, I had described 11 who could not eat adequately at the time of entry as required by the protocol, three Chabot approved despite psychiatric illness—another reason for exclusion—and one lacking social support, again as mandated by the written rules of the trial (there was some overlap, with two patients failing more than one entry criteria). And to my great disappointment, the OHRP letter made no mention of patients such as Patient #38, whom Dr. Chabot kept waiting for weeks before coming to a conclusion about eligibility.

The second paragraph appearing at the top of page 2 left me somewhat baffled:

> Columbia University Medical Center (CUMC) found that for 40 of 62 subjects it appeared that informed consent was not documented with a signed written consent form prior to the initiation of research activities . . . although it was

documented prior to the subjects undergoing other research interventions dictated by the protocol.

When I first read this, I was dumbfounded that *40 of 62 patients* ultimately entered had not been properly consented—proof within this one brief page of text that Chabot had not managed the admission process properly. But the OHRP letter seemed to imply that eventually Chabot obtained written consent for all of these 40 patients "prior to the subjects undergoing other research interventions dictated by the protocol." As I have previously discussed at some length, Dr. Isaacs and I identified three patients sent to us for treatment for whom no evidence existed of a completed consent form, contrary to Dr. Andreason's claim that at some point all approved patients signed the documents.

Nonetheless, 40 patients improperly consented? What was going on in Chabot's office? However, as far as I was concerned after all this time OHRP still had not done the job properly.

I was also surprised to read that "Columbia University Medical Center (CUMC) found that for 40 of 62 subjects it appeared that informed consent was not documented" as if the institution itself conducted the investigation, not the OHRP—a strange scenario, I thought, if truly the case. Did OHRP really stay on the sidelines, relying on the findings of an internal audit conducted by the very place under scrutiny? I could understand full well that with allegations of serious mismanagement levied against one of its top physician researchers, Columbia would appropriately wish to look into the situation itself, regardless of any federal probe. I had also filed a complaint with the Dean of Columbia against Chabot, Grann, and Fine after their attempt to publish in *JAMA* without my knowledge—an action that inevitably would have prompted some type of internal review of the study. But why would the OHRP, a governmental agency, refer to a Columbia evaluation as a basis for its findings, in essence allowing the fox to guard the henhouse? Shouldn't OHRP have pursued its own investigation, independent of what Columbia might or might not choose to do?

If, as the letter implied, Columbia took the lead, the situation became even trickier considering my relationship to that academic center, the nature of the therapy to be tested in this clinical trial, and the origins of OHRP involvement. Neither Dr. Isaacs nor I have ever been Columbia staffers, nor did we have any affiliation with that university in any way, other than as participants with the clinical study. Columbia owed us no loyalty whatsoever. Chabot, on the other hand, was (and is) a Columbia lifer, who completed his surgical residency there before working his way up to the important position of Chief, Division of General Surgery.

Not only were we complete Columbia outsiders, but we practiced an unconventional, nutritionally-based controversial therapy that, according to Dr. Antman, the Columbia administration approached with great caution and with little enthusiasm. I believed that the changes in both the protocol document and consent form over the years reflected some discomfort with me, my therapy, and this study. Then, to make matters worse, I, the outsider, the fringe practitioner, actually filed the complaint claiming mismanagement by Columbia staff.

Perhaps Columbia intended to conduct a relentless, hard-hitting, objective, unbiased probe of my allegations against one of its own respected professors regardless of my outsider status, the nature of the therapy Dr. Isaacs and I practiced, and we being the source of the complaint. And perhaps OHRP did not, in its decision-making process, depend primarily on Columbia's own internal audit of the clinical trial. But if Columbia did take the lead it is hardly irrational at least to wonder if its investigators might have wished to soften the findings, hoping to ward off a potential scandal—perhaps even lawsuits from me—and protect its stellar reputation against the allegations of an alternative outsider whom few of its senior staff apparently respected.

Despite my disappointment with the OHRP findings, at least Dr. Isaacs and I had been vindicated to a significant degree. However Columbia and the OHRP arrived at the number 40, the improper consenting of so many patients in a study consisting of only 62 total subjects, counting both arms together, did confirm, might I say, less than ideal management.

Unfortunately, nowhere did the writer, Dr. Andreason, identify Dr. Chabot as the culprit, the person solely responsible for the admission of Subject 113 or the problems with consent. Andreason did reference Chabot in two places, first at the top of the letter as the "Principal Investigator" of the trial and then again after the concluding paragraph in a list of those individuals copied. But Chabot's name did not appear in the body of the letter itself. Dr. Andreason mentioned me only once, in parenthesis in the study title on the first page. From our perspective, a casual reader perusing the document might easily think Dr. Isaacs and I were the guilty parties.

The letter ended cordially, as if Columbia and OHRP had worked well together, pursuing some flaws in the consent process and perhaps a single error in judgment in the case of "Subject 113." With appropriate corrective action, all, apparently, would be well. OHRP suggested no real punishment, no limitation on Chabot's research activity, only a plan for "corrective action."

After his signature at the bottom of the second page, Dr. Andreason listed the names of six individuals whom he had copied, including, in the order in which they appear: Mr. George Gasparis, Executive Director, Human Subjects Protection Program, CUMC [Columbia University Medical Center]; Dr. Andrew Wit, Chair IRB #1, CUMC; Dr. Neil Schluger, Chair IRB #3, CUMC; Dr. Chabot; Dr. Sherry Mills, NIH; and Mr. Joseph Ellis, NIH.

The name at the bottom of the list, Joseph Ellis, I recognized from documents I had seen as someone working within Dr. Zerhouni's office at the NIH. I wondered if he was involved in any way with the director's factually inaccurate December 2005 response to Congressman Burton. I didn't know who Dr. Mills might be, but the descriptions of her I found easily enough on the NIH website indicated, at least to me, that she was yet another mid-level professional NIH bureaucrat, moving from one position to another. Chabot, of course, I knew well, but I had never heard of the two other physician-members of the Columbia IRB copied by Andreason. The name heading the list, Mr. George Gasparis, Executive Director, Human Subjects Protection Program, CUMC, I immediately recalled from conversations with Dr. Chabot about the Columbia IRB.

According to what Dr. Antman had told me, initially the IRB seemed at least somewhat supportive of our project, giving its blessing without any great delay to the early protocol drafts and thus permitting the study to proceed at Columbia. This backing was hardly trivial, since at any academic center the IRB wields extraordinary power, responsible as it is for approving or disapproving each and every proposed research effort. At its discretion the IRB can also stop a clinical trial already in progress. Furthermore, the rules at Columbia specified that all ongoing research studies must undergo yearly reassessment, with the ever-looming threat that for whatever reason, the IRB could shut down a project midstream without much appeal possible.

During the first five years of our study, from 1998 until early 2003, the Columbia IRB, despite the unusual and controversial nature of my treatment and this trial, granted the yearly approval without apparent delay, even when the design changed from a randomized format to matched cohort. But in late 2003, Dr. Chabot informed us of drastic changes in the IRB staff, including the arrival of a new director with significant power, a Mr. George Gasparis, identified as neither a physician nor scientist. I did not make much of his lack of academic credentials, since IRB members usually arrive with a variety of professional backgrounds; many are health care workers and researchers from within the institution, but the group usually includes lawyers, so-called academic experts in "ethics" as well as interested lay people from the community.

Initially I thought personnel shifts must occur regularly at any medical institution, but some time later, Chabot warned us that many of the new IRB members viewed our clinical trial with great skepticism—even contempt. Such disdain I knew presented more than an annoyance since the IRB could stop our study at any time for any reason, under the guise of protection of human research subjects. According to Chabot, when our project next came up for its regular review, the IRB members barely voted to renew its approval, against some vociferous objections.

After reading the OHRP determination letter of March 2008, I searched the Internet looking for tidbits of interest about Mr. Gasparis, Executive Director, Human Subjects Protection Program. I did not have to look too far on the Columbia site, where I quickly located an official biography appearing in a section entitled "Bioethics." According to the document, Mr. Gasparis' academic training consisted of an undergraduate degree from George Washington University, though the writer failed to specify the field of concentration. However, I was somewhat startled, to say the least, to read about his previous employment:

> George Gasparis is the Asst. Vice President and Sr. Asst. Dean for Research Ethics at Columbia University Medical Center. He also serves as the Executive Director, Human Subjects Protection Program for both Columbia University and Columbia University Medical Center. In this capacity, he is responsible for developing and implementing a comprehensive human subjects protection program and for the administration for four IRBs at Columbia. Prior to his arrival at Columbia University in June 2003, Mr. Gasparis was the Director for the Division of Assurances and Quality Improvement at the Office for Human

Research Protections (OHRP). He started at OHRP (at the time OPRR) in 1996 as an Assurance Coordinator.[75]

This information about Gasparis' connection to OHRP certainly caught my attention. To begin with, I could only conclude that Gasparis must have participated in the investigation of my complaints, probably in a major way. The OHRP letter to the Columbia Dean itself proved that point, since his name appeared at the top of the list of those copied. One would also logically assume that the "Executive Director, Human Subjects Protection Program" would play a role in Columbia's response to allegations of misbehavior by its staff, involving patients enrolled in a federally funded research study. But I suspected he served as far more than a simple liaison with the government, since OHRP apparently turned the undertaking over to Columbia—as the determination letter implied. It would therefore not be irrational to suspect Gasparis may have at least coordinated Columbia's investigation of itself. It this was the case, I questioned the propriety of Gasparis, a former OHRP official, essentially overseeing his previous employer's investigation of the institution where he now worked.

Overall, the OHRP posting left me feeling somewhat distressed. How could Columbia or the OHRP or whoever did the actual work ignore the 16 patients whom I believed on the basis of available evidence should not have been entered into this study? Reasonable men and women might argue over some of these cases, but the majority simply did not meet the explicit written criteria of the protocol. And how could the OHRP, with evidence that in three cases no signed consent forms existed, state in their determination letter that all patients eventually signed all required documents? I wondered how Dr. Andreason, the official OHRP spokesman, could make this incomprehensible claim, given the documentation I had sent him proving otherwise? I began to wonder whether he had ever read any of the materials I had sent his office.

The day I first read the OHRP determination letter, in a less than cordial mood I e-mailed Dr. Borror, my original contact at OHRP:

> Needless to say, further comments will be forthcoming from myself and others regarding the determination appearing today on the OHRP website.

> Of all the issues I find most troubling about this study and this letter, at the top of page two, paragraph labeled (2) reads "We note that Columbia University

Medical Center (CUMC) found that for 40 of 62 subjects iti [sic] appeared that informed consent was not documented with a signed written consent form prior to the initiation of research activities involving humna [sic] subjects . . . **although it was documented prior to the subjects undergoing other research interventions.** [bold mine]

I then discussed my belief that the forms had never been signed, before continuing:

Chabot's admission appears not only in e-mails to our office but in the official minutes of the regularly schedule [sic] group meetings, copies of which I gave to your office. I would like to know how it is that after 22 months of OHRP investigation it is now possible for you to state that for these two patients consent "was documented prior to the subjects undergoing other research interventions."

I sent the e-mail off, then alerted Congressman Burton's staff of the online OHRP findings. In subsequent discussions with his aide I learned that he, like me, was not pleased by the brief OHRP response after a 21-month investigation, its disregard of so much solid evidence, and the lack of punitive action against Chabot or Columbia. He was sufficiently annoyed that he intended to write directly to Michael O. Leavitt, the new Secretary of the Department of Health and Human Services, the ultimate parent organization above OHRP, the NCI, and the NIH, suggesting his office now get involved.

When I heard nothing from Dr. Borror after four days I decided to contact her boss, Dr. Ivor Pritchard, identified on the OHRP site as the group's Acting Director. After all the delays, I did not have the patience for another long wait followed by an inconsequential carefully crafted response. This time around, four days was long enough.

In my letter to Dr. Pritchard, portions of which I excerpt below, I expressed my belief, based on my review of the trial's documentation, that the two patients (#9 and #16) had never signed consent forms. However, I did not mention the third patient admitted in 2002 who Chabot's office acknowledged had not completed the required document:

I have decided to write you directly regarding the above referenced determination letter.

Last week, I e-mailed Dr. Borror and Dr. Dahlberg regarding an obvious and absolutely incomprehensible error in the first paragraph at the top of page 2 of the OHRP letter. The pertinent section reads as follows:

> We note that Columbia University Medical Center (CUMC) found that for 40 of 62 subjects it appeared that informed consent was not documented with a signed written consent form prior to the initiation of research activities involving human subjects . . . although it was documented prior to the subjects undergoing other research interventions.

While the paragraph does state rather clearly that informed consent was handled repeatedly in an improper manner—though Dr. Chabot, the perpetrator, remains unidentified—in fact the conclusion of the sentence is false. In my e-mail to Dr. Borror of this week, I reminded her that patients #131 and 133 were never consented [to our knowledge] at any time, and died before we discovered that they had not been properly consented by Dr. Chabot.

We spent, as my extensive documentation given your office shows, 2.5 years trying to learn from Chabot's office what happened to the consent forms for these two patients to no avail. Only after I insisted Chabot give us an explanation did he admit, long after both patients were dead, that they had never been consented in writing [as we believed]. He later made the same admission at the regularly scheduled group meeting of staff personnel held on March 20, 2006, as documented fully in the official minutes composed by the NCI staff member assigned to the project. Copies of these minutes, as well as multiple e-mails from our office to Chabot's office that document the sorry history of the missing consent forms were provided to your office. Therefore it is inconceivable and disappointing that after all the evidence given your office, Dr. Andreason can write, regarding informed consent, for all patients "it was documented prior to the subjects undergoing other research interventions." In Subjects #131 and #133 written consent was never obtained [as far as we knew].

I am particularly disturbed by this error, because of the effort invested by my office to provide Dr. Borror and Dr. McNeilly with the appropriate documentation, including copies of relevant e-mails and the official meeting minutes. In addition I discussed these two specific patients with Dr. Borror during two separate phone conversations. I discussed these two patients specifically with Dr. McNeilly during phone conversations as well.

I would also add, as I have explained to Dr. Borror in conversations in addition to the written documentation provided, that [as far as we knew] Dr. Chabot continued to count these two patients as legitimate data points and as if properly consented throughout the greater time of the study until its near conclusion, at which time he suddenly removed these two patients from his official data sheet without any explanation. . . .

I am also somewhat surprised to read in the first sentence of that paragraph that "We note that Columbia University Medical Center (CUMC) found . . . etc." I find it most strange that the OHRP would reference Columbia's own investigation first, and your confirmation of their findings second, as if Columbia took the lead on an investigation of itself. Does the OHRP routinely allow an institution under investigation to investigate itself, in effect do you permit the fox to guard the henhouse? Was I mistaken in thinking that OHRP was conducting the investigation of Columbia staff, not Columbia?

I also note that the name "Mr. George Gasparis" leads the list of those copied on the OHRP letter. Mr. Gasparis, as the letter indicates, is currently Executive Director, Human Subjects Protection Program at Columbia. As you well know, prior to his arrival at Columbia in 2003, Mr. Gasparis served as Director for the Division of Assurances and Quality Improvement at none other than the OHRP. I would have thought that an OHRP insider now representing a private institution under investigation by the OHRP should have been distanced from the investigation, to avoid the obvious concerns about undue influence—particularly in a case such as this, in which the complainant, myself, is not a Columbia staffer. The lack of such disengagement becomes particularly worrisome since your own determination letter indicates that Columbia may have taken the lead on the whole investigation! Since Mr. Gasparis' name leads those copied, I would like to know in writing specifically what role Mr. Gasparis played in this investigation, as well as the name or names of those who actually conducted this investigation.

In my e-mail to Dr. Borror of this week I did not discuss a serious error of omission on page 1, second paragraph, in which Dr. Andreason references Subject 113,"enrolled into the study more than 8 weeks after undergoing biopsy of his pancreatic tumor."

While I appreciate the confirmation of my previous allegation regarding patients admitted beyond the eight week time period after biopsy, I am perplexed that the letter makes no mention of Subjects #129 and #133, whom Dr. Chabot also approved for entry to the nutrition arm though each was beyond eight weeks from biopsy. I discussed Subject #113 and #129 beginning on page 282 in my response to Dr. Zerhouni, sent to Dr. Borror in June 2006. Later, in my narrative account sent to Dr. McNeilly, beginning on page 9, I discussed all three patients at length, providing accompanying documentation in the form of copies of dated official biopsy reports and the clinical trial records confirming date of entry more than eight weeks after biopsy. Yet the letter makes no mention of either patient #129 or #133, nor does Dr. Andreason provide an explanation of why these two subjects have been ignored.

I request from you a full and detailed written explanation of why the official OHRP letter on page 1 failed to reference Subjects #129 and #133, despite the extensive documentation provided Dr. Borror and Dr. McNeilly confirming that these two had been admitted beyond the eight week cut off point for eligibility.

I request from you a full and detailed written explanation, since Dr. Borror has to date not responded to my e-mail, why the OHRP letter claims, with easily demonstrable inaccuracy, that all patients entered into this study were ultimately consented in writing.

I request from you a full and detailed written explanation why OHRP has chosen to ignore my extensive documentation including multiple e-mails and copies of the official NCI meeting minutes confirming the lack of written consent for these two patients long after both were dead. Frankly, these two errors hardly inspire confidence that your office conducted a thorough or accurate investigation.

I request from you a full and detailed written explanation why OHRP seems to be relying on Columbia's investigation of its own staff, rather than its own investigation of Columbia staff.

Finally, I note that my name appears on the OHRP document only once, in the title of the "Research Protocol" at the top of the letter. My name appears nowhere in the body of the letter, nor am I listed at the end as one of those individuals copied. I note that multiple staff at Columbia were copied, including Dr. Chabot. And though Dr. Chabot is listed as "Principal Investigator" at the top of the letter, nowhere in the body of the document does Dr. Andreason identify Dr. Chabot as the individual solely responsible for the inappropriate entry of Subject #113 or the 40 subjects who were improperly consented. Reading the letter, one might easily assume that I am the culprit, and Columbia must now pick up the pieces of my incompetence.

I request from you a full and detailed written explanation of why OHRP fails to identify Dr. Chabot as the individual responsible for the protocol violations, and I as the complainant. On a lesser note, I would like an explanation of why you chose to copy Dr. Chabot, but not me.

Ultimately, the clearly erroneous information included in an official OHRP letter . . . creates serious misleading inaccuracy that will not be ignored by me, and I hope, will not be ignored by you.

I look forward to your quick response.

Only six days later, on March 19, 2008, Congressman Burton sent off his letter to Secretary Leavitt at the Department of Health and Human Services, restating in detail some of the major issues at stake, particularly his concern over the lackluster OHRP performance. The letter began:

Dear Secretary Leavitt:

As you know, the National Institutes of Health's (NIH) 27 Institutes and Centers have been at the forefront of some of our Nation's most significant medical discoveries since their inception. Receiving financial support for research from NIH has long been looked upon by medical professionals as the gold standard because NIH is widely assumed to demand that the most rigorous research protocols and safety standards be adhered to.

That is why I am greatly disturbed by continuing reports alleging egregious mismanagement of research activity, and most recently, potential mismanagement of an investigation into human research protection violations involving Columbia University's NIH supported Research Project: Gemcitabine Compared With Pancreatic Enzyme Therapy Plus Specialized Diet (Gonzalez Regimen) in Treating Patients Who Have Stage II, Stage III or Stage IV Pancreatic Cancer. . . .

In 2006, I contacted various officials at the Department of Health and Human Services (HHS) and NIH—including then NIH Director Zerhouni—to ask them to investigate serious allegations of scientific misconduct by Columbia University's principal investigator Dr. John Chabot. Although I appreciate that an investigation of this nature takes time to complete, considering that the allegations involved the safety of human research subjects, it concerns me that it took OHRP nearly two years to make a final determination in this case. I am further troubled that Dr. Zerhouni took no action to suspend Dr. Chabot's research activities at Columbia University, or at least increase oversight of his activities, pending the completion of the investigation, when this matter was brought to his attention two years ago.

Including this most recent case with Columbia University, I understand that in the last decade or so three serious violations of human subject protections—involving NIH-funded research—have been uncovered. I am told that the first instance occurred in 1999 after an 18 year old patient died in a gene therapy trial at the University of Pennsylvania. It was subsequently learned that at least six patients had died across the country. The Food and Drug Administration became involved and immediately suspended research at a number of institutions until patient protections were assured. I believe that this was the correct course of action.

In contrast, the second incident apparently involved the Uganda AIDS Study. I understand that NIH would eventually admit to South Africa's Medicine Control Council a number of problems with the study including problems with the manner in which the study was conducted and an inability to confirm that voluntary informed consent by the trial participants was obtained. While the drug, nevaprine [sic] would eventually be vindicated, the study controversy was worsened when the whistleblower, Dr. Jonathan Fishbein, was fired, plunging NIH into a lengthy legal struggle which, I believe, it would ultimately lose.

It seems to me that this third violation of human subject protection involving Colombia [sic] University is more closely following the Uganda pattern rather than the University of Pennsylvania pattern. For example, the February 25th letter states that OHRP concurs with Columbia University Medical Center's own investigation which found that Dr. Chabot violated the enrollment criteria with one patient and failed to have documented informed consent in 40 of 62 subjects prior to the initiation of research activities. The February 25th OHRP letter is unclear, however, regarding who actually led the investigation—Columbia University Medical Center or OHRP. Did OHRP make a determination based solely on the conclusions presented by Columbia University Medical Center or did OHRP, in fulfillment of its oversight responsibilities, undertake its own investigation independent of Columbia University's?

445

OHRP seems to suggest that they did not do their own investigation. For example, the February 25th letter points out that documentation shows that (informed consent) documentation was obtained prior to the research intervention. I am told by individuals with intimate knowledge of the case that this is not an accurate reflection of the facts. In fact, it is my understanding that in documentation provided to OHRP are emails and meeting minutes that prove that two patients who subsequently died were enrolled and participated in the study, even though Dr. Chabot failed to obtain signed informed consent documentation. It is also my understanding that many other scientific and management irregularities occurred with this particular study and that NIH staff (at the National Cancer Institute and the National Center for Complementary and Alternative Medicine) were aware of these irregularities, and yet apparently took no action to ensure Dr. Chabot was complying with required Federal regulations governing the protection of human subjects. I believe that Dr. Gonzales [sic] himself—the developer of the Intensive Pancreatic Proteolytic Enzyme Therapy With Ancillary Nutritional Support protocol—repeatedly raised concerns about the study's compliance with research protocols.

This head-to-head comparison of an alternative cancer protocol to the conventional cancer approach was the first of its kind and showed great promise. The Columbia University researchers were reputed to be experts in clinical trial implementation and thus were entrusted to control this study. Their violations of Federal law need to be fully investigated and remedied by the Federal government not Columbia University.

As I stated before, there is an expectation among the scientific community and the general public that all NIH-funded studies are conducted with the scientific rigor and proper attention to all human research protections. I believe that a Department of Health and Human Services initiated "top-to-bottom" audit would not only be good for Columbia University but I believe good for all NIH-funded human research studies. Toward that end, I am respectfully asking you to consider taking the following actions:

> 1. A comprehensive independent audit of the OHRP's investigation into Research Project: Gemcitabine Compared With Pancreatic Enzyme Therapy Plus . . . This audit should also include a review of NIH's handling of the reports from Dr. Gonzalez (and this office) of alleged mismanagement and misconduct in this study.

2. An immediate review of Dr. John Chabot's eligibility for Federal research funding as a consequence of his failure to protect individuals in clinical research as acknowledged in the OHRP letter.

3. An immediate review of all NIH-funded clinical research, especially at Columbia University, to verify documentation demonstrating that all individuals involved in clinical research are adequately protected, and that the studies are being conducted in accordance with all applicable Federal guidelines.

Given the seriousness of this issue and its implications on future human research, I believe the above suggestions are the least we can do to ensure not only the safety of research subjects but the integrity of Federal research in general.

On April 4, 2008, Dr. Borror responded to me via e-mail, explaining OHRP's current position on the investigation:

We have received your emails to me and Ivor Pritchard of March 10 and 17, 2008 regarding our evaluation . . . .

We made our determinations in the letter you reference based on documentation provided to us by Columbia University Medical Center (CUMC) and other relevant sources. If you wish to see that documentation, you may file a Freedom of Information Act request; however, it is unlikely that the request will be filled until the case is closed. The issues that you raise in your emails involve the specific facts of the case that were communicated to us by CUMC. Because this case with CUMC is still open, it is our policy not to discuss the case in this level of detail with nongovernmental parties other than the institution. Please note that we plan to address the remainder of your allegations in a subsequent letter to CUMC, and may make additional determinations if appropriate.

As noted in "OHRP's Compliance Oversight Procedures for Evaluation Institutions," . . . it is standard procedure for OHRP to ask the institution to conduct an investigation of the potential noncompliance and to report those findings, along with documentation, to our office for review. It is also standard procedure for us to omit the name of the complainant from any public correspondence to protect their privacy and confidentiality, and to only cc the principal investigator on our correspondence with the institution, and not other investigators on the study.

We suggest that your questions about Mr. Gasparis' role in the CUMC investigation would be best directed to CUMC.

OHRP appreciates your concern about the protection of human research subjects. Please do not hesitate to contact me should you have any questions.

Dr. Borror's note left me somewhat confused. The February 25, 2008 determination letter posted on the OHRP website nowhere indicated that the investigation was still in progress. After reading that document multiple times, I could only assume their work was done—but apparently, perhaps because of my protest, it was not.

Chapter 38

NCCAM's New Chief

While I continued my dialogue with OHRP, in late April 2008 I learned that the NIH hierarchy had selected a permanent replacement at NCCAM for the deceased Dr. Straus. The new director, Dr. Josephine Briggs, was a physician with impressive academic credentials, catalogued in some detail in the official NIH press release announcing her appointment:

> Dr. Briggs received her A.B. *cum laude* in biology from Harvard-Radcliffe College and her M.D. from Harvard Medical School. She completed her residency training in internal medicine and nephrology at the Mount Sinai School of Medicine, followed by a research fellowship in physiology at Yale School of Medicine.
>
> She was a professor of internal medicine and physiology at the University of Michigan from 1993 to 1997. From 1997 to 2006 she was director of the Division of Kidney, Urologic, and Hematologic Diseases in the National Institute of Diabetes and Digestive and Kidney Diseases. From 2006 until her NCCAM appointment, she was senior scientific officer at the Howard Hughes Medical Institute (HHMI), Bethesda, Maryland.
>
> Dr. Briggs has published more than 125 research articles and is on the editorial boards of numerous journals.[76]

Her stellar resume seemed lacking in only one area, an indication of experience with, or expertise or even interest in, complementary and alternative medicine. No matter, the NIH document extolled her arrival, much as the NIH had earlier lauded the appointment of Dr. Straus in 1999.

> "We are pleased to have Dr. Briggs return to NIH to lead NCCAM," said Dr. Zerhouni. "She has been a leader in trans-NIH activities, and her in-depth understanding of NIH and translational research will bring new opportunities to the study of CAM."

> "I am honored to be selected to lead NCCAM, and I welcome the opportunity to develop further the NIH investment in this exciting field of biomedical investigation," Dr. Briggs said. "Alternative approaches to health and wellness are of enormous public interest, and we need a strong portfolio of science in this area. NIH has already taken significant steps to build research programs to explore the potential of CAM. I look forward to working with scientists and the CAM community as well as my colleagues across NIH to strengthen our understanding of the potential of CAM and to examine the opportunities for integration of proven CAM approaches into our nation's health care delivery."[76]

Each of the 27 individual Centers and Institutes of the NIH, such as the National Cancer Institute and the National Institute of Mental Health, operates semi-autonomously, with its own budget and staff, but always under the watchful eye of the NIH Director chosen by the President. And each of these various entities supports research in a restricted area of medicine, such as cancer or mental illness, with a director recognized for leadership in the field he or she was chosen to supervise. That is, the head of the NCI invariably has excelled in oncology research; the director of the National Institute of Mental Health has earned laurels for innovation in psychiatry.

In 2008, I reviewed the backgrounds of the then current NIH Institute directors, all of whom, with only one glaring exception, had garnered great respect in the medical specialty he or she was appointed to manage. For example, the Director of the National Institute of Allergy and Infectious Diseases, Dr. Anthony S. Fauci, internationally known for his HIV research, graduated from my alma mater, Cornell University Medical College, then joined the Institute he now heads in 1968 immediately after completing his residency at New York Hospital-Cornell. He quickly rose within the NIAID ranks, in 1984 becoming director, with his impressive research accomplishments recounted in his official NIH biography:

> Dr. Fauci has made many contributions to basic and clinical research on the pathogenesis and treatment of immune-mediated and infectious diseases. He has pioneered the field of human immunoregulation by making a number of basic scientific observations that serve as the basis for current understanding of the regulation of the human immune response.[77]

His choice as Director of NIAID seems absolutely appropriate.

The official National Cancer Institute website described its director (as of 2009), Dr. John E. Niederhuber in glowing terms:

> A nationally renowned surgeon and researcher, Dr. Niederhuber has dedicated his four-decade career to the treatment and study of cancer—as a professor, cancer center director, National Cancer Advisory Board chair, external advisor to the NCI, grant reviewer, and laboratory investigator supported by NCI. . . .[78]

I don't think anyone would question his choice to head the NCI.

In a press release posted on January 26, 2005, the official National Heart, Lung, and Blood Institute website summarized the achievements of its then new boss, Dr. Elizabeth G. Nabel:

> Elias Zerhouni, M.D., director of the National Institutes of Health (NIH), today announced the appointment of Elizabeth G. Nabel, M.D., as director of the National Heart, Lung, and Blood Institute (NHLBI). Dr. Nabel, who is currently the Scientific Director of Clinical Research in the NHLBI intramural program, will begin her appointment on February 1, 2005.
>
> "Dr. Nabel is a leading scientist and recognized expert in the development of novel genetic and cellular therapies for cardiovascular disease. Her research on vascular biology and the regulation of smooth muscle cell growth has provided important insights into the development of heart disease," said Dr. Zerhouni. . . .[79]

Further down, the document described her academic background:

> Dr. Nabel is a board certified cardiologist who has taken care of many patients with cardiovascular disease, including women with heart disease. She joined the NHLBI in 1999 as the Institute's Scientific Director of Clinical Research.

Among her many accomplishments as Scientific Director, she initiated a cardiothoracic surgery branch, a state of the art training and research program in cardiovascular surgery.[79]

Dr. Nabel seems eminently suited to lead the NHLBI.

I could go on, but I think I've made the point. It should not be surprising that the leaders of these various NIH Centers and Institutes have been chosen precisely because of their accomplishments in the particular area of research they now supervise. This hardly startling rule holds true for 26 of the 27 NIH Centers and Institutes—with the exception, of course, of NCCAM. According to their own statements in published reports, neither Dr. Straus—who took the helm of that Center in October 1999—nor his successor Dr. Briggs had or has knowledge of, experience with, or interest in any form of alternative medicine.

Such an anomalous situation suits the NIH, and the conventional media, just fine. In contrast, Dr. Wayne Jonas, who headed the old Office of Alternative Medicine from 1995–1998, had intensively studied various forms of "unconventional" medicine. Not that he wasn't also very traditionally educated, as I earlier reported: he completed his undergraduate education at Davidson College, medical school at Bowman Gray, residency in family practice while serving in the Army. After further training at Walter Reed, he served there with the rank of Colonel as Director of the Medical Research Fellowship.

An NIH document (NIH AIDS Research Program Evaluation AD HOC PANEL ON COMPLEMENTARY AND ALTERNATIVE MEDICINE THERAPIES RESEARCH) described Dr. Jonas' unusual background:

> Dr. Jonas served as Director of the Medical Research Fellowship at Walter Reed, where he taught research methodology and conducted laboratory research [in] immunology and toxicology.
>
> In addition to his conventional medical training, Dr. Jonas has received training in homeopathy, bioenergy therapy, diet and nutritional therapy, mind/body methods, spiritual healing. . . . He has conducted research in and written about a variety of research approaches and he contributed to a report to the NIH entitled "Alternative Medicine: Expanding Medical Horizons," a report about the history and current practices of alternative medicine modalities in the Unites [sic] States.[80]

452

When I first met Dr. Jonas back in 1990, while he still served as an Army officer, I thought he possessed a rare combination of skills, with expertise in both conventional and alternative medicine approaches. One would have thought that Dr. Jonas, with his rather unique background, would have been the ideal choice for the OAM director.

For the heads of the other 26 Centers and Institutes, such interest in the area of medicine they were to manage has always been not only lauded, but considered necessary. For Dr. Jonas, this rule was turned upside down. As he painfully learned, his very skill set in the subject matter of "alternative medicine" made him a target for the media, even among his colleagues, from whom the media took its cues.

I remember very well an early interview with Dr. Jonas appearing in the press shortly after he arrived at OAM, an interview that really turned out to be a very premeditated ambush. Dr. Jonas agreed to meet with the journalist thinking he would be discussing the new OAM research agenda, but the shrewd and calculating reporter seemed determined to make Dr. Jonas look as foolish as possible. In a confrontational tone, the writer questioned Dr. Jonas ad nauseum about his interest in alternative medicine and homeopathy, as if he had uncovered a hidden past of child molestation. Unfortunately, to my knowledge, the attitude of the media toward Dr. Jonas never deviated during his difficult three year stint at OAM. When he finally left in some frustration to return to Walter Reed, I felt a sense of relief, believing that this well-intentioned physician would no longer be targeted for ridicule. I knew him to be far too decent a man, far too serious a scientist, to need that headache.

The *Science* writer who worshipfully interviewed Dr. Straus after he assumed leadership of the new NCCAM in late 1999 continued the tradition, belittling the long-departed Dr. Jonas, though without mentioning him by name. In the second paragraph of his January 2, 2000 article, he wrote:

> The office's reputation didn't improve under the tenure of the next director, a homeopathic physician.[69]

True, Dr. Jonas audaciously had studied homeopathy, but the writer chose to leave out that as a Colonel in the Army he also taught research methodology at Walter Reed Army Medical Center, the military's pre-eminent medical institution, the hospital of Presidents and other political leaders.

What Went Wrong

An article appearing on the *Time Magazine* website on May 15, 2002, some four years after Dr. Jonas left OAM, lambasted him yet again for his interest in alternative medicine. The title "Wasting Big Bucks on Alternative Medicine" says it all:

> It's been nearly a decade since Iowa Senator Tom Harkin foisted a New Age entity known as the OAM . . . upon the National Institutes of Health. In the years since, the Congress has steadily increased its financial support. . . . All the while, most of the medical community has watched aghast as the agency I call Harkin's Folly murkily pursues its goals. . . .
>
> It was no accident, then, that the OAM, the NCCAM and their advisory committees have been loaded with New Age gurus like Andrew Weil, assorted mystics, quacks—like the one that treated Harkin's allergies. . . . Indeed, a recent director of the Center, Wayne Jonas, proudly listed in his resume the authorship of a book called "Healing with Homeopathy." Is it fair of me to say that Jonas, and many of those on OAM advisory committees, did not bring to the table an abundance of objectivity?[81]

So oddly, according to this writer an interest in alternative medicine on the part of the Director of the Office of Alternative Medicine—even authoring a book on the subject—was proof of bias and scientific incompetence.

In contrast, I have been unable to find anywhere any criticism in any media outlet aimed at any director at any of the other NIH Centers or Institutes because they had an interest—at times an all-encompassing fanatical interest—in the research discipline they supervised. Nor have I heard of a director at one of the other NIH Centers or Institutes belittled for a lack of objectivity because he or she might have actually published an article or book in the field. In all cases other than that of Dr. Jonas, in the minds of journalists and scientific colleagues, such accomplishments only *prove* ability, competence, and of course, scientific objectivity.

In my office, I have six editions of the classic oncology text *Cancer: Principles & Practice of Oncology*, including the first edition published in 1982, released during my fourth year of medical school. Dr. Vincent DeVita, at the time "Director, National Cancer Institute," with other academic luminaries has edited every edition in the book's long history. Dr. DeVita himself rose to fame in NIH circles during the 1960s as the developer of the MOPP multi-drug chemotherapy regimen for Hodgkin's disease, which turned this deadly malignancy into a very treatable illness. During the 1990s, Dr. DeVita moved on for a time to Sloan-Kettering, where he served as Physician-in-Chief, before assuming his current position as Director of the Yale Cancer Center. He continues as editor of each edition of *Cancer,* and continues to list, presumably proudly, that achievement on his resume. In the now 29 years since the first edition of the text appeared, I have never heard a journalist, or anyone else for that matter, criticize Dr. DeVita's interest in oncology, or assume that his association with a text in the field reflected a character flaw, a personality defect, or a lack of the objectivity needed to function as NCI Director (or Physician-in-Chief at Sloan-Kettering, or head of Yale's Cancer Center). Quite the contrary, the publication over the years has garnered only praise within the medical community, as proof of great scholarship and scientific insight. While I agree Dr. Jonas' book never intended to be exhaustive in the same sense as the DeVita text, its author nonetheless was and is a serious researcher and well-intentioned scholar who never should have been ridiculed for his legitimate scientific efforts.

The infatuation among journalists and scientists with the late Dr. Straus, and now Dr. Briggs, sadly reflects the bias that both groups seem to share. Expressed simply, these folks seem to believe as a first guiding principle that no form of alternative medicine could possibly be of value, therefore anyone with a serious interest in any aspect of this "witchcraft" cannot conceivably be a *real* scientist (like Straus, Briggs, or of course Killen), and only those with absolutely no interest or background in this field should run NCCAM.

Chapter 39

Some Vindication, But the Battle Goes On

During the second week of June, I received a lengthy response from Dr. Andreason, who had signed the official OHRP February 2008 report. In his letter dated June 3, 2008, Dr. Andreason addressed my additional charges and questions—for the most part, incorrectly.

Dear Dr. Gonzalez:

The Office for Human Research Protections (OHRP) has completed its evaluation of human subject protections in the research referenced above. During the course of our evaluation of your complaint we issued two determination letters to Columbia University Medical Center (CUMC). We would like to summarize the determinations that we have made regarding your complaint:

(1) Subject 113 was enrolled into the study more than 8 weeks after undergoing biopsy of his pancreatic tumor, which was inconsistent with the inclusion criteria stipulated in the institutional review board (IRB)-approved protocol. Subject 129 began enzyme treatment in the study 11 weeks after undergoing biopsy of the pancreatic tumor, which was inconsistent with the inclusion criteria stipulated in the institutional review board (IRB)-approved protocol that subjects begin treatment within 8 weeks of pancreatic tumor biopsy. Department of Health and Human Services (HHS) regulations at 45 CFR 46.103(b)

(4)(iii) require that the IRB review and approve all proposed changes in a research activity, during the period for which IRB approval has already been given, prior to initiation of such changes, except when necessary to eliminate apparent immediate hazards to the subjects. We determined that the enrollment of subjects 113 and 129, who did not meet all eligibility criteria, represented a change in the research activity that was implemented without IRB approval.

In his original letter to the Columbia Dean, Dr. Andreason had identified only a single patient, 113 using Columbia's numbering system, who had begun treatment beyond the eight-week cutoff. So at least OHRP now agreed that two patients admitted into the nutrition arm failed the eight-week rule, confirming yet another protocol violation committed by Dr. Chabot. Perhaps Dr. Andreason finally read the evidence regarding patient 129 I had presented in great detail in each of my two monographs. Regardless, I was disappointed that it took OHRP two years to get such a simple fact right.

The second paragraph began with a replay of the 40 patients Dr. Chabot approved who had not been properly consented, followed by a lengthy reply to the many issues I had raised in my most recent letter to OHRP. Note that in the following excerpt from Dr. Andreason's letter I have edited out some sentences that repeat verbatim portions appearing in the earlier version:

(2) It was found that for 40 of 62 subjects it appeared that informed consent was not documented with a signed written consent form prior to the initiation of research activities involving human subjects . . . although it was documented prior to the subjects undergoing other research interventions dictated by the protocol. . . . We determined that the informed consent for the 40 of 62 subjects referenced by CUMC was not documented prior to the start of research activities, nor was the requirement for documentation waived by the CUMC IRB for subjects in this study. Included in this count of 40 subjects were subjects 131 and 133 for whom you alleged that a consent form had never been signed. You alleged that this failure to ever have the subject sign a consent form had been documented in a meeting with the National Cancer Institute (NCI) on March 20, 2006. The NCI minutes for this meeting stated,

"Number of subjects in the enzyme arm and missing consent forms: The Columbia staff investigated this issue. Two consent forms from subjects entered in the enzyme arm are missing. Their follow-up into this issue revealed that there are notes in both subjects' medical charts indicating that they were consented and in at least one of these cases, it is recalled that the patient requested to take the consent form with them and planned to return it. It appears that both of these patients 'walked off' with their forms. The IRB was informed of this and as both charts note that subjects were consented, the IRB left it up to the investigators to decide about inclusion of the data. . . ."

We therefore cannot prove the allegation that consent forms were never signed by subjects 131 and 133; however, we maintain our original determination that both of these subjects were among the 40 of 62 subjects engaged in research activities prior to the documentation of their signed consent in violation of HHS regulations. . . .

(3) You alleged that subject 133 was enrolled in the enzyme arm of the study beyond the allowable 8-week post-biopsy period stipulated in the IRB-approved protocol, in violation of HHS regulations. . . . The information submitted to us indicates that subject 133 was classified as not enrolled. It appears that the principal investigator did obtain identifiable private information about subject 133 prior to providing documented informed consent as stated in (2) above; however, we found no evidence proving that subject 133 was improperly enrolled in the enzyme treatment research arm of the protocol beyond the 8-week period following the subject's diagnostic biopsy as was alleged. We therefore determined that there was no proven violation of HHS regulations. . . .

(4) You alleged that a minimum of 72 subjects were to be enrolled under the IRB-approved protocol, but that the study was terminated with only 62 enrolled subjects, in violation of HHS regulations. . . . CUMC reported that the Data Safety and Monitoring Committee (DSMC) for this protocol recommended that the study be terminated due to predetermined stopping criteria. . . . We therefore determined that there was no proven violation of HHS regulations. . . .

(5) You alleged that while patients who could not eat adequately at the time of enrollment were to be excluded under the IRB-approved protocol, study subjects 103, 114, 118, 121, 127, 131, 132, and 147 were enrolled even though they could not eat adequately at the time of enrollment, in violation of HHS regulations. . . . CUMC provided excerpts and copies from research medical

records that stated that "appetite" or "eating" was adequate for these subjects at the time of enrollment. We therefore determined that there was no proven violation of HHS regulations . . . regarding this allegation.

(6) You alleged that while patients who lived alone were to be excluded under the IRB-approved protocol, subject 111 was enrolled even though she lived alone, in violation of HHS regulations. . . . Review of the study record found that the subject disclosed that she lived with her son at study entry. Subject 111's self-assessment . . . questionnaire rated her perception of emotional support from her family with the highest mark. Ten days prior to her death a research chart note stated that her social support had not been what she had indicated at the time of her entry into the study. At the same time period however, there were other records of conversations with the subject's son and daughter regarding the subject's medications and preparation for hospice care. We therefore determined that there was no proven violation of HHS regulations . . . regarding this allegation.

(7) You alleged that while patients with significant histories of psychiatric illness were to be excluded under the IRB-approved protocol, subjects with significant histories of psychiatric illnesses were included in the study, in violation of HHS regulations. . . . We note that the protocol exclusion criteria stated that a subject may be included if they have "No serious medical or psychiatric illness preventing informed consent or intensive treatment (e.g. serious infection)." Based on our review, it appeared that subjects with previous histories of psychiatric illnesses were properly evaluated for their ability to cooperate with the protocol and provide informed consent. We therefore determined that there was no proven violation of HHS regulations . . . regarding this allegation.

Corrective Action: The CUMC IRB met with the principal investigator and he has acknowledged the non-compliance with the requirements of 45 CFR part 46 in this case with regard to the timing of the documentation of informed consent for 40 of 62 subjects. We note that the principal investigator has committed to seeking documented informed consent prior to the initiation of any research activities or IRB review and approval for waiver of the requirements for documenting informed consent as appropriate under 45 CFR 46.117 in the future. We note that CUMC has cooperated fully with our evaluation of this matter.

We acknowledge that CUMC has instituted a comprehensive educational training program for ethical conduct of human-subjects research. We also acknowledge the CUMC IRB collaboration with both OHRP and private resources to further develop content for education training materials.

We find the education programs described in CUMC's response adequately address the above determinations and are appropriate under the CUMC Assurance and anticipate no further involvement in this matter.

Sincerely,

Paul J. Andreason, M.D.

As a start, I was somewhat perplexed by point (4) above, beginning "You alleged that a minimum of 72 subjects were to be enrolled under the IRB-approved protocol, but that the study was terminated with only 62 enrolled subjects, in violation of HHS regulations." In my March 14, 2008 letter to OHRP director Pritchard, I had not raised this issue, though it had been thoroughly discussed in earlier documents I submitted to his office.

Nonetheless, despite my disappointment at the litany of denials—denials with which I strongly disagreed—OHRP still did find that 42 patients had been admitted improperly. That was an extraordinary number of protocol violations for a study ultimately consisting of 62 total patients. And in this OHRP letter we have official government confirmation that the "principal investigator," that is, Chabot, acknowledged "non-compliance" with federal requirements in his processing of multiple patients. Though the earlier February 25, 2008 report described numerous breaches of the protocol rules, the culprit was nowhere identified. Now, that had changed. Chabot's admission to his own IRB, as documented here by OHRP, contradicted his repeated claims over the years that he had never entered a single patient who did not satisfy the various entry criteria.

This revised document also indicated that in response to OHRP instructions, Columbia had developed some type of retraining program for its staff in the tenets of research methodology. In the earlier February 25, 2008 letter to Dr. Shea at Columbia, Dr. Andreason had only requested that Columbia design a plan for "corrective action." Now we learned that with its "comprehensive educational training program for ethical conduct of human-subjects research" in place, Columbia had complied with the OHRP order. This outcome was, I thought, also a victory of sorts, and an ironic one at that, requiring the academic researchers at the eminent Ivy League medical center to undergo reeducation as a result of complaints brought by the perceived fringe alternative practitioner.

While progress had been made, I wasn't yet ready to celebrate or capitulate. True, Chabot finally had admitted to significant managerial lapses, as reported in an official—and very public—government document. I doubted at this point he would ever again try to publish an article about the study, with proof of his errors in judgment so prominently displayed for all to read on the OHRP website. Nonetheless, Dr. Isaacs and I agreed the denials in Dr. Andreason's letter required challenging. Once again, I would try to set the record straight.

Chapter 40

My June 15, 2008 Letter to Dr. Andreason

S ome two weeks after receiving Dr. Andreason's letter, I replied at length.

June 15, 2008

Paul J. Andreason, M.D.
CAPT, USPHS
Compliance Oversight Coordinator
Division of Compliance Oversight
Office of Human Research Protections
The Tower Building
1101 Wooton Parkway, Suite 200
Rockville, Maryland 20852

Re: Gemcitabine Compared With Pancreatic Enzyme Therapy Plus Specialized Diet (Gonzalez Regimen) in Treating Patients Who Have Stage II, Stage III or Stage IV Pancreatic Cancer.

Project Number: P30-CA13696

Dear Dr. Andreason:

Thank you for your letter dated June 3, 2008. I am pleased that your investigation at least partially vindicates my concerns about Dr. Chabot's mismanagement of this clinical study, concerns that the NIH hierarchy and staff chose to ignore for years. Nonetheless, your letter contains what I believe to be errors in fact and interpretation, as well as serious omissions requiring comment. I will address the errors first, then secondly, the omissions.

In terms of errors, in the following I address the subjects in the order in which they appear in your letter, with your paragraph notations: (2), the issue of informed consent: (3) a patient admitted beyond the 8-week post-biopsy period; (4) entry of inadequate numbers of study subjects: (5), admission of patients who could not eat adequately: (6) admission of subject 111 lacking the required family support: and finally, (7) admission of patients with psychiatric illness.

Errors or Misrepresentation of Fact in OHRP Documents

Patients admitted without signed informed consent. On Page 2, paragraph (2) you catalogue the 40 of 62 patients entered into the study improperly consented, who reading your letter one would assume at some point after the initial processing did sign the required forms. You also reference subjects 131 and 133 whom I have alleged never signed any consent form. You include, in your discussion of this point, the excerpt from the official minutes of a group meeting held at Columbia March 20, 2006. Though we declined to attend the session, the group did review at our suggestion the issue of the missing consent forms. Your statement reads:

> Included in this count of 40 subjects were subjects 131 and 133 for whom you alleged that a consent form had never been signed. You alleged that this failure to ever have this subject sign a consent form had been documented in a meeting with the National Cancer Institute (NCI) on March 20, 2006. The NCI minutes for this meeting stated:
>
> 1. <u>Number of subjects in the enzyme arm and missing consent forms:</u> The Columbia staff investigated this issue. Two consent forms from subjects entered in the enzyme arm are missing. Their follow up into this issue revealed that there are notes in both subjects' medical charts

indicating that they were consented and in at least one of these cases, it is recalled that the patient requested to take the form with them and planned to return it. It appears that both these patients "walked off" with their forms. The IRB was informed of this and as both charts note that subjects were consented, the IRB left it up to the investigators to decide about inclusion of this data. The investigators conducted the statistical analyses both with and without these two subjects and there is no effect on the statistical conclusions.

You then conclude "We therefore can not prove the allegation that consent forms were never signed by subjects 131 and 133. . . ."

As you know I had discussed at some length the history of the missing forms in Chapter 20 (beginning on page 166) of my "Response to Dr. Elias Zerhouni" manuscript, which I provided your office some two years ago, and hereafter identified as the "Zerhouni manuscript." I again discussed this issue at length in my document submitted to Dr. McNeilly of OHRP in September 2007, under the heading "Patients with no evidence of signed informed consent."

I would like to make several points about the above:

1. Never during the 2.5 years we tried to elicit some response from Dr. Chabot regarding the missing consent forms for the two subjects 131 and 133 did he ever state or imply or write in any communication to us that these two patients had actually *signed* the forms. Furthermore, the statement from the official minutes of the March 20, 2006 group meeting nowhere states that Dr. Chabot claimed that the patients had *signed* the forms, only that they had been "consented" and "walked off" with the forms. We had been told and knew that Dr. Chabot as part of the entry process, discussed orally with the patient present in his office the risks and benefits of entering the study, hence performing oral "consent." Such oral consent does not imply signing of the consent forms.

2. We have never seen the actual notations allegedly made in the charts of subjects 131 and 133 documenting the alleged "consent" that occurred. However, we do have in our possession an e-mail dated August 19, 2004 sent to us by Dr. Chabot's assistant, Carolyn DeRosa, a year after we had first tried to find out what had happened to the forms for these two patients. In her e-mail she discusses the specific form for subject 131:

Linda/Michelle:

As noted previously, there are no consents in the charts for patients #9 and #16 seen on 2–7–03 and 2–10–03. There is however, a note by JC [John Chabot] in the chart that the patient #16(133) was given the consent form at the time of the office visit.

So according to Dr. Chabot's own assistant who reviewed the chart at our request Dr. Chabot's notation in the chart of subject 133 only states the patient "was given the consent form" and nowhere claims the patient actually *signed* the form.

Furthermore Ms. DeRosa's own review of the charts in response to our queries says nothing about a notation in the chart of subject 131 regarding the consent form. One can only assume, since she had searched the charts precisely to look for information on the consent that might or might not have been completed, if a notation actually existed for subject 131 she would have told us, as she did in the case of subject 133. Furthermore, if either patient had actually signed the forms Dr. Chabot would have been obligated to document the event in the charts, and no such notations to that effect apparently exist. . . .

I had assumed that you would have actually reviewed the records of subjects 131 and 133 yourself, to learn what the alleged notations actually said. Apparently you did not, but the evidence from Dr. Chabot's own office seems rather strongly to argue against any notation confirming these two patients signed the forms, and certainly seems to indicate that no forms were signed.

I have enclosed a copy of this e-mail document with this letter.

3. Legal precedent, as I realize you well know, long ago established that in the case of a record missing from the medical chart that cannot be located, the event documented in the missing record never happened. I realize OHRP may operate under a different legal standard in its investigations, but certainly the lack of evidence of any signed forms, the lack of any notation to my knowledge alleging signing of the forms in these two cases seems from a legal perspective, to give strong grounds for arguing legitimately that neither subject 131 or 133 signed consent forms at any time.

Furthermore, having studied this issue and reviewed the NIH and NCI regulations relevant to this issue at some length, I have been unable to find any provision that states it is proper operating procedure in a Federally funded, Federally supervised clinical study to allow a patient to walk off with the original of a signed consent form under any circumstance. The NCI's own regulations state:

Section 50. 27 Documentation of Informed Consent

(a) . . . informed consent shall be documented by the use of a consent form approved by the IRB and signed and dated by the subject or the subject's legal representative at the time of the consent. A copy shall be given to the person signing the form.

As the above regulation mandates, a *copy* of the signed form is to be given to the patient. The original always stays in the official chart. Dr. Chabot's admission that patients "walked off" with the forms constitutes a violation of NCI regulations, which to my surprise you and the OHRP, judging by your determination letter, failed to address. And this violation differs considerably from the issue you do discuss, the patients not initially properly consented, but then subsequently consented.

Am I to conclude that OHRP in defiance of Federal regulations now claims it is perfectly fine for a Principal Investigator to allow prospective clinical study candidates to "walk off" with their consent forms without copying such forms—and then, in the continued absence of such forms, send the patient for experimental treatment?

I dispute your statement "We therefore can not prove the allegation that consent forms were never signed by subjects 131 and 133. . . ." I think a review of the actual charts for these two patients, all relevant communication between Dr. Chabot's office and my office including the above referenced e-mail, and an interview with Carolyn DeRosa might prove nicely that neither subject 131 or 133 signed any consent forms at any time.

I would like to know, for the official record did you or any OHRP staff ever read the actual notations in question for subjects 131 or 133 before reaching your conclusions? I would like to know, for the official record, did you or any OHRP staff ever speak with Ms. DeRosa?

I remain absolutely perplexed that neither the official OHRP determination letter of February 25, 2008, nor your June 3, 2008 letter to me mentions the third patient, —, who by the admission of Dr. Chabot's own office staff never signed a consent form. This patient was first seen in our office July 17, 2002 and died September 28, 2002, on hospice. During this period of treatment, we assumed this patient had been properly consented. Only after her death did Dr. Chabot's office inform us the patient had never signed the consent form, and consequently would be excluded as a valid data point. We were told once again that Dr. Chabot had allowed the patient to "walk off" with the unsigned forms, which were never returned to his office.

I discuss this patient on pages 168–169 of my "Zerhouni" manuscript so the evidence regarding her history was made available to you.

Why has your office done absolutely nothing to address this patient entered for treatment on a Federally funded, Federally supervised clinical trial who according to Dr. Chabot's own office never signed the required consent form? The fact that Dr. Chabot, realizing his error, may have disqualified this patient after she had already been treated and had died, does not excuse this protocol violation. And this protocol violation certainly differs in nature and severity from the violations documented in the OHRP determination letter for the 40 subjects initially entered without proper consent but, according to you, then subsequently consented.

And why has the OHRP once again chosen not to discuss specifically Dr. Chabot's admitted practice of allowing patients accepted into a Federally funded, Federally supervised clinical trial to "walk off" with their consent forms, whether signed or not, without making copies for the chart, then sending the patients on to us for treatment as if they had been fully and properly consented in the absence of evidence of signed forms?

A patient admitted beyond the 8-week post-biopsy period. In paragraph (3) of your letter you discuss my allegation that Dr. Chabot approved subject #133 for entry beyond the 8-week post-biopsy period as stipulated in the official protocol for the study. You write:

> This information submitted to us indicates that subject 133 was classified as not enrolled.

I documented this patient's history in great detail on pages 4–7 of my "McNeilly" document. He was first seen in our office February 6, 2003, seven weeks after the biopsy of December 20, 2002. Dr. Chabot sent the patient to us to begin the treatment process, though he decided not to admit the patient into the trial until the Columbia Pathology Department had reviewed the biopsy slides.

Records of phone conversations and my own e-mail correspondence with Dr. Chabot confirm that as late as March 5, 2003, Dr. Chabot had not contacted the patient regarding his eligibility, nearly 11 weeks since the biopsy. Neither the patient nor I knew if Dr. Chabot had formally qualified him for the study. Unfortunately, the patient never began treatment, claiming to us that he didn't want to start the therapy until he heard from Dr. Chabot, and died in April 2003.

Though I repeatedly e-mailed Dr. Chabot about this patient as the records prove, neither Dr. Chabot nor any of his staff ever informed us the patient had not ultimately been admitted. Only when Dr. Chabot sent us his final data sheet in April 2006, did I learn this patient was not included as a study subject, at a time when Dr. Chabot knew I had complained up the NIH ladder about his mismanagement of the study. But prior to that data, he never once indicated to us in any document or conversation that patient 133 had not been enrolled. What proof do you have that this patient was not enrolled?

In an e-mail dated April 21, 2003, two months after the patient had been seen in our office, Cara DeRosa, Dr. Chabot's assistant, e-mailed our office, asking if we had a copy of this patient's signed consent form. The relevant section reads:

> Also, do you keep consent forms on file for the nutritional arm. If you do, I need a copy of the last page of the consent form for: #9(131)'s and #16(133). My number is 212–305–0787 if you need to speak with me.
>
> With warm regards,
>
> Cara.

If this patient was never entered, why did Dr. Chabot's own assistant contact our office searching for a copy of the signed consent form for entry into the study? . . .

Entry of inadequate numbers of study subjects. As to paragraph (4) of your letter, the Columbia Data Safety and Monitoring Committee (DSMC) argued that the study should be stopped before full enrollment of 72 patients since in their opinion chemotherapy already showed such an advantage over my treatment. But the DSMC based its conclusion . . . that the study had been run properly with no protocol violations, and represented a fair evaluation of my treatment. In my lengthy "Zerhouni manuscript" I document in detail the various problems with the trial that made a reasonable interpretation of the data meaningless, including the admission of multiple nutritional patients unable or unwilling to comply with the prescribed treatment, the poor compliance documented among nutrition patients, the unequal numbers admitted into each group, the uneven rate of entry of patients into the group, with most nutrition patients entered during the early years of the study, and 48% of chemotherapy patients admitted in the waning several months of the project, when Dr. Chabot knew I had complained about the management of the study.

None of my serious concerns about the management of the study had ever been disputed at any time by anyone, until Congressman Burton relayed my complaints to NIH Director Dr. Zerhouni in his letter dated November 4, 2005. From that point on, as documented in Dr. Zerhouni's misguided response of December 22, 2005, all involved in the study including Dr. Chabot and the NCI staff . . . claiming the study had been managed flawlessly, that I was the problem and that I had complained because I was disappointed with the data.

As my "Zerhouni manuscript" makes clear, after the December 13, 2004 group meeting I detailed the various problems in a letter sent to the various study personnel. In response, in an official letter addressed to Dr. Chabot and dated January 27, 2005, Dr. Linda Engel of the NIH/NCCAM confirmed my complaints. I excerpt the relevant section from my "Zerhouni" manuscript below:

> **My January 7, 2005 letter:** In response to the survival statistics presented at the December meeting and Dr. Killen's proposal the trial be stopped, I wrote my 29 page, single spaced January 7, 2005, letter (see appendix), sent to all involved, including Dr. Chabot, Dr. White, Dr. Smith, Dr. Engel and Dr. Killen. I also copied Dr. Antman, who at this point had moved on to the NCI. In this document, I described in great detail, on a fact by fact, issue by issue and patient case by case basis, the flaws in both design and management of the project that I believed made valid assessment of my treatment impossible. I specifically addressed the attempts by oncologists to sabotage the project; the perpetual delays in the study; the entry of unsuitable patients; the effect of non-compliance among the nutrition patients; and finally, the disparity in stage distribution between the nutrition and chemotherapy arms. I did not in that document review the financial burden placed on my office due to the reimbursement lapses.

470

Dr. Engel's January 27, 2005 letter: In response to my charges, Dr. Linda W. Engel, Special Assistant to the Director, NCCAM, and the Program Officer at NCCAM responsible for overseeing the project grant, wrote directly to Dr. Chabot on January 27, 2005 copying me and Dr. Isaacs. In her letter, Dr. Engel states her purpose clearly: "We thought it important to clarify for you (Dr. Chabot), as Principal Investigator of the study, key points raised in the letter (of Dr. Gonzalez) in order to ensure that they are clearly articulated for the entire team, and so that the record is appropriately corrected." I wasn't quite sure what record she sought to correct, since in her letter she disputes none of my charges, as the following excerpts clearly indicate:

> There have been numerous and very difficult scientific, operational, and procedural challenges in carrying out this trial. These have been well documented and frequently discussed.

> The results of the trial, as contained in the most recent interim analysis, are both surprising (control arm) and disappointing (experimental arm), particularly in comparison with the historical data on which the protocol was based. . . .

> In spite of everyone's best efforts, it appears as if the current design and implementation of the study may have resulted in accrual into the two study arms of patient populations that are not comparable. As a consequence, it is very difficult (if not impossible) to ascertain treatment effect with certainty.

> Given all of the challenges, the surprising outcomes, and the uncertainties about balance between the two arms, it is highly likely (if not certain) that reviewers of the data from this study will raise substantive and legitimate concerns about the comparability of the two populations. As a consequence, it is virtually certain that the controversy surrounding the study will not be settled by the data from it.

Dr. Engel then discussed the value of continuing the study as it has been designed and implemented:

> The December 13 discussion with the team was very illuminating in that nothing materially altered this assessment. With respect to the specific matters raised in Dr. Gonzalez' letter, we will make only two brief comments:

> We discussed at considerable length his concerns about the probable accrual of patients unable to comply fully with the nutrition arm of the protocol. It was our impression that everyone in the room basically agreed that, despite best efforts, there is in fact, reason to be concerned about this issue, and that it clouds interpretation of the data. Even if we assume, however, that this is the explanation for the disappointingly poor outcome of patients on the nutrition arm, accrual of 15 or 20 additional patients by the nutritional arm of <u>this comparative study, as it is designed and currently being implemented,</u> would only be appropriate if there is a chance that the interim results would change.

> Regardless, Dr. Engel's document, written in her official government capacity, disputes not a single one of my concerns expressed in my 29 page letter and agrees explicitly with the most grievous.

The DSMC decided to stop the study believing the two groups were comparable, and the data completely legitimate. Based on what I have been told by Dr. Chabot himself, he had not informed the DSMC of the study's many problems, Dr. Engel's concern about the incomparability of the two groups and the flawed nature of the study's data, as confirmed by the NIH's own evaluation.

I think it [inappropriate] of Dr. Chabot to allow the Columbia DSMC to make determinations about the trial and specifically its stopping point without informing them of the numerous real problems that rendered comparison of the two groups and interpretation of the data impossible. And since the NIH claimed, to repeat, "In spite of everyone's best efforts, it appears as if the current design and implementation of the study may have resulted in accrual into the two study arms of patient populations that are not comparable," I cannot agree with your statement "Termination of the study in response to the DSMC recommendation was appropriate. . . ."

I would like an explanation from you of how you arrived at your conclusion that the Columbia DSMC acted properly, in view of the NIH's own conclusions about the data as expressed in Dr. Engel's January 27, 2005 letter. It is inconceivable to me you could have come to your conclusion after having read that letter.

Have you actually read Dr. Engel's January 27, 2005 letter? If not, why not?

Admission of patients who could not eat adequately. I find your conclusions expressed in paragraph (5) incomprehensible for a number of reasons. You reference 8 patients for whom we reported inadequate appetite, a reason for exclusion from the study as outlined in the protocol entry requirements. You report in your letter to me all could eat sufficiently, stating that "CUMC provided excerpts and copies from research medical records that stated that 'appetite' or 'eating' was adequate for these subjects at the time of enrollment." You do not specify the source of this information, but presumably there are two—patient comments, and Dr. Chabot's own written comments.

We warned from the beginning—a warning no one involved with the study thought preposterous — that patients might be so anxious, even desperate, to get into this clinical trial based on the positive pilot study results, they would easily say what they needed to say to get into the study. To compound the situation, Dr. Chabot's office made the error in judgment of sending the protocol requirements for entry to prospective patients who contacted the Columbia offices seeking information about the trial, in effect handing them on a silver platter a study manual informing them what they needed to say to gain admission. Global or general statements made by prospective study candidates related to their appetite or eating could not be taken seriously.

The entry process required insightful and comprehensive dietary and food recall questioning, as both the late Dr. Wynder, a world expert in the field, and I insisted at the initiation of the project. Unfortunately, Dr. Chabot, the Principal Investigator and solely in charge of evaluation of study candidates after 2000, to my knowledge never had any training in dietary recall or dietary evaluation, nor did he have any experience with my complicated treatment approach. So, the difficult job of assessing study candidates fell to a physician with neither the experience nor the expertise for the job of determining the suitability of patients for my particular treatment.

Furthermore, as your findings rather conclusively document, Dr. Chabot couldn't perform the most basic aspects of entry processing such as informed consent properly. Even if we for a moment disregard the three patients entered for whom no evidence exists of signed informed consent, you found Dr. Chabot qualified 40 patients who had not been properly consented. We also know that in three cases by his own admission he allowed patients to walk off with the consent forms displaying carelessness, a lack of basic management skills, and a disregard of common sense. Why would you then assume that Dr.

473

Chabot, a surgeon untrained in nutrition or dietary evaluation or nutritional therapeutics beyond what a surgeon learns, would be suddenly capable of evaluating the appetite and eating habits of patients seeking admission into this trial . . . ?

Remember too, that in December 2006, Dr. Chabot attempted to publish an article in *JAMA* claiming the study had been run properly and that all patients had been appropriately entered. He further claimed that I was not listed as a coauthor because I had refused to cooperate with the paper, when in fact I knew nothing about the article, and have in response as you know filed a complaint against Dr. Chabot with the Columbia Dean.

With all this in mind . . . I am somewhat astonished that you apparently hold statements in Dr. Chabot's records sacred without a second thought, and apparently disbelieve mine. I would like an explanation why you selectively take as legitimate the records of Dr. Chabot, and disregard mine?

In my "Zerhouni" manuscript, on pages 283–292, I discuss 10 patients I believed Dr. Chabot had qualified improperly who could not eat adequately at the time of entry. Perhaps a reasonable scientist might dispute several cases, and even I discounted one in my "McNeilly" manuscript upon restudy of the records, but for two the issue is beyond dispute, hence my astonishment at your findings. These would be subjects 118 and 131, discussed not only in my "Zerhouni manuscript," but also in the "McNeilly" document—neither of which I suspect, based on your comments, you read.

Below, I excerpt selected sections from my discussions of these two patients [in "McNeilly"], to reinforce the poor appetite and inadequate food intake in each at the time of entry. Note that in both manuscripts I used our own office number scheme, with Patient #8 the same as Chabot's 118 and Patient #9 the same as Chabot's 131.

> Patient #8(118): This patient, discussed at length beginning on page 283 of my [Zerhouni] monograph, should never have been admitted. I devoted considerable space to his story in my monograph because his entry represented to me such a glaring violation of the written protocol, and because Dr. Chabot, in an April 22, 2006 letter to me, [misstated] this patient's history. . . .
>
> I first met with Patient #8 on January 16, 2001, before he had been seen by Dr. Chabot or approved for the study. Beginning on page 3, my note from that session clearly documented the patient's poor appetite:

The patient reports that his surgeon, Dr. M— also told him that che-motherapy would not be particularly helpful and actually suggested he think of alternatives. One of the biggest problems is that the patient's appetite has been "terrible." A week ago one of his doctors (and he's not sure which one) started him on Megace 2-tsp day. With this his appetite has improved although it's still down. He reports a 20–25 lb. weight loss.

After my session with Patient #8, I immediately called Dr. Chabot, arguing that the patient needed to be disqualified. I reference this conversation in the "Assessment" section at the end of my note from that day:

The patient was tentatively approved for the clinical trial but he doesn't meet the criteria at this point. . . . He has no appetite and he's on Megace for appetite. An inability to eat precludes his entrance into the trial. I discussed this with Dr. Chabot.

In the "Plan" section I wrote:

I am willing to start the patient on a program but I'm going to have to discuss with the various investigators whether he's appropriate for the clinical trial.

First, I want to comment that once again out of a sense of fairness, I agreed, as I had in the case of other study candidates whom I believed did not meet the entry criteria, to treat the patient for free if he didn't qualify for the study.

Importantly, in this single note, before Patient #8 had been seen or approved by Dr. Chabot, in three separate places I documented his terrible appetite, and in two places my belief he did not qualify. I also documented that I discussed the patient's poor appetite, and my belief he should not be admitted into the study, with Dr. Chabot directly.

I then e-mailed Dr. Chabot the day of my initial meeting with Patient #8, describing very clearly my belief that this patient should not be approved for entry:

Since then he's lost 25 pounds, admitted he wasn't eating, couldn't eat and had no appetite until his local MD put him on Megace a week ago. He is eating some now, but we have never had any success with a patient staying on the program who had to be put on Megace because of appetite. . . . I know from my experience he's already missed his window and I doubt he will stay on the program ten days.

The following day, Patient #8 was scheduled to see Dr. Chabot for his intake interview, before returning to my office for his second session to review the prescribed protocol. Dr. Chabot did call me after his session with Patient #8, informing me he would order blood work before making a final determination about eligibility. The written protocol required that certain blood parameters fall within a specific range, and Dr. Chabot wanted to make sure the patient's lab results allowed for entry. But in my mind, the blood work issue had nothing to do with the patient's poor appetite, which should have disqualified him at once.

Dr. Chabot instructed me nonetheless to proceed with my second session on January 17, 2002, as if Patient #8 had been approved. I would have seen Patient #8 regardless of his eligibility for the study, as my note indicates:

> Patient #8 came in with his family. We spent 2 hours reviewing his protocol. I spoke with John Chabot as well regarding his eligibility for the protocol.

> Dr. Chabot agrees that we need to check his blood work and have more recent blood work. I explained this to Patient #8. He wants to do the program regardless. I won't charge him, if he's not eligible. . . .

When the bloodwork came back within the accepted range on January 22, 2002, 5 days after our second meeting, I suspected Dr. Chabot would approve the patient, despite his poor appetite.

My note from that day reported:

> Patient #8's blood work came in. It actually looks within the parameters of the clinical trial.

> I called Mrs. Patient #8 and told her that we don't have a final decision. I'm waiting on Dr. Chabot. . . . he is eating.

My comment on his "eating" did not mean to imply a normal food intake, only that he was getting some food down, or at least, he was according to his wife. I also want to remark that during my first session with the patient and his wife, she cried several times when she thought her husband might not be eligible for the trial because of his poor appetite.

This case couldn't be clearer: the patient had a 25-pound weight loss prior to entry into the study, an appetite described as "terrible", so terrible his local doctors had already prescribed Megace, used only to stimulate appetite in terminal cancer patients unable to eat normally.

I would like to ask you, as both a physician and an OHRP representative, how you can tell me that this patient's "appetite" or "eating" was adequate . . . at the time of enrollment?

> Patient #9(131): This patient should never have been admitted into the trial. I first met Patient #9 in my office, when he arrived for his initial visit, on February 5, 2003, before Dr. Chabot had interviewed, and approved him. At times, due to scheduling conflicts, Dr. Chabot would ask us to begin our treatment process even before his first meeting and final decision about eligibility.

> On page 2 in the body of my note from that day I clearly expressed my concern that this patient appeared to be too ill to comply with the program, and should not be admitted:

>> Currently, he does not seem to be doing well. Frankly, I think he is too sick to enter into the clinical trial. He has developed chronic, dull lower back pain that is resolved with Darvocet. His appetite is down. He lost about 20 pounds in the last six weeks. . . . His appetite is very poor and it sounds like he is starting to deteriorate.

> In the "Assessment" section at the end of the note, I repeated my concern.

>> Widely metastatic pancreatic cancer. He (sic) last blood work is already a month old. I suspect it is much worse than it was. Liver function tests were elevated at the time. In the last week, there has been significant deterioration in his clinical status. I do not believe he is going to be strong enough to do the program. I think it is too late. I think he is probably not going to last very long. I will e-mail Dr. Chabot at Columbia and let him know about my feelings on this patient.

> I did e-mail Dr. Chabot that same day, February 5, 2003 to express my concerns about the patient's eligibility:

>> I saw Patient #9 today for his first session, you will be seeing him Friday. . . . However, he looked like a patient who is about to crash very soon. From my experience, I know he isn't going to make it. Over the

past week, he and his wife both said there has been a significant deterioration, he is having trouble eating, he is getting pale, he gets short of breath going up stairs (his lung sounded clear on exam so I suspect it's anemia). His window of opportunity has passed.

The following day, February 6, 2003, I met with the patient for two hours to review the prescribed program. At that point, though Dr. Chabot had not yet interviewed nor approved Patient #9, I followed his instructions and prepared the patient as if he had been entered. Nonetheless, in my note from the day, I again expressed my strong belief that the patient did not qualify, though I offered to treat the desperate patient off protocol and for free. I wrote:

> My feeling is that he is too sick and I suspect his liver functions tests will have worsened since they were done a month ago. He is going to discuss these issues with Dr. Chabot. He wants to do the program regardless of whether he is on the clinical trial or not and I agreed of course to do that.

Despite my strong objections, Dr. Chabot insisted the patient be admitted.

I have included a copy of a note from my files dated February 18, 2003, just 12 days after our second visit, documenting a phone conversation with Patient #9 in which he admitted he couldn't eat. My note reads:

> Patient #9 complains he cannot eat. I thought he was far too sick to do the program. He is trying to get the pills down but it is difficult.

In an e-mail to Dr. Chabot two days later, on February 20, 2003, I again expressed my frustration that this patient had been admitted into the trial. Once again, I gave Dr. Chabot the benefit of the doubt, suggesting perhaps patients were misleading him regarding their true clinical status, in order to gain entry into the study. I hoped a non-confrontational approach might encourage him to work harder to do his job correctly. In any event, I wrote:

> I am concerned about Patient #9. He called after five days on the supplements to tell me he has no appetite and "can't eat." This was my concern when I first worked him up. I think patients like this are so desperate to get on the clinical trial they mislead you about their eating. We've had three patients recently who couldn't do it.

In a chart note dated March 10, 2003, reporting another phone conversation with Patient #9, I repeat my belief he should never have been entered. By this time, the patient's local doctor had prescribed Megace because of his lack of appetite:

> I called Patient #9 to see how he is doing. He is not doing well. I do not think he should have ever been entered into this clinical trial. He cannot eat. His local doctor put him on Megace because he cannot eat. His pain is poorly controlled with morphine and Darvocet.

Then in an e-mail to Dr. Chabot dated April 28, 2003, I again questioned the admission of this patient:

> I had started to get suspicious about patient Patient #9 from —. I hadn't heard from him for weeks. I called several times leaving messages, but no call back. Today his wife called saying he had died two weeks ago, not doing his program.

> As it turns out, for the record, within days of returning to — after his meetings with us his oncologist locally started him on Megace because he "couldn't eat." This was my concern about entering him into the study because he had lost some 20–25 pounds in the weeks before coming to New York and he and his wife said to us he couldn't eat well.

My notes at the "time of enrollment" clearly document this patient's declining overall performance status, and his declining appetite. In my note from February 5, 2003, I document a 20 pound weight loss in six weeks, more than 3 pounds weekly, and record "His appetite is very poor." In my e-mail to Dr. Chabot that same day, I documented that "he and his wife both said there has been a significant deterioration, he is having trouble eating." Then, shortly after returning home, his local doctors started him on Megace because of his poor "appetite" and poor "eating."

I would like to know from you, as both a physician and an OHRP representative, how you can tell me that this patient's "'appetite' or 'eating' was adequate . . . at the time of enrollment?"

I would also like to know whether you actually read any of the documentation I provided your office?

Admission of subject 111 lacking the required family support. In paragraph (6), you begin by stating:

You allege that while patients who lived alone were to be excluded under the IRB-approved protocol, subject 111 was enrolled even though she lives alone, in violation of HHS regulation. . . . Review of the study record found that the subject disclosed that she lived with her son at study entry. . . .

The protocol requirement for supportive family read as follows:

> 3.3. Since the Enzyme-Nutritional Therapy will be administered by the patients at home, they and their families must be willing to undertake the required work.

> 3.5. Non pregnant, non lactating
> Able to eat solid food, three meals per day. . . .
> **supportive live-in spouse or other family member**

So the protocol clearly states that entry requires live-in family members who are first, supportive of our nutritional therapy, and second, "willing to undertake the required work" of the treatment, such as shopping for food and cooking.

In my "Zerhouni" manuscript on pages 295–296, I discuss this patient as follows:

> **A patient lacking family or social support:** Dr. Chabot approved one patient, #15, for entry into the nutritional arm of the study although she lived alone, with no evidence of family support whatsoever, live-in or otherwise, as required by the *written* eligibility criteria 3.3 and 3.5 listed above. Consequently, she should have been rejected from the study. Since for advanced patients, a lack of live-in family help, for both emotional and practical reasons, guarantees poor compliance and treatment failure, she would have been better off proceeding with chemotherapy.

I discuss this patient on page six of my January 7, 2005 letter:

> Patient 15 misrepresented her family situation, had in fact no family support whatsoever, and quit after trying for two weeks.

This patient was followed by Dr. Isaacs, not by me, and I do incorrectly state above that she lived alone though Dr. Isaacs' initial records did reveal that she lived with her son. But the issue wasn't whether she lived alone or not, but whether she lived with family members supportive of the nutritional therapy and willing, as the entry criteria required, to help with the work of the treatment. As it turned out though the patient did live with her son he did not assist with his mother's therapy. To the contrary, the patient essentially functioned as his caretaker, cooking him meals even as her own health rapidly deteriorated.

In my "McNeilly" manuscript pages 47–49 I discuss this patient and her family situation at some length as follows:

> Dr. Isaacs first met with the patient on September 22, 1999, after Dr. Chabot had already approved her entry into the study. As described on page 1 of Dr. Isaacs' note from that day, Patient #15 reported a poor appetite as well as a 20-pound weight loss. Because the patient also claimed more recently improved food intake, we did not argue against acceptance on the basis of poor appetite.

> On page 2. . . . Despite a list of somewhat formidable social problems, Patient #15 also reported, as Dr. Isaacs documented, "Family is supportive," and that she had an active church life.

> After Patient #15 returned home, she seemed unable to follow the program adequately. Dr. Isaacs began to question the patient's alleged "supportive" social network described during their initial meetings. In a note dated October 20, 1999, Dr. Isaacs documents a phone conversation in which the patient admitted not only did she have no "help," but that she essentially, as sick as she was, had taken on the responsibility for caring for family members, including her adult son.

> > She has no help—she is doing all this herself. She is tired, has a hard time getting help. But in further discussions, she is making meals for her grown son who lives with her even though he neither expects nor demands this.

> > She is sleeping through enzyme doses—perhaps doing ½ the doses.

> > I explained that doing what sounds like perhaps ½ of the program <u>will not</u> work. She needs to ask people to do small specific tasks for her. . . . I encouraged her to make a plan to get help.

> As the patient deteriorated, Dr. Isaacs eventually helped arrange for hospice care. In her note from November 15, 1999, Dr. Isaacs documented a phone conversation with a hospice nurse, who discussed the absent family:

> > She apparently spends the whole day alone at home, there is no one in the family to help with medications or food.

The hospice nurse faxed us a copy of his note describing the home visit with the patient. In the "Intervention/Plan" section at the bottom of the page, he mentioned twice that the patient seemed to be at "home alone":

> Pt confused, @ home alone, pt drifting off to sleep during conversation . . . PT describing very scared, being home alone. . . .

The following day, November 16, 1999, Dr. Isaacs, as recorded in her note from that day, discussed the situation with the hospice doctor:

> Spoke (with) hospice director. . . . He attempted to see the patient today, but no one responded to knocking. Apparently a social worker was able to see the patient later, she said she was asleep. They feel she needs their inpatient unit.

In an e-mail to Dr. Chabot dated November 17, 1991 [sic], Dr. Isaacs reported the lack of social support in this patient's case:

> Unfortunately, from the beginning she never did her program fully . . . her social support was not as she had indicated before she came in, in fact, she had no assistance whatsoever and was sleeping through most of her doses of supplements. It also turned out she did **not** have a local physician (note: as required by the protocol) to help with her care contrary to what we believed. . . .

> The patient is not cooperating with the hospice nurses, or anyone else according to her son.

I would like to make several pertinent points about the admission of Patient #15 into the study. Even if Patient #15 misrepresented her social situation to gain entry into the trial, once we learned the truth of her situation, she should have been disqualified at once. Dr. Chabot, however, insisted that Patient #15 be counted as a properly entered "Gonzalez patient."

In your letter, you reference the self-assessment questionnaire filled out by the patient, in which she "rated her perception of emotional support from her family with the highest mark." She simply wasn't telling the truth as she later would admit.

You then write that "Ten days prior to her death a research chart note stated that her social support had not been what she had indicated at the time of her entry into the study." Your statement here perplexes me completely. As the above chronology documents, by October 20, 1999, only 4 weeks after Dr. Isaacs first met with her, the patient already admitted she had little at home support:

> She has no help—she is doing all this herself. She is tired, has a hard time getting help. But in further discussions, she is making meals for her grown son who lives with her even though he neither expects nor demands this.

Your letter to me continues "at the same time period however, there were other records of conversations with the subject's son and daughter regarding the subject's medications and preparation for hospice care."

First of all, the daughter lived in another city and hardly represented a live-in family member who could assist with the work of the treatment. Furthermore, our records show a much different scene than what you claim, with absent children, the patient left alone for long periods of time without help, to the point the hospice director himself went to the house, but was unable to gain entry to see the patient. To what records are you referring that prove your point?

Though our records conflict with your conclusions, even if the son and daughter cooperated with hospice care as you claim, how does such cooperation with hospice care at the end of the patients' life translate into cooperation with an intensive nutritional dietary program at the beginning of the treatment process? Entry criteria 3.3 and 3.5 make no mention of "support" with hospice care, they specifically refer to support and assistance with our treatment, neither of which this patient's family provided. The criteria, as you can see, are quite explicit, requiring their families "must be willing to undertake the required work." Your logic eludes me, completely.

Admission of patients with psychiatric illness. I find paragraph (7) at best ludicrous. I will, in response, excerpt pages 292–293 from my "Zerhouni" manuscript, in which I discuss patient 129, one of three we believe should have been excluded based on psychiatric disability.

> **Patients entered with psychiatric illness:** At least three patients accepted into the nutrition arm of the study—#14(129),16(133) and 23(148)—suffered mental illness severe enough to preclude appropriate compliance and should have been excluded based on the written criteria of section 3.9. I want to emphasize that I insisted this provision be included for the benefit of candidates with such problems. We know from our experience that those battling psychological disability cannot stick with the therapy, and for their own good need to find a more suitable approach.

Below follow descriptions of these three patients from my January 7, 2005 letter, beginning on page 6:

> Patient 14's(129) course was uniquely peculiar. Because of a long history of severe depression and suicidal ideation, Dr. Chabot did not immediately approve her for the trial, but instead requested she be seen by a psychiatrist for further evaluation since active mental illness is grounds for exclusion. Nonetheless, Dr. Isaacs did agree to see her and begin the treatment process before a final decision about eligibility had been made, so the patient could get started with the program. Unfortunately, the psychiatric work-up dragged on for a month, and though seen by us 12/20/02, she was not officially accepted into the trial until 1/24/03, **a full five weeks later.** During this period, the patient did not begin any aspect of the therapy because, as she told us, she didn't want to follow the regimen if she wasn't going to be a part of the study, and therefore had to pay for the supplements herself. Her husband also inquired if the supplements would stimulate her rapidly deteriorating appetite (they don't). Though quite debilitated, she thereafter struggled to follow the treatment plan and did survive 40.6 weeks from the time of her initial biopsy. In this case, her lack of urgency about the situation caused a critical loss of valuable time.

I don't know how a psychiatrist could claim, after a single one-hour evaluation, that this patient, with a long history of severe depression and suicidal ideation did not suffer mental disability. Perhaps he meant that she wasn't acutely psychotic . . . however, the written protocol does not limit exclusion to such flagrant conditions, but any **"medical or psychiatric illness preventing informed consent or intensive treatment."** The patient's own behavior during the five week period after her first visit with Dr. Chabot, during which time she did no part of the treatment, indicates to us cognitive difficulties sufficiently severe to make adherence to the nutritional regimen impossible. And by the time she decided to begin the treatment, her appetite had deteriorated to the point she could not possibly follow the regimen. All of this was brought to the attention of Dr. Chabot, but he still insisted she be entered and that we treat her. We believed then and believe today that this patient would have been better served had she been rejected from the study after the first visit with Dr. Chabot, so she could begin chemotherapy, a treatment that would not have required her active participation.

You state, rather remarkably, that "Based on our review, it appeared that subjects with previous histories of psychiatric illnesses were properly evaluated for their ability to cooperate with the protocol and provide informed consent." I find your statement preposterous, in view of the fact that though seen by Dr. Isaacs and instructed to begin our regimen while she awaited the outcome of the alleged psychiatric evaluation, she chose to do nothing, follow no therapy of any kind for five weeks, compromising her chance of response to any treatment, including ours. . . .

As I am sure you know, the Women's Health Initiative long-term study of dietary and nutritional factors excluded patients with depression, because such patients were considered unlikely to adhere to the prescribed regimen (Ann. Epidemiol. 2003;13:S18-S77, page S20). In the case of our study, the behavior of subject 119 while she was seeking entry showed clearly she could not comply with the therapy, and should have warranted exclusion.

Since you are not only a physician but a representative of the Office of Human Research Protection, with the emphasis on "Human Protection," I would like you to explain the benefit of admitting a patient with an advancing terminal cancer into a clinical study with a history of psychiatric illness who was so paralyzed she did no therapy for five weeks?

Serious Omissions of Mismanagement
In OHRP Documents

I find equally as troubling the omissions, areas of mismanagement that OHRP apparently chose to ignore. Below, I discuss the most egregious; patients kept waiting for many weeks before Dr. Chabot rendered his decision about eligibility, different standards for stopping treatment, and Dr. Chabot's serious conflict of interest.

Patients kept waiting for many weeks before Dr. Chabot rendered his decision about eligibility. Your omission that I find most disturbing relates to the many patients Dr. Chabot, when he alone evaluated prospective study candidates and alone determined eligibility, kept waiting for weeks at a time before rendering his decision. During this period the patients, often frantic, pursued no treatment as their terminal disease continued to advance. For subjects with an estimated prognosis without treatment measured in only months, we believe this tardiness jeopardized any possibility of response to our regimen.

What Went Wrong

In my "McNeilly" manuscript, I document at length a number of such patients. Below, I excerpt the most troubling episode, that of subject 108 (our #38).

Shortly after this episode, on March 12, 2001, the man who was to become Patient #38(108) contacted our office, explaining to my staff that he had been diagnosed with pancreatic adenocarcinoma on February 27, 2001, some two weeks prior to his call. After investigating various treatment options, both conventional and alternative, Patient #38 decided to pursue our therapy. He didn't seem to be aware of the clinical trial when he first called our office, so my office staff member, as required, referred him to Dr. Chabot. We heard nothing again about the case until Patient #38 sent us an urgent fax on April 5, 2001, 24 days after his original call to our office. As we instructed, he had contacted Dr. Chabot's office, but still awaited a decision about his eligibility. Knowing his life hung in the balance, he had grown frantic as the days passed with no response from Columbia. I include his letter in its entirety:

Dear Dr. Gonzalez:

I am urgently in need of your assistance.

I am a—year-old male living in — diagnosed with pancreatic adeno-ductal carcinoma on February 27. I researched the treatment options available and decided that the proteolytic enzyme treatment you offer is the best option for me. I contacted your office and was told I had to apply for the clinical trial at Columbia Presbyterian Medical Center.

I contacted Dr. John Chabot's office on March 23 regarding the trial, providing initial information on my case. <u>Since then, I've encountered one delay after another in getting approval for the clinical trial—even though I believe I meet all the eligibility requirements.</u>

Attached is a summary of my contacts with Dr. Chabot's office for the clinical trial.

I want to stress that the program co-coordinator, Michelle Gabay, and her assistant Suzanne, have always been extremely positive and courteous.

I was originally told by Michelle that scheduling an appointment would "only take a few days" once I was approved. However, the "paper work" obstacles have dragged on for almost three weeks now—

putting me in the agonizing position of having to (put) my treatment program on hold.

I need to know where I stand regarding the clinical trial. <u>I would prefer to see you directly, and as quickly as possible.</u> I am prepared to come to New York, at any time.

Dr. Gonzalez—can you please help me with this?

As we reviewed the records Patient #38 sent us, we found a copy of a fax he had sent to Dr. Chabot ten days earlier, on March 26, 2001, pleading for some response. When he didn't hear from Columbia, Patient #38 suspected Dr. Chabot had rejected him because of his specific tissue diagnosis, which in reality did not disqualify him from the study.

Dear Dr. Chabot:

I am most anxious to participate in the clinical trial using the pancreatic proteolytic enzyme therapy. I have researched Dr. Gonzalez' treatments and results and am convinced this is the right treatment program for me right now. In fact, I have been utilizing elements of his program while waiting for the past two weeks to see if I qualify.

I believe I qualify in all essential respects for the trial. <u>Please do not exclude me from the program because my diagnosis is adenoductal carcinoma.</u>

<u>Since I must go through the clinical trial screen program in order to see Dr. Gonzalez, you are my only hope for getting this treatment—which I desperately need.</u>

When Dr. Chabot failed to respond to this desperate fax after ten days, Patient #38 then decided to contact us directly on April 5, 2001.

I would like here to comment briefly about the above communications. Note that after two weeks of his first contact with Columbia, in frustration Patient #38 pleaded his case in writing directly to Dr. Chabot, but received no reply, not even after another ten days. . . .

I would also like to mention for the record that in his letter to Dr. Chabot of March 26, 2001, Patient #38 clearly identified Dr. Chabot as solely responsible for patient screening, and for all decisions regarding eligibility. He repeated in his fax what we had told him, that Dr. Isaacs and I could see no patient, whether on trial or off, until Dr. Chabot completed his evaluation. I find it extraordinary to hear today, six years later, that now Dr. Chabot insists that somehow Dr. Isaacs and I participated in any way in the intake process after July of 2000.

We did call Dr. Chabot's office on Patient #38's behalf, hoping to push Dr. Chabot into a decision. . . . Finally, on April 16, 2001, 35 days or exactly five weeks after his first contact with Columbia, Dr. Isaacs met with Patient #38 to begin the treatment process. Since our veto power had been revoked, we had no choice but to proceed. However, even if we still had a vote in entry decisions, we probably would have agreed to treat Patient #38 on trial without complaint. As in the case of Patient #15, who waited some four weeks to hear back from Dr. Chabot about her eligibility, Patient #38 had been through enough stress dealing with Dr. Chabot. We would not have chosen to make his life more unpleasant than it already was.

Though Patient #38 tried valiantly to follow his program, he eventually died in May 2002, some 13 months after his first meeting with Dr. Isaacs. We suspect his chance for response had been unfortunately compromised by the inexcusable five-week delay before Dr. Chabot finally admitted him for treatment. . . .

Though all the study administrators from the various institutions seemed fixated that Dr. Isaacs and I, if not watched carefully night and day, might somehow in some way influence the study's outcome, not once did any of them express concern about the obvious bias against us created by Dr. Chabot's slow pace of evaluating trial candidates, even when Dr. Isaacs and I discussed the issue. After all, as Dr. Chabot dawdled up at Columbia, many patients eventually admitted into the trial lost weeks of valuable treatment time, perhaps setting the stage for treatment failure. . . .

Different standards for stopping treatment. Neither the OHRP Determination letter of February 25, 2008, nor your June 3, 2008 letter to me discuss Dr. Chabot's different standards for stopping treatment as applied to the two arms of the study. I discuss this issue at length in my "Zerhouni" manuscript on pages 250–254 which I include below, so there can be no misconception about this issue. Dr. Chabot's interference with patients assigned to the nutritional arm represents yet another protocol violation that helped render the data meaningless:

Different standards for stopping treatment: If a patient on the GTX regimen doesn't appear to be responding, if the disease appears to progress on CT scans for example, Dr. Fine and his colleagues don't give up, stop treatment, suggest another approach or call hospice; instead, he adjusts the regimen, changes the doses, alters the sequence of the drugs. Based again on his own published comments, he seems only to get more determined, not less so with evidence of worsening disease.

This never-give up attitude presumably applied and applies to the chemotherapy patients of our current clinical trial under Dr. Fine's supervision. Over the years I have never heard Dr. Chabot criticize Dr. Fine for his doggedness, in fact he seems quite impressed by the resolve of his Columbia colleague. Yet as I read through the actual written documents of our clinical trial, it seems to me that Dr. Chabot believed our patients needed to be handled quite differently, as if once again two standards governed the trial, in this case, one for Dr. Fine, one for us. It appears perfectly acceptable that Dr. Fine, faced with disease progression, only gets more aggressive with his drugs, but that at the first sign of worsening, our nutrition patients should be sent elsewhere for different treatment.

During the March 20, 2006 meeting, Dr. Smith finally—about six months late—questioned Dr. Chabot about the issues raised in my lengthy September [2005] e-mail written in response to errors in the summary from the June meeting. In a section entitled **"The PI (Principal Investigator) phone calls to physicians and hostility to the trial**," Dr. Chabot discusses his contacts with the physicians charged with monitoring our patients. Here, the notes state,

> If there was any concern about the supportiveness, that is if the patient mentioned anything to him or if it didn't appear that there was a cooperative physician, he would give them a call to assess whether they were interested in having their patients on this trial, whether they have a problem, and whether they are willing to care for the patient on the trial. *In some situations, Dr. Chabot found that the patient had a physician supportive of their patients' participating in the enzyme arm but upon recognition of increased disease, the physician then acted to facilitate the patient moving to other therapy.* [Italics mine]

In the cases we've been able to document, physician opposition began before the alleged disease progression . . . Furthermore, the comments make even less sense if we consider that Dr. Chabot as far as I know based on his own earlier statements only called the few physicians he did call at the time of patient intake—not weeks or months later when the disease might have progressed

But if we, for the sake of discussion, assume Dr. Chabot's perspective as stated above is valid, certain points can nonetheless be made. In our private practice, if radiographic studies indicate that a patient's disease might be worsening, we don't quit, unless the patient wishes to change course. Instead, we do exactly what Dr. Fine does—we adjust the treatment. We might increase the dose of enzymes, increase the number of enzyme doses per day, the number of days on the supplements (our patients always must cycle off the pills after a period of time), we might alter other aspects of the program, such as the diet or the frequency of coffee enemas, that can influence progress. It's not unusual, in our experience, to see tumors initially enlarge before stabilizing and eventually hopefully regressing, sometimes just with time, sometimes with fine-tuning of the regimen. My well-known patient M., diagnosed with biopsy proven, metastatic pancreatic cancer that had spread into his lungs, liver, adrenals and bones, had no reduction, and some evidence of progression, in his many tumors after eighteen months on therapy. I changed his supplement and enzyme doses, but thereafter, he refused further scanning until five years later when I urged him out of my own scientific curiosity to have some testing done. He relented, and at that point, CT studies showed total regression of his once deadly disease. Had I given up on him early on, panicked and sent him packing, he would have died.

Ironically, the written protocol, which Dr. Zerhouni and Dr. Chabot repeatedly reference in their defense . . . specifically allowed Dr. Isaacs and myself to alter the treatment, not send the patient elsewhere, when scans indicated possible tumor enlargement or spread. In section 11.0 **"REMOVAL OF PATIENTS FROM PROTOCOL THERAPY,"** the document clearly states:

11.1 **Enzyme-Nutritional Protocol Therapy:**

> **Response or Stable Disease:** Continue full treatment with full doses of enzymes and adjunctive nutrients, diet and detoxification routines.
>
> **Disease Progression:** Modify the doses of enzymes and other nutrients according to the protocol but do not discontinue protocol

> therapy except at the patient's request. Describe tumor progression including tumor measurements on flow sheets.

The *written* protocol criteria could not be more clear, giving us the right—assuming the patient agreed—to modify our treatment, just as Dr. Fine could do with his chemotherapy regimen. Consequently, it was neither acceptable nor appropriate for an outside physician who knew nothing about our therapy or the trial requirements to make decisions about stopping the regimen or pushing any of our patients into a different treatment plan—unless again, the patient so requested. But in his comments, Dr. Chabot isn't talking here about a change of heart on the part of the patient, he's specifically permitting the monitoring physician to make the decision. Such outside interference constitutes plain and simple a violation of the written criteria for the trial, not an appropriate medical intervention for the patient's benefit. Dr. Chabot should know this, and as Principal Investigator he should not be justifying with such ease an obvious breach of study regulations—particularly since he seems perfectly happy with Dr. Fine's never-give-up attitude. It's interesting to read Dr. Zerhouni's lecturing Congressman Burton about the absolute need to abide by the criteria as written, then have him ignore, even bless, Dr. Chabot's disregard for those very inviolate rules. Unfortunately, Dr. Chabot's two sets of standards in this case, one for Dr. Fine and one for me, not only reflects a serious bias—and disregard for the written protocol—but also influenced, as his own statements demonstrate, the treatment course of nutrition patients.

Dr. Chabot's serious conflict of interest. Finally, neither the OHRP Determination letter of February 25, 2008 nor your June 3, 2008 letter to me address Dr. Chabot's conflict of interest that should have precluded him from serving as Principal Investigator on this study. I discussed this issue at length in my "Zerhouni" manuscript, pages 254–261. To sum up that issue briefly, Dr. Chabot's role as Principal Investigator required that he have no direct involvement in either of the treatments being evaluated in this study, the GTX chemotherapy regimen, or my nutritional therapy. However, Dr. Chabot, as the published literature confirms, proved hardly to be a disinterested third party referee. On the contrary, he had worked closely with the Columbia team under Dr. Fine developing the very GTX regimen used against my treatment in this study. His involvement with Dr. Fine and with the GTX research represented a conflict of interest . . . which should have required he step down as Principal Investigator.

After 24 months of investigations, why did you not address this issue, when I provided your office with the documentation to prove such a glaring conflict of interest? I find your indifference particularly peculiar, since in some respects, Dr. Chabot's significant ties to the chemotherapy regimen used in this study represent in many ways the most serious of violations, since he should not have been running this study in the first place.

Based on what appears to be either disregard or ignorance of the facts in this case expressed in your June 3, 2008 letter to me, I would like to know for the record whether you yourself ever read any of the documentation I provided your office.

I would like to know for the official record whether you and your OHRP colleagues fulfilled their mandated profession and ethical responsibility by conducting your own thorough investigation of the issues raised in this case. Or did you, as I suspect, rely primarily if not exclusively on the internal review conducted by Columbia staff . . .

I look forward to your prompt response.

Sincerely,

Nicholas J. Gonzalez, M.D.

Cc: Congressman Dan Burton
      Dr. Ivor Pritchard
      Dr. Kristina Borror

I sent the letter off, concentrated on my practice, and waited.

On another front, nearly five months after Congressman Burton's March 2008 letter to Secretary Leavitt of the Department of Health and Human Services, Joxel Garcia, M.D., M.B.A., Assistant Secretary for Health, responded with a one-page note dated August 4, 2008:

> Dear Mr. Burton:
>
> Secretary Leavitt has asked me to thank you for your letter regarding research conducted at Columbia University and to respond to you directly.
>
> The Office for Human Research Protections (OHRP) has completed an evaluation of the matter referenced in your letter. OHRP made the determinations in the letter you reference based on documentation provided to them by Co-

lumbia University Medical Center (CUMC) and other relevant sources. The issues that you raise in your letter involve the specific facts of the case that were communicated to OHRP by CUMC. Please note that OHRP addressed the remainder of the complainant's allegations of noncompliance with 45 CFR Part 46 in the June 2, 2008 letter to CUMC, and made additional determinations.

It is standard procedure for OHRP to ask the institution to conduct an investigation of the potential noncompliance and to report those findings, along with documentation, to OHRP for review. OHRP then makes determinations based on that documentation and other relevant sources.

There has been no change in Dr. John Chabot's eligibility to receive Federal research funds based on OHRP's determinations to date. Dr. Chabot's continued eligibility will depend on the outcome of OHRP's evaluation and the findings of any additional determinations it may make.

Let me assure you that the National Institutes of Health (NIH) takes its stewardship responsibilities very seriously and requires institutions to carry out research with human subjects in accordance with the ethical principles and rules embodied in HHS regulations for the protection of human subjects found in 45 CFR Part 46 and other applicable Federal statutes and regulations. NIH obtains assurance from every organization receiving NIH funding for human subjects research that it has an OHRP approved Federal Wide Assurance and that research involving human subjects has been reviewed and approved by an appropriate Institutional Review Board. . . .

This Department and its agencies appreciate and share your commitment to the protection of human research subjects. Should you or your staff have any additional questions regarding this matter, please feel free to contact Dr. Kristina Borror, Director of OHRP's Division of Compliance Oversight. . . .

The letter arrived as Congress departed Washington for its five-week summer break, but Monica Knab, Mr. Burton's aide assigned to the case, informed me she felt the response inadequate—particularly in view of the very light punishment meted out to Dr. Chabot. She believed Chabot's repeated denial of management lapses over the years, even to the NIH Director despite evidence proving otherwise, called for stronger penalties, even banishment from future government funding. Perhaps, Ms. Knab suggested, Congressional hearings might provide the ultimate remedy, to help sort out what really happened to this $1.4 million federally financed trial that failed to resolve the questions about my treatment it was set up to answer.

Nearly three months would pass before Dr. Andreason replied to my June 2008 letter. In a brief, two paragraph note dated September 4, 2008, he claimed that OHRP had done all it could do within their jurisdiction:

> We acknowledge that your letter of June 15, 2008 is clear that you are not satisfied with the outcome of our actions in this case; however, your June 15, 2008 submission does not provide us new substantive information regarding allegations of non-compliance with human research-subjects protections regulations at 45 CFR 46. Our compliance oversight case with Columbia University School of Medicine regarding the above research will therefore remain closed.

Dr. Andreason did not respond to my simple question posed to him, had he ever read any of the manuscripts or documents I sent OHRP? Without a straightforward answer, I assumed that he had not, and wouldn't say so in writing.

Chapter 41

What Does the Data Really Mean?

A fter eight years of work and $1.4 million in government funds spent, many have asked me if the study showed anything at all about the efficacy of our treatment. Even after we describe Dr. Engel's 2005 letter or OHRP's confirmation of Dr. Chabot's mismanagement, some still wonder if any valid data can be salvaged. By the strictest standards of a properly run clinical trial, the answer is a definite "no." With so many patients entered into the nutrition arm who could not or would not adhere to the prescribed therapy, with so many acknowledged protocol violations, in our opinion no legitimate assessment can be made. Dr. Engel concluded as much in her January 2005 letter, when all but one of the nutrition group had been admitted:

In spite of everyone's best efforts, it appears as if the current design and implementation of the study may have resulted in accrual into the two study arms of patient populations that are not comparable. As a consequence, it is very difficult (if not impossible) to ascertain treatment effect with certainty.

Given all of the challenges, the surprising outcomes, and the uncertainties about balance between the two arms, it is highly likely (if not certain) that reviewers of the data from this study will raise substantive and legitimate concerns about the comparability of the two populations. As a consequence, it is virtually certain that the controversy surrounding the study will not be settled by the data from it. . . .

The December 13 discussion with the team was very illuminating in that nothing materially altered this assessment. With respect to the specific matters raised in Dr. Gonzalez' letter, we will make only two brief comments.

We discussed at considerable length his concerns about the probable accrual of patients unable to comply fully with the nutrition arm of the protocol. It was our impression that everyone in the room basically agreed that, despite best efforts, there is in fact, reason to be concerned about this issue, and that it clouds interpretation of the data.

In one respect, Dr. Chabot's *JAMA* paper actually helped confirm just how non-comparable the two groups really were. Until I read this document, neither Dr. Isaacs nor I knew very much about how the chemotherapy group came to be. True, at times Dr. Chabot shared with us general information about these patients, such as their overall survival, but he had not told us much about how they were selected. For example, we weren't at all sure if the majority (or all) came through the Columbia system, or whether some or many might have been treated at other institutions. In the Chabot *JAMA* report, I learned for the first time that all those admitted for chemotherapy were indeed Columbia patients of Dr. Fine and his colleagues, an important fact to know for a number of reasons. First, it meant every patient entered into the chemotherapy arm would have been provided the most aggressive supportive care available at a tertiary care academic center, with enormous resources in place to keep each alive as long as possible. This approach, as I hope I have made clear, differed considerably from the unhelpful, indifferent and at times hostile attitude of the local doctors toward many of those treated by Dr. Isaacs and me.

The fact that Dr. Fine and his Columbia team supervised all those approved for chemotherapy provided a clue to another important question—just how Dr. Chabot managed to enter 11 into this group during the waning months of the study, when he had admitted a grand total of 12 during the first six years. But now, from the *JAMA* submission, we knew that these last 11 chemo entries were all Columbia patients of Dr. Fine. We could only assume that Dr. Chabot, with time running out and investigations in progress, worked hard with his Columbia friends and colleagues to fill the under-represented chemotherapy arm.

We also had learned from the published literature that Dr. Fine, during the same period as our trial, supervised a number of other studies at Columbia testing his GTX regimen. We wondered if any of these 11 patients approved for chemotherapy in our project at the last minute were newly diagnosed, or whether they had been recruited from other studies running concurrently at Columbia.

Unfortunately, we still had no answer to another perplexing question. As I have previously discussed, the written protocol required all patients in both groups be entered within eight weeks of diagnosis. Even the OHRP, as laggard as they seemed to have been in their evaluation, acknowledged that Dr. Chabot approved two patients, Patients #14(129) and #34(113), well beyond that cutoff, at 11 weeks and 10 weeks from the date of biopsy.

We had also documented that Dr. Chabot repeatedly qualified candidates for the nutritional arm who, though technically admitted within eight weeks of diagnosis, he kept waiting for prolonged periods before determining their eligibility, thereby causing a loss of valuable treatment time. I have earlier discussed in some detail the stories of Patients #15 and #38, kept on hold by Dr. Chabot four and five weeks respectively before he informed each of their status, during which time neither patient pursued any therapy. Such delays seemed hardly inconsequential for patients diagnosed with advanced pancreatic cancer and with life expectancies measured in weeks and months.

In our own practice, Dr. Isaacs and I do not treat everyone who wishes to pursue our regimen, but select those we feel from our experience we can help and seem best suited for our self-administered nutritional approach. We carefully evaluate each prospective patient, routinely turning down those we don't think would benefit. As part of our initial assessment, we first review pertinent medical records, then request all potentially suitable patients undergo an interview with one of my staff members. Only then do we make our final decision, usually within 24 hours, so these people will not be kept waiting while we ponder the case. To this day, we still don't understand why Chabot frequently needed four and five weeks to determine eligibility.

Unfortunately, Patients #15 and #38 were hardly anomalies. As it turned out Dr. Chabot approved many candidates for the nutrition arm who had been diagnosed many weeks earlier, even if technically falling within—though often barely—the eight-week cutoff from biopsy. The following chart lists those nutrition subjects whose tissue diagnosis dated four or more weeks prior to their initial consultation with us.

Patient #	Time From Biopsy to Consultation in Our Office
1	43 days (6 weeks)
2	52 days (7.5 weeks)
3	34 days (nearly 5 weeks)
8	31 days (4.5 weeks)
9	45 days (6.5 weeks)
11	50 days (7+ weeks)
12	30 days (4+ weeks)
13	33 days (4.5 weeks)
14	77 days (11 weeks)
15	42 days (6 weeks)
16	49 days (7 weeks)
17	28 days (4 weeks)
19	44 days (6+ weeks)
20	52 days (7.5 weeks)
21	46 days (6.5 weeks)
22	28 days (4 weeks)
28	52 days (7.5 weeks)
29	43 days (6+ weeks)
30	40 days (5.7 weeks)
32	36 days (5+ weeks)
33	43 days (6+ weeks)
34	71 days (10+ weeks)
35	36 days (5+ weeks)
36	64 days (9+ weeks)
38	56 days (8 weeks)
39	43 days (6+ weeks)

As the above chart illustrates, for 26 of the total of 39 patients entered into the nutrition arm, the time from biopsy to initial consultation with us exceeded four or more weeks, and in 17 cases, it exceeded six or more weeks. With so much valuable time lost between diagnosis and entry into the trial, many of the nutrition patients were from the onset simply too sick to comply.

And I think it's important to revisit the case of Patient #13 listed above, diagnosed with liver metastases. Chabot not only approved him for entry more than four weeks after his biopsy, but upon returning home and before he could begin his treatment Patient #13 underwent emergency surgery for an intestinal obstruction unrelated to his pancreatic disease. Postoperatively he developed pulmonary emboli that required intensive treatment and hospitalization for a full five weeks, during which time he pursued no aspect of the prescribed regimen. Once home, he did valiantly try to begin his therapy—some ten weeks from his biopsy—but found compliance difficult. Nonetheless Dr. Chabot insisted this patient be considered a properly entered, properly treated Gonzalez failure.

For all 39 nutrition patients I calculate an average delay between biopsy diagnosis and their first visit with us of 36 days, or slightly more than five weeks—not insignificant for a disease as relentlessly aggressive as pancreatic adenocarcinoma.

But just how important, in the larger scheme of things, were these lapses between biopsy and admission into the study? Did routine delays of four, five, six, even in one case 11 weeks really affect these patients' clinical status that much, and ultimately, their chance for response to our therapy? For our trial subjects, all diagnosed with advanced pancreatic cancer, these lost weeks when they received no therapy did in our opinion often mean the difference between treatment success and failure. I could think of no more appropriate reference to prove my point than Dr. Zerhouni's letter of December 22, 2005, written to Congressman Burton. In this document the NIH director made the case strongly and convincingly that the status of patients diagnosed with pancreatic cancer can change dramatically within days—though he paradoxically used this fact in a misguided defense of Chabot's management of the study.

Specifically, in the second paragraph of the third page, he first incorrectly denied that Chabot had admitted patients who failed to meet the entry requirements. Then in answer to my complaint that Chabot had approved many patients too ill to comply, Dr. Zerhouni wrote:

Due to the nature of pancreatic cancer, it is not unusual for patient status to change within days or weeks. Patients who meet the requirements at the time of enrollment may experience changes in their ability to meet the criteria over time.

Precisely because, as Zerhouni's own words confirmed, patients with pancreatic cancer often deteriorate so rapidly, they needed to be approved for our study promptly, not routinely four, five, six, seven, or even 11 weeks after diagnosis.

We do not know how soon after biopsy, on average, Chabot accepted the chemotherapy patients into the trial since he never shared that information with us. With long experience in our private practice evaluating patients diagnosed with pancreatic cancer, we have a pretty good idea how quickly conventional oncologists mobilize—often, they are arranging to begin treatment within 24–48 hours after confirmation of disease. Recently, a patient with advanced pancreatic adenocarcinoma who worsened despite chemotherapy called our office, desperate to begin our regimen. He explained that he had begun treatment the very day he was diagnosed, before he had a chance even to consider alternatives such as mine. His is not an unusual story.

We suspect for those patients diagnosed at Columbia—known for its aggressive approach to the disease—this rule would have applied. Of course, some of the chemotherapy group may have been initially diagnosed at an outside hospital, then referred to Dr. Fine, but even in these cases, we doubt that the lag time between biopsy and the beginning of treatment routinely amounted to six or more weeks—even 10 and 11 weeks—as was true with the nutritional patients. Unfortunately, we just do not know the whole story. But if the average delay between diagnosis and entry into the study differed significantly between the two groups, such a discrepancy would make comparison even more meaningless for a disease as aggressive as pancreatic cancer, with its brief window of opportunity for treatment response.

Having said all this, can we glean any meaning out of those few nutrition patients who actually did comply with the prescribed regimen? Here, I believe the answer is yes, particularly if one considers for a moment how the field of cancer chemotherapy, a multi-billion business in the U.S., first came to be. Ironically, the current cancer-drug industry owes its existence to nitrogen mustard, the poison gas used with deadly effect in World War I. The Wikipedia section of the "History of cancer chemotherapy" summarizes the initial efforts to apply these deadly chemicals against cancer:

> The beginnings of the modern era of cancer chemotherapy can be traced directly to the discovery of nitrogen mustard, a chemical warfare agent. . . . Two pharmacologists, Louis S. Goodman and Alfred Gilman were recruited by the United States Department of Defense to investigate potential therapeutic applications of chemical warfare agents. Autopsy observations of people exposed to mustard gas had revealed profound lymphoid and myeloid suppression. Goodman and Gilman reasoned that this agent could be used to treat lymphoma. . . . They first set up an animal model—they established lymphomas in mice and demonstrated they could treat them with mustard agents. Next . . . they injected a related agent, mustine . . . into a patient with non-Hodgkin's lymphoma. They observed a dramatic reduction in the patient's tumour masses. Although this effect lasted only a few weeks, this was the first step to the realization that cancer could be treated by pharmacological agents.[82]

Early in our study, when the first signs of rampant non-compliance among the nutrition patients surfaced, Dr. Antman referred to the origins of modern cancer treatment, as described in the above quote. She made the point that cancer chemotherapeutics developed because of a single patient who responded dramatically, even if only briefly, and not dozens and dozens who did well in carefully controlled clinical studies. But that single episode of tumor regression was surprising enough to capture the attention of the entire oncology research community.

So, she assured us, if our therapy yielded a couple of unusual responders in terms of unexpected prolonged survival, even a single such case that no one else could match, that finding alone should legitimately encourage interest from the academic world in our approach. She believed that such a "tail" of outstanding survival as she called it, would be scientifically significant.

In the text of his *JAMA* paper, Dr. Chabot made no reference to such long-lived survivors in the nutrition group, but hidden away after the main text of the article, he included seven pages of charts. The second to the last of these consisted of a graph tracking the survival, measured from the date of entry into the trial, of every patient admitted into each arm. Here we learned that the longest-living chemotherapy patient at the time this paper was submitted to *JAMA* in late 2006 appeared to be alive approximately two years, four months, after entering the study—certainly unusual longevity for a patient with advanced pancreatic cancer treated with drugs.

The graph also revealed that the two longest-surviving patients of all those approved for the trial were ours, both diagnosed with advanced stage IV disease. One, with liver metastases, initially complied well with stabilization of malignancy after 14 months, but ultimately abandoned the regimen at the urging of her oncologist. She nonetheless lived two years and six months from her admission into the study. Since Chabot approved this patient 7.5 weeks after her biopsy, her overall survival from diagnosis actually measured nearly two years and eight months. The second, the most compliant of all nutrition patients and the longest survivor in the entire study as of the *JAMA* submission, died three years and four months after being qualified—11 months longer than the longest living chemotherapy patient. He was approved for treatment with us 43 days, or slightly more than six weeks after biopsy, so counting that time his overall lifespan from diagnosis approached three and a half years. His clinical course was ultimately complicated by multiple lengthy hospitalizations during his last months not due to his cancer but because of problems with a mesh surgically implanted into his abdominal wall to correct an inguinal hernia. Unfortunately, the mesh became infected, but for some time his local doctors mistakenly attributed his worsening condition to his malignant disease. By the time the situation had been correctly diagnosed, the infection had infiltrated extensively throughout the abdominal wall tissues. In a debilitated state, he finally underwent surgery for removal of the mesh, but during his long and arduous recovery he complied only sporadically with his nutritional therapy and eventually succumbed.

Yet in the body of his *JAMA* paper Dr. Chabot nowhere reported that the two longest survivors, and by a substantial margin, were ours. One needed to examine the graphs to learn of this, and the graphs, I might add, came with little narrative explanation. The fact that at the time of the paper's submission these two had outlived any in Dr. Fine's chemotherapy group was not an inconsequential finding, since they were up against aggressively treated patients given access to the most intensive supportive care in the history of conventional cancer medicine.

To put the survival of our two patients in perspective, one need only review the Gemzar data from 1997 that helped establish the drug as the standard of care worldwide for the treatment of pancreatic cancer. In that trial of 126 total subjects receiving two different forms of chemotherapy, not one lived longer than 19 months. Yet based on meager improvements in average survival and quality of life compared to older drug regimens, Gemzar earned FDA approval and is today a billion dollar industry worldwide. Our leading survivor lived more than twice as long, our second 11 months longer than the longest-living Gemzar patient. And our nutrition group consisted of at most 39 patients (or 35 as reported in the Chabot *JAMA* submission), compared to the 126 total treated in the Gemzar study, to make the comparison more striking. But again, in his paper Dr. Chabot did not mention any of this. On the contrary, in his discussion Dr. Chabot lauded the efficacy of his chemotherapy, without attributing any response in any of our patients.

So the "tail," to use Dr. Antman's term, of unusual survivors did exist, indicating a significant response to treatment in at least two of the small group of nutrition patients who complied. These two outlived by far all the 126 entered into the Gemzar study and at the time of the *JAMA* submission had survived longer than any of those treated with chemotherapy in our own trial.

Since the entire field of modern cancer chemotherapy began when a single patient responded for several weeks to a toxic chemical, one would think that our two long-term survivors would generate some interest. These particular patients also make the point we have so often repeated, that survival correlates with compliance. Patients diagnosed with pancreatic cancer who comply often respond, those that do not follow the treatment plan—the majority entered into the study, for example—do poorly.

I have to this point discussed the many patients Dr. Chabot admitted for treatment with us whom we believe did not meet the explicit entry criteria. But there is one patient Dr. Chabot refused to enter we think actually qualified, Sarah Ann Cooper (who wrote this book's Foreword).

In December of 2000, after a period of intermittent abdominal distress, Ms. Cooper underwent a CT of the abdomen that revealed a 3.4 cm mass in the head of the pancreas, but no evidence of distant spread. After a series of additional tests and referrals to various doctors, in early February 2001 she underwent CT scan guided biopsy of the tumor, which proved to be a very aggressive, poorly differentiated adenocarcinoma. The pathology slides were sent for review to the Mayo Clinic, where the diagnosis was confirmed. Shortly thereafter Ms. Cooper learned about the clinical trial and contacted our office wishing to set up an appointment.

After speaking with my staff she agreed to follow up with Dr. Chabot to begin the evaluation process. After passing Dr. Chabot's initial assessment of her case, Ms. Cooper flew to New York for her interview at Columbia and her appointments scheduled with Dr. Isaacs. Her Chabot session had actually been sandwiched between her first and second visits in our office, so Dr. Isaacs met with her before her meeting at Columbia. This initial consultation with Dr. Isaacs went well, so well we thought we finally might be accruing a patient who could and would follow the prescribed nutritional regimen.

But during his interview with Ms. Cooper, Dr. Chabot decided the tumor might be surgically resectable, a reason, he insisted, to exclude her from the trial. Though Ms. Cooper made it clear to Dr. Chabot and later to us that she would not proceed with surgery under any circumstances, he refused to admit her. Ms. Cooper, having flown in from the West with such high expectations, was devastated, thinking she could not receive our treatment unless approved for the clinical trial. Dr. Isaacs subsequently assured her otherwise, explaining also that we would treat her for free after all she had been through (though she would have to pay for the supplements which we do not sell).

Dr. Isaacs and I were disturbed by the turn of events for a number of reasons. First of all, Chabot was supposed to review the medical records of all prospective study candidates before setting up his New York interview to avoid putting those who didn't qualify through unnecessary stress. Based on our preliminary assessment, she seemed like an ideal candidate, with a great attitude, a previous interest in alternative approaches, and a determination to follow our regimen. So after the second session with Dr. Isaacs, I called Dr. Chabot, arguing that she should be approved for the study. The operability of the tumor hardly seemed certain, and Ms. Cooper would refuse surgery under any conditions. Unfortunately, Dr. Chabot wouldn't relent, so Ms. Cooper came under the care of Dr. Isaacs as a private patient without ever undergoing surgery.

She subsequently fared very well, as she diligently followed her nutritional regimen. Over her many years on the therapy, CT scan studies confirmed gradual though not complete regression of the tumor. Today, more than eleven years since her diagnosis of aggressive pancreatic cancer, she is in excellent health, enjoys her life fully, and continues following a modified version of the regimen.

Why has Ms. Cooper done so spectacularly well? Fortunately she was diagnosed early in the course of her disease before it had, at least by CT studies, spread beyond the pancreas. She could eat normally—unlike the majority of patients entered into the clinical trial—and she followed the program as prescribed. She knew what she wanted to do, took full responsibility for her decision to refuse surgery, never looked back, had faith in our approach and never questioned her choice of treatment. Ms. Cooper, believing that Dr. Isaacs would do the best she could to help her whatever the outcome, repeatedly expressed her gratitude to us for making this therapy available to those who want it.

Her manner typified the patients we see in our private practice, in contrast to many of those admitted into the clinical study. Yes, I acknowledge that she was diagnosed at an earlier stage than many of the trial patients, who were simply too ill to comply adequately. Above and beyond that point, many of those Chabot sent to us for treatment just didn't have her resolve, easily giving up with the first problem, or when their oncologist—or some family member—questioned their choice of an unconventional approach. Without faith in us or what we do, many were quick to quit.

Why would this be, why would this clinical trial have attracted, as I believe it did, patients so different in terms of attitude than those we normally see in our private practice? In retrospect, Dr. Isaacs and I suspect that at least in some cases, patients who normally would never have considered an alternative treatment sought entry into the study precisely because of the official NCI grant, which in their minds perhaps gave us some sort of academic respectability, and not because of a basic belief in what we do. Ms. Cooper, on the other hand, though wishing to participate in the study, contacted us primarily out of her interest in nutritional approaches. Yes, she was upset when Chabot rejected her from the trial, thinking she could not then receive our treatment. Otherwise she fundamentally could have cared less about the NCI, the NIH, our "respectability" or Dr. Chabot's opinion, all of which she thought was a distraction from her focus, to start our treatment as soon as possible. With an attitude like that, she has surely been a pleasure to work with over the years.

A patient such as this—certainly a remarkable survivor, now more than eleven years from diagnosis—should warrant at least some interest by the so-called experts. Based on my past experience I expect my critics, who seem by their nature never to be satisfied, will choose to ignore this case or instead say, "even if the Gonzalez regimen does work sometimes, it's so difficult to follow it's simply not practical. Even if we accept his claim that most patients entered into the clinical study didn't comply that just proves it's too difficult for wide application." I've heard statements like this before, when colleagues have been faced with patients such as Sarah Ann Cooper they can't easily explain away.

The therapy really is not that difficult to implement. For most cancer patients, it is no great chore to eat food, or take two hundred pills spread throughout the day, or undergo the daily coffee enema routine. Though I myself have never been diagnosed with cancer, I follow a fairly rigorous preventive program myself. I eat organically, juice if not daily at this point frequently, take 100 pills a day, do the detox routine including the coffee enemas I prescribe for my patients, and work long days, seven days a week, year in and year out. It isn't that difficult at all, if one's mind is in the right place for it. On the other hand, if someone thinks drinking carrot juice or eating whole grains or swallowing pills equates to inhumane torture, it will be difficult.

Our dietary and nutritional therapy does require patients be able to eat normally, that is just the reality of our therapy which we readily acknowledge. We also recognize that pancreatic cancer, involving a major digestive organ, often disrupts appetite significantly, perhaps more than other cancers. Consequently, patients in the advanced terminal stage of the illness—as were the majority Dr. Chabot entered into this trial—often cannot comply, whatever their mindset, because of their inability to eat. But we believe, based on our 24 years of experience, that most cancer patients, even those with advanced disease, could follow our program successfully, and should have it available to them as an option.

Chapter 42

More Letters and More Meetings

In early October 2008, I learned from Monica Knab that Congressman Burton was not happy with the Department of Health and Human Services' (DHHS) response to his letter, particularly the director's apparent acceptance of the incomplete OHRP investigation as adequate. The Congressman was concerned enough that he subsequently contacted the Inspector General (IG) of the DHHS, Daniel Levinson, the official with the power to authorize audits, investigations, and inspections of institutions and individuals engaged in government sponsored research. In a letter dated October 31, 2008, after summarizing the study's history Congressman Burton requested the IG open a formal evaluation of the trial's management:

> I believe it is important for Congress, the American public, and the medical community to have confidence in Federally-funded medical research. To that end, we need to know whether or not the NIH is fulfilling its mission and Congressional mandates with vigor and competence, and whether or not NIH is performing its oversight responsibility at optimal levels. NIH's management of this particular clinical trial has underscored a very real concern of many members of Congress, the public and the research community. Given the seriousness of this issue and its implications on future human research, I respectfully request that your office review the case to determine if reports alleging

mismanagement of this particular NIH research activity and potential NIH mismanagement of the investigation into human research protection violations have any merit.

As we waited to hear from the Inspector General, Beth Clay, my Washington consultant friend, suggested that I contact Dr. Briggs, NCCAM's new director, and request a face-to-face meeting with her to review my concerns about the trial's outcome. Ms. Clay suspected that the NCCAM and NCI staff may not have thoroughly briefed Dr. Briggs about the managerial lapses that had derailed our study, so she might not even be aware of the OHRP findings. Ms. Clay—who had in the past worked at both the NIH and the old OAM— thought it would be in my best interest to give Dr. Briggs the full picture of what had happened. Despite Dr. Briggs' lack of prior interest in or experience with alternative medicine, many leaders within the field, Ms. Clay explained, considered her fair-minded and intent on supporting legitimate research evaluations of unconventional treatments. If true, such an attitude, we both agreed, would contrast greatly with that of her predecessor.

In November 2008 I wrote to Dr. Briggs, proposing, at her convenience, a meeting at the NCCAM offices in Bethesda. She responded quickly in writing, expressing her openness to the idea, and eventually we set the date for December 12, 2008. She did not object when I asked if I might bring the patient who lived in the Washington area and had accompanied me to the session with Senator Harkin a year earlier. By 2008 this patient had already survived for five years on my therapy after a diagnosis of stage IV adenocarcinoma of the lung unresponsive to previous aggressive chemotherapy. I thought his unusual story might have some impact on Dr. Briggs.

Meanwhile, in late November 2008, after hearing nothing from the Office of Research Integrity (ORI) for some time, its director, Dr. Dahlberg, finally wrote me, stating in part:

> The concerns you raised about the research included problems with the consent process, changes in the protocol, and conflict of interest on the part of Dr. Chabot. OHRP's investigation into the human subjects concerns clearly reflects the seriousness with which they took your allegations. We are also committed to serious consideration of allegations of misconduct. However, in this case, your allegations against Dr. Chabot do not fall within ORI's legal jurisdiction.

Then, after describing government policies on research misconduct, he continued:

> ORI, as a matter of long-standing policy, does not consider informed consent issue [sic] to fall within its jurisdiction, and the OHRP letter indicates that the matter has been appropriately dealt with. I also emphasize that "research misconduct does not include honest error or differences of opinion." As you have not raised substantive issues involving intentional falsification or fabrication of research data that could be proven by a preponderance of the evidence, ORI does not have jurisdiction in this case, nor are we permitted by law to address any of your other concerns about the research.

At this point, no statement from a government official surprised me. Nonetheless, I didn't understand Dr. Dahlberg's letter since I had previously raised with him the serious, multiple misstatements and inaccuracies apparent in the *JAMA* submission which by his own statements above would seem to warrant an investigation by his office. So, I buckled down, completing yet another letter to Dr. Dahlberg, this one dated November 24, 2008. I began the 16-page document with an introductory section summarizing my concerns, including my belief Dr. Chabot had misrepresented fact and data:

> Dear Dr. Dahlberg:
>
> Thank you for your letter dated November 17, 2008. I understand full well that you can only investigate issues that fall within your explicitly defined jurisdiction. I also appreciate that the OHRP has been given the mandate to evaluate issues of informed consent. I also recognize that OHRP, however unsatisfactory I may find their overall investigation of the matter, clearly did find Dr. Chabot mismanaged the entry of multiple patients into the trial.
>
> Nonetheless, your letter left me somewhat perplexed, to say the least. It is precisely because of the differences in jurisdiction between you and OHRP that I first contacted you in 2006. I do not comprehend your ignoring in your letter, and apparently in whatever investigation proceeded under your supervision, serious issues. . . . Because I had earlier raised these issues with you directly at some length, your letter is indeed very troubling.
>
> These issues include [inaccurate] statements about me, my participation in the study, and the data, appearing in Dr. Chabot's attempted publication from December 2006.

I will discuss these points in some detail, but here, for your convenience, I outline the major areas you chose not to address:

Dr. Chabot's attempt to publish an article about the trial without notifying me of its existence or his plans for it.

Dr. Chabot's false statement in his manuscript that "The patients in both the control and experimental arm were carefully **enrolled** *(bold Chabot's) according to* **strict** *(bold Chabot's) entry criteria," when in fact official trial records of which he was keenly aware had already documented that Dr. Chabot admitted multiple patients who did not meet the "strict entry criteria" including three admitted for whom no evidence of signed informed consent exists. Of course, OHRP's determination that 42 of a total of 62 patients had been improperly entered confirms Dr. Chabot's managerial lapses.*

Dr. Chabot's failure to note in his manuscript the carefully documented fact, as confirmed in an official NIH letter to him, that a significant number of nutrition patients had been unable or had chosen not to comply and that, to quote the NIH, **"there is in fact, reason to be concerned about this issue, and that it clouds interpretation of the data."**

Dr. Chabot's failure to note in his manuscript official NIH staff conclusions further confirming that due to the management problems the two arms of the study could not be compared and that the study most likely had yielded no meaningful data.

Dr. Chabot's failure to discuss in his manuscript the vast difference in the level of care available to the chemotherapy patients treated at Columbia, and our patients.

Dr. Chabot's failure to note in his manuscript that despite the significant managerial lapses on his part, and the entry of so many nutrition patients who failed to comply adequately with the prescribed regimen, the two longest survivors in the study, both good compliers, were my patients (in the nutritional arm).

Dr. Chabot's false statement in his manuscript "Dr. Gonzalez expressed concern related to patient selection and elected not to continue participating in the study. . ." when in fact I never withdrew from the study, as the record of the trial clearly proves.

Dr. Chabot's false statement that "Although repeatedly invited to discuss the manuscript and to serve as co-author, Dr. Gonzalez declined to participate in manuscript preparation" when in fact I had not been invited to review any manuscript, knew nothing of the manuscript, and in fact six months before its attempted publication I had warned Dr. Chabot not to attempt any future publication with federal investigations of mismanagement in progress.

Dr. Chabot's inappropriate downstaging of five nutrition patients, all appropriate at stage IV, to lesser stages, so they appear to have been less sick in the final data chart made available to us in April 2006. In addition, in that document he also eliminated two stage IV patients from the nutrition arm . . . In this way, Dr. Chabot [helped correct] . . . the glaring staging disparity between the chemotherapy and nutrition patients, with most chemotherapy patients at an earlier stage and most of ours at stage IV. This disparity, which helped render meaningful comparison between the two groups impossible, we had earlier carefully documented and made known to all involved including Dr. Chabot.

Below I discuss each point in some detail: I request you read all that follows carefully, and answer the questions that I include toward the end of the letter.

I sent off the carefully documented letter and prepared myself for another long wait, assuming as per usual I would not hear back from Dr. Dahlberg for some time.

Meanwhile, the December 12, 2008 meeting with Dr. Briggs went ahead as planned at NCCAM headquarters, located in one of the many buildings on the impressive, sprawling NIH campus in Bethesda. When I first arrived with my patient at Dr. Brigg's offices, I chuckled when I saw Dr. Killen's name appearing near the top of the NCCAM directory, identified as the Acting Associate Director.

But Dr. Killen did not attend our meeting, nor was he mentioned, though Dr. Briggs did bring along another NCCAM scientist, Dr. Andrea Sorkin. I found Dr. Briggs to be gracious, intelligent, and well spoken, lacking any evident hostility toward me. Though our talk proved quite pleasant, as Beth Clay suspected, Dr. Briggs seemed unaware of the many problems and managerial lapses that had plagued our study, even of Dr. Engel's letter or the OHRP investigation. She admitted that she had not been extensively "debriefed" about the trial, to use her word, before stating she hoped that we would all look "forward" rather than backward. With a research interest in diabetes, Dr. Briggs did agree that clinical studies investigating dietary and nutritionally-based treatments for serious disease required a more flexible design than the standard approach of comparing the effects of Drug A to Drug B. She thought such a simplistic format might not be suitable for evaluating complex nutritional regimens such as mine—the very issue I had first raised with Dr. Antman in 1997, as we worked on the first version of the written protocol and as she pushed a conventional chemotherapy study model onto our trial. Dr. Briggs also seemed intrigued by my patient's personal fight against advanced cancer with my treatment. After some 40 minutes she concluded our session by saying she hoped I would be willing to share my experiences with others at NCCAM and the NIH, so we might all learn from the mistakes made during this eight-year effort.

We parted amicably. Several days later I wrote Dr. Briggs, thanking her for her time, and enlarging upon some of the points we had discussed. She responded with a two-paragraph note dated December 30, 2008, in which she in turn thanked me for coming down to Bethesda:

> I very much enjoyed our conversation. It is clear to me that you have a deep commitment to your patients and to exploring innovative methods to help with this terrible disease.

> In 2009 we are beginning our new strategic planning process, which will include the input from our many communities on areas of focus and priority. As that process goes forward, I hope that you will share your thoughts on how we might conduct clinical trials more effectively.

Despite the pleasantries, and my subsequent offer in writing to share my experiences with her staff, I would not hear from her again.

In late January 2009, Inspector General Levinson wrote to Congressman Burton, informing him that he had referred the matter of the clinical trial to their Office of Investigations for review. Beth Clay thought the reply a good sign, an indication of a sincere interest in the case, since with limited available resources the IG's office pursued only a small number of complaints sent them.

Shortly after, in a brief, one-page letter dated February 2, 2009, Dr. Dahlberg of ORI responded to my most recent communication. Though he finally seemed ready to take my allegations seriously, Dr. Dahlberg—to my surprise—informed me that any further probe into the issues I had raised would need be conducted by the institution involved, in this case Columbia:

> The Division of Investigative Oversight (DIO) within the Office of Research Integrity (ORI) has received your letter of November 24, 2008. While your

letter contains information that could lead to an inquiry into research mis-conduct, that inquiry and the related fact finding must be conducted by the institution.

So if I wanted to pursue further action, I would have to rely on Columbia, as had OHRP, to investigate itself. As I read his note, I wondered why ORI even existed, if it could do nothing independently. While this time around Dr. Dahlberg may not have dismissed my complaints—indeed a refreshing change—I hardly felt confident Columbia would move aggressively based on charges leveled by me. After all, though the Dean's office had acknowledged receipt of my December 2006 letter written after Chabot's aborted attempt to publish in JAMA, I had not heard a word from Columbia in the two years since. The lack of response over an issue as important as scientific integrity did not inspire much confidence. So after mulling over my options, I decided to leave the matter, at least for the time being, in the hands of the Inspector General's office in Washington.

Chapter 43

Hollywood Comes to the Rescue

Quite unexpectedly, one afternoon in February 2009 Julie Turkel, identifying herself as the assistant to the actress and writer Suzanne Somers, contacted my office wishing to speak with me. I took the call, and after some pleasantries Ms. Turkel explained that Ms. Somers wished to talk to me informally, if I were willing, to introduce herself and discuss a book she planned to write about promising alternative approaches to cancer. If this initial conversation went well, again with my approval, at some later date Ms. Somers would interview me at greater length for the book. After that second conversation, she would then want to talk directly with a number of my patients diagnosed with poor-prognosis cancer who had done well under my care.

Like most Americans, I was quite familiar with Ms. Somers, though I had never spoken with her. I knew that she had starred in two very successful television series, the #1 hit *Three's Company* beginning in the late 1970s, then during the 1990s *Step by Step* in which she played the mother of a combined extended family. I had also read that after leaving *Three's Company* in the early 1980s she developed a very successful Las Vegas nightclub act.

In addition to her performing work, she had authored a series of best-selling books covering a variety of alternative medicine topics such as anti-aging, weight loss, and bio-identical hormone therapy, more than one making its way to the vaunted *New York Times* bestseller list. Ms. Somers was also well known, even to me, as a very successful businesswoman. Unlike so many Hollywood stars who rise and fall quickly with little to show for the effort, she had managed her money astutely, starting a number of profitable commercial ventures. And I was already aware Ms. Somers had survived a bout with breast cancer some ten years earlier, which she treated with a combination of conventional and alternative approaches.

In late February I spoke by phone with Ms. Somers herself for about half an hour, as our introductory talk, and from the outset I found her to be very intelligent, very gracious, and very well-informed about my work. In our conversation, she relayed her own cancer history that began with a diagnosis of localized breast cancer treated initially with surgery followed by a course of radiation. The effects of these interventions proved so debilitating that she subsequently refused the recommended chemotherapy, instead beginning her foray in the world of alternative medicine. Though she never had consulted me, she worked with a number of well-known unconventional physicians who guided her in terms of diet, nutrition, supplements, and bio-identical hormones.

She had done well for some ten years, avoiding any recurrence of her disease, when in the fall of 2009 she became acutely ill, to the point she ended up in the emergency room of a Los Angeles hospital. When CT scans seemed to confirm widespread metastatic cancer including multiple tumors in her lungs, her doctors insisted she begin chemotherapy at once. Though in a state of shock, she decided to hold off—fortunately for her. As she explained to me, it turned out she had no recurrence of her long-dormant malignancy, but a severe fungal infection, Valley Fever (coccidioidomycosis), that once properly diagnosed was treated effectively with appropriate medication. Determined to extract some good out of her terrible experience and the initial misdiagnosis, as she recovered she decided to tackle for her next book that most explosive of subjects, alternative cancer therapies. She told me she thought it was time treatments such as mine, largely ignored or vilified by the conventional medical world, received some type of recognition.

Her editor at Crown, a division of Random House, supported the project enthusiastically, proposing an initial printing of some 500,000 hardcover copies—a very substantial number that would be supported by an aggressive publicity campaign. Though Ms. Somers understood such a book would inevitably generate considerable controversy and undoubtedly bring on the wrath of the conventional medical world, she believed the issue so important that she was willing to endure attack. Despite such predictable opposition, she expected that based on the success of her previous books, this one would have an enormous impact.

As our discussion continued, Ms. Somers told me that she had followed my work and research efforts for years with great interest. As a former cancer patient, she said, the fact that I existed gave her a sense of peace, knowing that even in its advanced stage the disease can often be beaten nutritionally. Though her combination approach had kept her own malignancy at bay for years, she said that if she ever experienced a recurrence she would be on a plane to New York the same day.

As we talked, I could tell that she clearly had done her homework: "I know everything about you," she remarked at one point, only half jokingly, and appeared aware of my NCI clinical trial, which she heard had been mismanaged by the conventional team of scientists assigned to supervise the project. This unfortunate outcome, she said, hadn't surprised her, since "The last thing the conventional medical wants is a non-toxic non-drug therapy that works out there in the world."

Ms. Somers explained in some detail her plan for the structure of the book, which she envisioned beginning with her own story, including the recent scare that fortunately proved to be a false alarm. The remaining chapters would be devoted to interviews with eight different practitioners, three of whom would be featured at some length including myself and Dr. Stan Burzynski of Houston.

As our conversation came to a close, she said she wished to interview me at a later date for a full two hours, allowing us to get into the details, the nuts and bolts of my treatment approach. Then, she hoped to speak with 10–12 of my cancer "success stories." I agreed to proceed, explaining that I should not have any difficulty finding appropriate patients willing to talk about their experiences publicly.

Later that day, I discussed the project with Dr. Isaacs, who, like me, found the whole situation ironic. At that point, in February 2009, we had spent more than ten years of our lives trying to work with the academic medical world at the highest levels, at Columbia, the NCI, and the NIH, hoping only for a fair, legitimate, honorably run evaluation of my treatment. But with the clinical trial undermined at each step, we had given up our dream that our therapy would find a home within the conventional research community. As our only viable option, we were resigned to continuing our private practice, treating patients one by one, never expecting any kind of approval or support from anybody. Then out of nowhere Suzanne Somers came into our lives, with a major book in the works inevitably destined to bring national focus, for better or worse, to our treatment approach. Paradoxically, Dr. Beard's legacy, our years of hard research, our therapy that we found so useful, would not gain recognition through the usual academic channels, but—if everything worked out the way Ms. Somers planned—as the result of a best-selling book by a non-scientist.

As all this was transpiring, at the suggestion of Congressman Burton's staff in March 2009 I wrote to Inspector General Levinson myself, describing in some detail the history of the study and the issues that troubled me: the overall mismanagement of the project; our early concerns about the study's supervision and Dr. Engel's January 2005 letter; the failure of Dr. Zerhouni to address the trial's failings; my complaints to OHRP and ORI; Chabot's *JAMA* submission of late 2006; and the failure of OHRP and ORI to evaluate my allegations fully. I included copies of relevant records to support my case, and not long after, in early April 2009, the Inspector General's office responded with a letter that seemed to me more strongly worded than its previous communication to Congressman Burton. I wondered if the enormous amount of documentation I provided had convinced the IG's office to take the matter seriously.

In his reply, the IG described his office's responsibilities, as well as the planned course of action:

> The Office of Investigations is tasked with investigating matters of health care fraud in their respective jurisdictions. This matter has been forwarded to our Office of Investigations, Special Investigations Branch where the referral will be assigned to an investigator who will review the issue and determine the most appropriate course of action.

In a subsequent phone conversation, the Inspector in charge of the case, German Melo, assured me that his office considered my complaints worthy of further consideration.

Meanwhile, Ms. Somers interviewed me as planned for a full two hours, then over a period of several weeks talked at length with 12 of my patients, all diagnosed with poor-prognosis or terminal cancer who had done well under our care. Each had experienced, by the standards of conventional oncology, very unusual long-term survival and in most cases evidence of regression of disease as documented by sequential radiographic studies. Among the group I included two patients originally diagnosed with metastatic pancreatic cancer whose tumors completely resolved while following only our nutritional regimen. I also suggested Ms. Somers contact Arlene Van Straten, a 73-year-old woman from the mid-West, diagnosed in 1982 with adenocarcinoma of the pancreas and biopsy-proven liver metastases. After a consultation at the Mayo Clinic in Rochester, Minnesota, the oncologist assigned to the case argued against conventional treatment, which he said would do little. At that point, Mrs. Van Straten began investigating alternative approaches, learned about the Kelley regimen in a book purchased at a local health score, and began the treatment under the supervision of a chiropractor trained in the method. My own connection to Mrs. Van Straten dated back to 1985, when I had first interviewed her as part of my original investigation of Kelley's therapy conducted under Dr. Good. I found her memorable from our first conversation, feisty, independent, and completely grateful for the life the Kelley program had given her.

In 2009, 27 years since her original diagnosis of terminal pancreatic cancer, she and I continued to be in touch by phone and by mail. Though she hadn't technically been my patient, I suggested to Ms. Somers that Mrs. Van Straten's extraordinary long-term survival would make for an interesting case history. Ms. Somers immediately agreed, some days later reporting back to me that her conversation with Mrs. Van Straten had been "sensational."

After this flurry of activity, for a time the situation on all fronts seemed quiet. I assumed the Inspector General's investigation was proceeding on course as per usual in such cases, slowly, but hopefully seriously. I continued working on the series of books that I first started some years earlier, at a time Dr. Isaacs and I still had hopes the clinical trial would prove to be a fair and legitimate effort. We put the final touches on the first volume, entitled *The Trophoblast and the Origins of Cancer*, which we planned to publish in the fall of 2009. In this monograph, we demonstrated how contemporary molecular biology helps prove much of what Dr. Beard claimed 100 years ago, particularly his belief that the early placenta represented the ideal model of cancer biology and behavior.[83] We also prepared for publication the second in the series, *One Man Alone: An Investigation of Nutrition, Cancer, and William Donald Kelley,* my evaluation of Dr. Kelley's therapy that I completed while an immunology fellow.[74] For more than two decades I had given up any idea of publishing the book, so strong were the biases against unconventional approaches to cancer. But now, after the passage of 23 years, the death of Dr. Good in 2003 and Dr. Kelley in 2005, Dr. Isaacs and I decided it was time, finally, to get the manuscript out into the world, rewritten and with a lengthy introduction by me from the perspective of 2009. And of course, I continued working on the third lengthy volume, describing the ten-plus year history of the Columbia-NCCAM-NCI project.

Chapter 44

The Journal of Clinical Oncology Article

T hroughout the spring and early summer, when I heard nothing further from Dr. Briggs, the Columbia Dean, NCCAM, or the NCI, I assumed the various institutions involved had put a stop to any proposed publication about the clinical trial, at least until the ongoing IG investigation reached some sort of conclusion. We also suspected that after the *JAMA* incident, Chabot would not try and place his paper in some other journal, particularly without letting us know first. But, as we were soon to learn, we had significantly underestimated the Columbia team.

As a safeguard, so we would not be blindsided by Chabot, Dr. Isaacs had subscribed to an e-mail alert system available through the National Library of Medicine. This service notifies clients via e-mail whenever an article written by a particular author of interest appears in the medical literature. We had requested warnings for Chabot but throughout the early summer we received no NLM communications advising us of any activity by the Columbia group.

During the afternoon of August 20, 2009, I happened to go into the office where Dr. Isaacs sat at a computer checking e-mails, when she said, sounding somewhat startled, "I can't believe it, they managed to publish the article." Immediately suspecting what she meant, I went to her desk and read on the screen an NLM message informing us of a new paper authored by Chabot and his Columbia cohorts appearing that day in the online version of *The Journal of Clinical Oncology* (*JCO*), the official publication of the American Society of Clinical Oncology, and considered by some to be one of the premier oncology journals in the U.S. Entitled "Pancreatic Proteolytic Enzyme Therapy Compared with Gemcitabine-based Chemotherapy for the Treatment of Pancreatic Cancer," the article listed Chabot as the lead author, followed by Wei-Yaun Tsai, Robert L. Fine, Chunxia Chen, Carolyn Kumah, and to our great disappointment, Karen Antman. We knew immediately what we were dealing with, the *JAMA* submission or some variation thereof, but this time around, no Dr. Pasche or Dr. DeAngelis had intervened. I was disappointed that without first contacting me *JCO* would publish an evaluation of my treatment supported by a grant awarded because of my efforts.

From the *JCO* website we easily retrieved the complete article, which I quickly reviewed. With some anger and a fair amount of disgust, I recognized that it did appear similar, though not identical, to Chabot's *JAMA* submission from late 2006. Once again, in the introductory "Methods" section Chabot reported that all patients had been properly entered, in accordance with the "strict clinical criteria for eligibility." As I searched through the document, nowhere did he mention or even allude to the two-year OHRP investigation or its findings confirming that he had approved 42 of 62 total patients improperly. It was as if that federal investigation, the results of which remain to this day posted on the official OHRP website for all to see, never happened.

Nowhere did Chabot reference Dr. Engel's January 2005 letter, in which she clearly stated the official NIH position that so many nutrition patients did not or could not adhere to the prescribed treatment, that the epidemic non-compliance "clouds interpretation of the data." As had the *JAMA* submission, the *JCO* article read as if all patients admitted into the nutrition arm followed the regimen appropriately and simply failed to respond to treatment, ignoring the vast number who did not comply at all, or who did so minimally.

The conclusion essentially mirrored what had been written for *JAMA*, that the survival of the chemotherapy patients far exceeded that of ours, by a factor of three. In other respects, Chabot had significantly modified his earlier paper: for example, this time around he claimed 55 patients ultimately had been entered into the trial, with 32 assigned to the nutrition arm, 23 treated with chemotherapy. These numbers differed from the total of 58 he had described for *JAMA* in 2006, and even more so from the 62 patients reported as officially approved in the OHRP determination letter of June 2008.

It's easy to track the changes over time in Chabot's statements. In the "Results" section for *JAMA* he had written:

> Of 70 patients with pancreatic cancer who expressed interest in the study, 8 did not meet the eligibility criteria . . . Of the first four eligible patients, three refused to be randomized and withdrew. One additional patient signed a consent form, which was misplaced due to a change in staffing. . . .

> Fifty-eight patients, 23 on the control arm and 35 on the experimental arm, enrolled in the study and were available for analysis.

If we identify as disqualified the eight who "did not meet the eligibility criteria," the additional three who withdrew and the one discounted because of the consent issue, we have a total of 12 who were excluded from consideration. This leaves us with the alleged number of 58 patients (70 minus 12) admitted into the study, as reported in the above paragraph.

But some three years later, for *JCO* this paragraph had been considerably modified:

> Of 70 patients with pancreatic cancer who expressed interest in the study, 15 patients were excluded; nine did not meet the trial inclusion criteria; and one additional patient signed a consent form that was misplaced because of a change in staffing. Five additional patients had a delay in enrollment of greater than 8 weeks from the date of diagnosis and, thus, were ineligible.

Chabot now claimed only 55 patients had been approved, though I had no idea what had happened to the other three included in his *JAMA* submission (or the other seven described in the OHRP determination letter). And I had no idea how he justified changing the number of enrolled patients years after the study's completion—such data should be fixed for all time, not fluid.

Regardless, he once again told the story of a single "consent form that was misplaced because of a change in staffing," ignoring the other two patients with no evidence of signed consent he sent to us for treatment. He had also contradicted his own statement appearing in the official minutes of the March 20, 2006 group meeting when he reported that two "patients 'walked off' with their forms," not that they were lost, and of course he had ignored the total of

40 patients he improperly consented by OHRP accounting. In this regard, it is important to keep in mind that the OHRP posted its last determination letter about the trial in early June 2008, more than a year prior to the *JCO* publication, so Chabot certainly knew of the findings.

This paragraph I found confusing for another significant reason. Chabot reported that "Five additional patients had a delay in enrollment of greater than 8 weeks from the date of diagnosis and, thus, were ineligible." First of all, the story had significantly evolved from the earlier *JAMA* effort of late 2006, in which Chabot did not mention any patient who violated the eight-week rule—even though at the time he knew he had approved patients beyond this interval because I had told him so on more than one occasion. He had, after all, sent his article to *JAMA* some time after my June 30, 2006 letter to him warning against publication anywhere with federal investigations in progress. In that document I reported for the written record that he had admitted patients diagnosed more than eight weeks after their biopsy—a fact he never disputed with me in any way. Though he had ignored these trial subjects in his *JAMA* paper, perhaps the very public OHRP determination findings had forced him to address this serious managerial failing for *JCO*.

Regardless, I wasn't sure where Chabot got the number "five" from, since we knew of only three patients accepted into the nutrition arm eight or more weeks after biopsy. OHRP itself had acknowledged only two such protocol violations for the entire study, both identified in our group, and their official determination letter said nothing about any chemotherapy patients admitted beyond eight weeks. So while I can identify two—or perhaps three—of the five Chabot reported, I don't know who the other two—or is it three—might be.

The statement also seemed to imply that all five, whoever they may have been, initially sought entry into the trial but were disqualified and presumably never treated after Chabot appropriately determined none of them satisfied the eight-week requirement and sent them away. But as clearly stated in their June 3, 2008 letter to me and as posted on their website, OHRP had already made the point that Chabot formally *approved and sent for treatment* two nutrition patients who had been diagnosed more than eight weeks after biopsy. These two had not been deemed "ineligible" as he claimed for *JCO* but had been considered by Chabot as acceptable—or at least until OHRP published their findings and he then had a chance to rewrite his earlier article.

The pertinent paragraph from the June 2008 OHRP document read, in part:

> Subject 113 was enrolled into the study more than 8 weeks after undergo-
> ing biopsy of his pancreatic tumor, which was inconsistent with the inclusion
> criteria stipulated in the institutional review board (IRB)-approved protocol.
> Subject 129 began enzyme treatment in the study 11 weeks after undergoing
> biopsy of the pancreatic tumor, which was inconsistent with the inclusion cri-
> teria stipulated in the institutional review board (IRB)-approved protocol that
> subjects begin treatment within 8 weeks of pancreatic tumor biopsy.

As we have argued, Dr. Isaacs and I identified a third nutrition patient we believe
Chabot approved more than eight weeks after the confirmatory biopsy, who
for reasons unknown to me OHRP considers as never having been admitted in
the first place.

In any event, I find Chabot's *JCO* apparent claim that he excluded these five
patients particularly ironic if we consider the case of Patient #34. As I earlier
documented, Chabot instructed us to treat this particular trial candidate as
part of the nutrition arm even though I advised him via e-mail that the eight-
week cut-off from biopsy had already passed.

As I read the *JCO* article closely a second time, I noticed the near total absence of
any reference to me, in fact I found my name only once in the entire document,
in the "Introduction," where Chabot wrote in passing:

> The Scottish embryologist John Beard first proposed pancreatic proteolytic
> enzyme treatment in 1906 and soon after published a monograph, entitled *The
> Enzyme Therapy of Cancer*. In 1981, Nicholas Gonzalez began to evaluate the
> use of proteolytic enzyme therapy.

I laughed to myself when I read the "Methods" subsection within the
"Abstract," where Chabot described some unnamed physician supervising the
nutrition patients, vaguely stating:

> All patients were seen by one of the investigators at Columbia University, and
> patients who received enzyme therapy were seen by the participating alterna-
> tive practitioner.

In contrast, for *JAMA* in 2006 Chabot mentioned me by name 11 times,
and made it quite clear that I was in charge of treating those entered into the

nutrition group (though of course few assigned to us followed the prescribed treatment program). Below, I include several of the relevant sections extracted from this submission:

In the "Abstract," the basic summary appearing at the beginning of the paper:

> Enzyme therapy patients were seen by Dr. Gonzalez and all patients by one of the investigators at Columbia University.

Then later, in the section entitled "Design":

> Patients in the experimental arm received proteolytic treatment under the care of Dr. Gonzalez. . . .

In the very next section, entitled "Proteolytic enzyme treatment":

> The enzyme treatment provided by Dr. Gonzalez included orally ingested proteolytic enzymes, nutritional supplements, detoxification, and an organic diet.

In the peculiar end note—deleted from the *JCO* article—Chabot incorrectly reported I had withdrawn from the study and refused to participate in the preparation of the manuscript. Here, he referenced me by name no less than *five times*:

> The Pancam study was proposed to the National Institutes of Health by Dr. Gonzalez and Dr. Wynder in 1997. In 1998, Columbia University's Herbert Irving Comprehensive Cancer Center was awarded a supplement to its National Cancer Institute Cancer Center Grant to implement Dr. Gonzalez's study protocol. Over the subsequent 7 years, Dr. Gonzalez served as a coinvestigator, attended all quarterly research team meetings at Columbia (in person or by telephone), and played an active role in study implementation, admitting and following all the patients accepted to the enzyme arm. In 2005 after the study was already closed to enrollment, Dr. Gonzalez expressed concern related to patient selection and elected not to continue participating in the study or its research meetings. Although repeatedly invited to discuss the manuscript and to serve as co-author, Dr. Gonzalez declined to participate in manuscript preparation.

Moving on, I noted that in the fifth paragraph of the *JCO* "Results" section, Chabot reported that the two longest-living patients had received chemotherapy:

> The longest survivors were one chemotherapy-group patient who died at 39.5 months and one chemotherapy-group patient who was censored at 37.5

months (ie, the closing date of the data analysis) and, at the time of manuscript submission, was still alive at 40 months.

Oddly there was no mention anywhere of our two long-term survivors, particularly our patient who lived 40 months from his diagnosis and 38.6 months from entry into the trial.

Certainly, three and four-year lifespans for patients diagnosed with inoperable pancreatic cancer and treated *only* with chemotherapy far exceeds any previous published data. As discussed earlier, in the Gemzar studies from 1997 of the 126 patients randomized to receive one of two single-agent drug regimens, no one lived longer than 19 months—but the improvement in median survival with gemcitabine to 5.6 months, as meager a benefit as it may have been, was considered a significant advance.

As Dr. Isaacs and I discussed these long-term survivors described by Chabot for *JCO*, we wondered how they—or in fact how any of the chemotherapy patients—might have been treated. In its basic form, the GTX regimen developed at Columbia, and given to most of the chemo group in our study, consisted of the three drugs Gemzar, Taxotere and Xeloda. We understood this, of course. But we had learned from our review of the literature (and not from any information provided by Chabot) that the Columbia GTX approach to pancreatic cancer had evolved over the years of our study to include not only aggressive chemotherapy, but frequently radiation followed by surgery. The GTX proponents, including Drs. Fine and Chabot, claimed that the drugs often shrank initially inoperable stage II and III tumors sufficiently so that curative surgery might then be possible. With aggressive preoperative radiation added to the mix, considerably more patients became surgical candidates. The Columbia team has reported that patients undergoing such surgery after GTX chemotherapy, particularly when combined with radiation, fared better than those never deemed operable.

The rules for our trial did allow for palliative radiation as needed for pain control, but not as a component of the primary treatment for the disease. Nor did the written protocol permit surgery *with curative intent*. As a first principle our trial was set up to exclude any subject with disease that might have been *surgically* curable. The very title of our project appearing on every one of the many protocol drafts that I have read made that point directly: "Evaluation of Intensive Pancreatic Proteolytic Enzyme Therapy with Ancillary Nutritional Support in the Treatment of *Inoperable* Pancreatic Adenocarcinoma." So a stage II or III patient with initially unresectable disease whose tumors shrank after GTX with (or without) preoperative radiation to the point he or she underwent curative surgery technically would have been ineligible for our particular trial, since surgery *with curative intent* was not part of the allowed treatments. Dr. Isaacs and I were certainly never told at any time that if any of our stage II or III patients experienced tumor regression, we might send them for surgery. The whole point of our study was to compare the effect of our regimen versus aggressive *chemotherapy* (and not chemotherapy with added radiation) in patients with *inoperable* pancreatic cancer.

An article appearing in the *Journal of Gastrointestinal Surgery* in January 2008, entitled "Neoadjuvant chemotherapy and radiation for patients with locally unresectable pancreatic adenocarcinoma: feasibility, efficacy and survival" coauthored by Chabot and Fine, discussed the Columbia experience with the GTX regimen in some detail.[30] Here, the authors made clear their goal of shrinking tumors sufficiently to allow for "curative" surgery in patients initially considered inoperable. This illuminating article made several points relevant to our study. Again it showed—in fact proved—that Chabot and Fine worked very closely together at Columbia on GTX for most of the duration of our study, an association that should have precluded Chabot from serving as Principal Investigator on our trial.

The abstract reported that from October 2000 to August 2006, right during the time of our own project, "245 patients with pancreatic adenocarcinoma underwent surgical exploration" at Columbia. Of these, 78 had previously completed "neoadjuvant" chemotherapy with GTX "for initially unresectable disease," with the hope of shrinking the tumor to allow for surgical resection. In addition, 75% of the GTX group had also undergone a course of radiation to help reduce the tumor burden still further. Those patients proceeding with surgery after receiving chemotherapy and radiation survived considerably longer, according to the authors, than those who were never considered appropriate surgical candidates.

This *Journal of Gastrointestinal Surgery* article included for analysis a hodgepodge of patients treated at Columbia, some of whom appeared to be part of a clinical study, some of whom were not. We wondered if any of the 23 patients Chabot admitted into the chemotherapy arm of our trial had been part of this larger Columbia cohort discussed in this article—and if any of the 23 might have been treated with radiation in addition to chemotherapy, or after receiving chemotherapy with or without radiation, had undergone surgery with curative intent in violation of the entry criteria of our study. Unfortunately, we have no way of knowing how the chemotherapy patients in our trial were actually treated since Dr. Chabot never once discussed the details of their care with us.

Overall, the *JCO* article left Dr. Isaacs and me somewhat perplexed, appearing as it did without any warning to us. But I knew we had to act quickly to undo the potential damage to our reputations this article represented. The repercussions could be far reaching, to say the least.

I decided to take direct action and phoned the editorial offices of *JCO* in Alexandria, Virginia, explaining to the pleasant receptionist answering the phone who I was and why I had called. I said, quite bluntly, that without any warning to me *JCO* had published an article that inaccurately portrayed my treatment approach in a most negative way. I then expressed my wish to speak with someone in a position of editorial authority.

The receptionist immediately connected me to Mr. Chris Bohn, identified only as one of the editorial staff who could appropriately deal with my concerns. I came right to the point with Mr. Bohn, who seemed nice enough, stating that in my opinion *JCO* had published a misleading article by Chabot, an allegation I could easily document. He seemed totally dumbstruck when I explained that contrary to the implication that the trial had been impeccably run, a completed federal probe by OHRP confirmed serious supervisory failings on Chabot's part—information absent from the *JCO* paper. I discussed Dr. Engel's letter, of which he knew nothing. He seemed particularly flummoxed when I told him that some two years earlier Chabot had submitted essentially the same article to *JAMA*, whose editors—unlike those at *JCO*—responded quickly and properly after talking to me, rejecting it outright.

After listening to me for some time, Mr. Bohn suggested that I put together a comprehensive account detailing the situation from my perspective and send it to his office, ideally that same day. Several hours later I forwarded to him a lengthy e-mail describing the study's shortcomings, with a link to the OHRP determination letter. I also provided as attachments several documents including scanned copies of Dr. Engel's January 2005 letter and Chabot's *JAMA* submission.

The following day, Ms. Terry Van Schaik of *JCO*'s editorial offices contacted me by phone, informing me that *JCO*, based on the information I had provided, would open an investigation of my allegations and that from here on in, I should address all correspondence to her. After our conversation, I sent her additional documents, including my June 30, 2006 letter to Chabot warning him not to publish with federal investigations in progress, my December 2006 letter of complaint to Dean Goldman at Columbia, and my June 15, 2008 letter to Dr. Andreason at OHRP, written in response to the most recent OHRP findings.

I also e-mailed Ms. Van Schaik two chapters from an earlier draft of this book, "Summary of Major Problems Affecting the NCI-NCCAM Study" and "Failure of Handling Informed Consent." This information, I thought, would provide a thorough accounting of the many serious and well-documented problems plaguing the study that Chabot failed to address in his article. In addition, I sent her an expanded analysis of the clinical trial, more comprehensive than the earlier e-mail I had completed for Mr. Bohn. I made the point that though the *JCO* paper obscured my involvement, the NCI originally awarded the grant for the project because of my efforts before I had even heard the name Chabot, and that I had remained fully engaged throughout the study's long history. This version emphasized Chabot's failure to reference the OHRP findings and his undeclared conflict of interest, of which *JCO* seemed completely ignorant. I stated for the record I thought the *JCO* review process had failed utterly, in contrast to the quick and appropriate action taken by *JAMA* when the Oncology Editor became suspicious of Chabot's submission to that journal.

In these initial communications, I sought to remain collegial, assuming the editors had been innocently misinformed and hoping the overwhelming amount of evidence I had now provided would force them to respond quickly. While their investigation proceeded I did request that out of fairness to me they take down the Internet posting of the Chabot article, and halt publication of the print version. I suggested to Ms. Van Schaik that Chabot's failure to mention the findings of an official federal investigation confirming his mismanagement indicated to me he had not been forthcoming to the *JCO* editors. Though in my opinion this omission alone justified removing the article from the *JCO* website, to my annoyance it remained in place with no mention of my complaint or the investigation in progress.

In addition to our e-mail correspondence, in the days that followed I spoke directly by phone a number of times to an apparently bewildered Ms. Van Schaik, who admitted she felt somewhat overwhelmed by the amount of information I had submitted to her. When asked to provide some details about the proposed *JCO* action, in an e-mail sent August 25, 2009 she replied that *JCO* would follow its usual protocol for evaluating complaints of misconduct lodged against the authors of a published paper. At my request, she sent me a flow chart describing their procedures in cases of alleged malfeasance.

On August 27, 2009, I wrote Ms. Van Schaik again, expanding on several points made in previous e-mails, and once again requesting the online version of the article be taken down. I might understand the *Journal*'s reluctance to act quickly if my complaints and allegations had been based solely on my personal opinion, but OHRP, an official government office, had already completed a two-year evaluation of the project proving multiple protocol violations.

In an e-mail dated August 27, 2009, Ms. Van Schaik responded:

> Please understand that JCO is taking your allegations very seriously. However, the volume and nature of the allegations—while well known to you—are new to us, and require time and effort on our part to investigate and respond to. To do so, we are following the procedures the Journal has established for allegations of author misconduct.

I thought her reply condemned *JCO*'s editorial process far more than anything I myself might say. If the documentation I provided was new to the *JCO* staff, it was only because they had in my opinion, not reviewed the article properly. Although Chabot, perhaps learning from his earlier *JAMA* experience, had virtually erased my ties to the project, by August 2009 many if not most academic oncologists knew about me and the NCI-NCCAM clinical trial. Somewhere along the review process one might think someone at *JCO* would have been intrigued that I was not listed as a co-author on a paper evaluating my own treatment, based on a grant awarded because of my efforts. For whatever reason the process had failed, resulting in what I considered an inaccurate article about my treatment on the *JCO* website. Certainly, I found the comparison with *JAMA*'s handling of essentially the same article to be stunning.

I decided to reason with Ms. Van Schaik yet again, hoping good sense might prevail. In an e-mail dated August 28, 2009, I wrote:

> Thank you for your recent e-mail. I am beginning to understand that you at JCO are taking the situation seriously. My doubts, perhaps skepticism to date

reflect only my experiences over the past seven years, since Dr. Isaacs and I first began to suspect the study was being improperly managed. . . .

I then discussed my concern over the slow pace of the proposed investigation of my complaint, before concluding:

> I will also restate what I stated in a prior e-mail. Your peer reviewers, and the peer review process, failed you miserably. Even though Chabot, presumably based on his JAMA experience, tried to downplay my involvement in the study, my name still appears, and few academic oncologists are unfamiliar with my work. For them not to call me before approval was negligent, did you [sic] editors no great service, and set this whole ugly scenaraio [sic] in motion.

By that point, on all correspondence I had been copying Dr. Daniel Haller, an oncologist at the University of Pennsylvania who served as the editor-in-chief of *JCO*. I hoped perhaps he, as a physician, would appreciate the seriousness of the situation.

In an e-mail dated August 31, 2009, Ms. Van Schaik replied, informing me of the timeline for the *JCO* investigation:

> Although I am not able to give you an exact length of time needed to conduct our investigation, we will act as expeditiously as possible and estimate the process could take up to 90 days.

In turn, I quickly sent a less than collegial e-mail dated the same day, August 31:

> Your response is completely unacceptable. . . .

> by continuing to publish a false article after being presented with the true facts, you are ratifying and participating in the falsity. You do not have to rely on my opinion of the falsity nor would I expect you to. But in the JCO article you have published, in the first paragraph under the section entitled "Results" Chabot reports on one patient he claims—though his own documented statements refute this claim—whose signed consent form was misplaced and that five patients were admitted beyond the eight week cut off. There is no mention here, or anywhere else in the article of the other 39 patients who were improperly consented, as a Federal investigation confirmed. This finding is on the OHRP website for the world to see, it is not a secret. . . .

> Neither Chabot nor his Dean countered nor denied a single claim in my lengthy letter of complaint, a copy of which I sent you. . . .

> Dr. Linda Engel's letter of January 2005 was the official NIH assessment of the data, at a time nearly all nutrition patients had been entered. This isn't my opinion, this is an official NIH assessment which you have in your possession.

Nonetheless, the *JCO* editors once again ignored my request that the article be taken down from their website, and I still didn't know the status of the print version, presumably scheduled to appear in the next hard-copy issue.

To complicate matters, on September 8, 2009, the NCI posted a four-paragraph discussion of the Chabot *JCO* paper on its "Cancer Bulletin" site, a comprehensive review of current literature in the field. Entitled "Chemotherapy Provides Longer Survival than Enzyme Therapy for Pancreatic Cancer," the article stated:

> In a clinical trial testing an experimental enzyme regimen against gemcitabine-based chemotherapy for advanced pancreatic cancer, patients receiving chemotherapy lived an average of 9.7 months longer.[84]

The NCI entry continued in some detail, treating the *JCO* publication as a legitimate report of a well-managed study that compared patients treated with chemotherapy to those the reader would assume fully complied with the experimental "Gonzalez" regimen, with my name included. To my surprise, the unnamed author quoted at length Dr. White of the NCI, who lauded the trial without reservation. By this point in September 2009, one would have expected Dr. White of all people to know full well of Chabot's managerial failings, the OHRP findings, the incomparability of the two groups, the fact that few nutritional patients had complied, and the absence of meaningful data. But reading the NCI posting, one would know none of this:

> The report was "a good attempt to bring as much rigor to the analysis as was feasible, given the inability to do a randomized controlled trial," said Dr. Jeffrey D. White, director of NCI's Office of Cancer Complementary and Alternative Medicine. "The study used a concurrent control with identical eligibility criteria and a statistical approach to check if significant bias was allowed in the lack of randomization. That is a good strategy for other studies having similar difficulties with randomization."[84]

As jaded as I had become after all these years, I still thought his statements incomprehensible in view of what actually had happened under his guidance during the study's very troubled history.

I responded with a lengthy e-mail to the Cancer Bulletin editor, forwarding along with my note several of the detailed e-mail summaries I had previously sent to *JCO*. Then, not to my surprise, because at that point, nothing surprised me, without any qualifying statement the NCCAM website provided a direct link to the *JCO* article. Under the heading "Questions & Answers: The Phase III Gonzalez Protocol Trial," the very brief entry read:

> **Updated August 2009**
> The results of the study are available from the Journal of Clinical Oncology.[85]

I responded quickly on September 9, 2009, e-mailing the NCCAM public affairs office to express my concerns, attaching a somewhat revised and enlarged version of the summary and timeline of the trial I had prepared for the *JCO* editors.

I also wrote Dr. Briggs directly, suggesting that the NCCAM reference to the article be removed from the site, or that qualifying information be added:

> at least include some basic facts, such as the fact the Office of Human Research Protections found Chabot had improperly admitted 42 of 62 patients, including 40 not properly consented and that Columbia was required to institute training programs in research methodology for its staff. . . .

> I would have thought that NCCAM of all places would have been proud that it was the alternative practitioners, Dr. Isaacs and myself, who insisted the study abide by the requirements of appropriate clinical trial methodology, while the conventional academicians, including Dr. Killen, did absolutely nothing to address our many legitimate complaints.

Three days later, on September 12, 2009, James Mathews, the NCI Cancer Bulletin editor, responded to the e-mail I had sent to him:

> As a matter of newsletter policy, our research highlights are drawn exclusively from peer-reviewed scientific journal articles, so we will continue to monitor JCO and other outlets closely for reports, updates, editorials and/or corrections related to this particular study. We will follow up as appropriate in light

of any developments. In addition, I have forwarded your correspondence to Dr. Jeff White, director of NCI's Office of Cancer Complementary and Alternative Medicine, who is quoted in the Bulletin highlight. We will, of course, immediately amend Dr. White's statement if he feels such action if warranted.

I thought Mr. Mathews' note not unreasonable, though I could not understand why, if the NCI website included a discussion of the *JCO* article, the editors would be unwilling to link to the official OHRP determination letter.

I subsequently received a more defensive e-mail response from Chris Thomsen of NCCAM:

> The NCCAM website was updated in August 2009 to include a simple citation and link to the peer-reviewed publication in the online *Journal of Clinical Oncology*. Our website does not contain any discussion of either the article or the treatment regimens including in the study.

> Should JCO publish further information regarding the paper, we will update our website to include that citation as well.

It made no sense to me that NCCAM would provide no mention or link to the OHRP website for the findings of an official federal investigation of a study that the Center itself had funded. As far as the NCI and NCCAM were concerned, it seemed the OHRP investigation simply didn't matter. And, Dr. Briggs never responded to my e-mail about the NCCAM posting.

With Internet chatter about the *JCO* article beginning only days after its appearance, Dr. Isaacs and I knew we needed to get the truth into public view quickly. So, we created a comprehensive section on my own website (www.dr-gonzalez .com), including a long document of some 9000 words refuting the *JCO* article, point by point. I also provided scanned copies of the January 2005 Dr. Engel letter, my 2006 complaint to the Dean of Columbia, and my response to Dr. Andreason's final OHRP findings. I also linked directly to the OHRP site.

We did subsequently learn from our own investigations and not from any communication from *JCO* that the print version of the Chabot article did not appear as we assumed had been originally planned in the September 2009 issue. If the journal had already been printed, its dismantling and the physical removal of the Chabot paper would have been an expensive proposition for a technical publication with some 26,000 subscribers.

In fairness to Suzanne Somers I told her about the Chabot article within hours of its posting on the *JCO* website. She needed to know that I was probably heading into a time of great controversy, so if she thought it best she could delete my section from her manuscript. She was not surprised by the turn of events, and insisted the book—entitled *Knockout* and scheduled for an October 20, 2009 release with a major publicity push—would stay as written, with my chapter intact.

In early October, Ms. Somers sent me several advance copies which I read avidly, with much appreciation for what she had done. In this well-researched and well-written work the chapter on our therapy turned out to be the longest by far, with the most case histories, nine to be exact, structured in interview format. In view of our recent experiences with the academic medical world, I felt a particular gratitude toward Ms. Somers.

After *Knockout's* release, Ms. Somers seemed to be everywhere in the media, on *Good Morning America*, on the *Today Show*, on other major TV venues, on the radio. Within days, *Knockout* hit #1 on the *New York Times* bestseller list for advice books, not surprisingly generating considerable praise as well as controversy. I appeared with Ms. Somers and Dr. Burzynski on the *Larry King Show* in Los Angeles, along with two less than happy conventional physicians, including Dr. Otis Brawley, an oncologist associated with the American Cancer Society. For some reason, the two "opponents" determinedly focused their attack on Dr. Burzynski, so that the *JCO* Chabot article never even came up.

In late October, Ms. Somers hosted a wonderful party at her mountaintop Palm Springs retreat, a stone house in French country style situated on some 60-plus acres of land that included a large organic garden. Ms. Somers had invited all the doctors she had interviewed and their spouses, as well as her extended family and select friends. That evening proved to be a high point of the year, a much needed respite from the cancer wars, a time of celebration among colleagues like Dr. Burzynski and my old pal Dr. Jonathan Wright, the nutritional physician from Washington State whom I hadn't seen for years. After a superb organic meal, Ms. Somers entertained us all, some 50 or so in number, with her nightclub act. She performed with her seasoned band on a stage sitting between some jagged cliffs that formed a natural amphitheater right on her property. The evening was perfect, a reverie away from the front lines, but of course too short.

Back in New York after the party, I returned to my ongoing battles with *JCO*. Despite my initial hope that the editors would exhaustively and objectively rethink the Chabot article, to my disappointment no one from the *Journal* contacted me for clarification or further proof of my allegations. As the months came and went with no word from the *Journal*, no request for supporting documents or further explanations, I began to doubt we would find the outcome satisfactory. How, I thought, could *JCO* adjudicate the serious issues I had raised without communicating with me, the complainant? Dr. Isaacs and I began to wonder if perhaps *JCO* had turned its investigation over to Columbia, whose staff—perhaps including Mr. Gasparis, the ethics expert—hardly felt, as I had been told, any great love for me or my controversial treatment. But if Chabot hoped to bury me with his article, Ms. Somers' book continued a rip-roaring success, bringing us recognition we sadly realized would never come through the usual institutional channels.

Meanwhile, since I had heard nothing from Mr. Melo of the Inspector General's office, during the waning weeks of 2009, several times I tried to reach him by phone. I left messages, but he did not initially respond. When we finally connected just before the Christmas holidays, he told me the information I had sent him warranted some sort of investigation be pursued. However, he did not believe the Columbia or government supervisors of the project had committed criminal acts—the main focus of the IG, he explained—so he would be referring the case to an NIH department he believed more suited to the task. As our conversation concluded, he promised to send a follow-up letter in January 2010, outlining his suggested plan of action.

Though Inspector Melo had not dismissed any of my allegations, I was nonetheless disappointed he would not be pursuing my complaints. I didn't press the issue, but wondered if he would now forward my file back to Dr. Dahlberg, who had already confessed that he could do nothing himself, thus finally completing the do-nothing circle.

As January 2010 came and went, the promised letter from Melo never arrived and our doubts about *JCO*'s intent seemed increasingly justified, since after five months no one from the *Journal* had contacted me. Subsequently, and not to our surprise, on March 15, 2010, we received an e-mail alert informing us that Chabot's article was about to be published in the print version of *JCO*— without any warning to me. After receiving the message, we searched the *JCO*

Internet site, where we found the newly-revised article already posted, replacing the August 2009 online version.

This new edition appeared to be nearly—but not completely—identical to the earlier on-line document. I did discover one important addition in the "Results" section, included I suspected as a further explanation for the patients OHRP identified who had been admitted beyond the eight-week cutoff from biopsy:

> Of 70 patients with pancreatic cancer who expressed interest in the study, 15 patients were excluded (Fig 1); nine did not meet the trial inclusion criteria; and one additional patient signed a consent form that was misplaced because of a change in staffing. Five additional patients had a delay in enrollment of greater than 8 weeks from the date of diagnosis and, thus, were ineligible. Several of these subjects were originally treated as part of the trial due to extenuating circumstances at the time of evaluation resulting in excessive elapsed time between diagnosis and therapy. Subjects often traveled great distances to be considered for this trial, and on several occasions, obtaining data at long distance or the requirements for subject travel (eg, travel to New York around the time of September 11, 2001) resulted in excessive delay. Data from these subjects are not included in the data reported in this article, in order that the analysis apply to subjects that strictly meet the inclusion criteria.

First of all, this paragraph included the same statement "one additional patient signed a consent form that was misplaced because of a change in staffing," that appeared in the earlier August 2009 *JCO* website post as well as in the *JAMA* submission from late 2006. But at the March 20, 2006 group meeting Chabot himself, as I have previously shown, said something completely different, claiming that signed consent was missing for not one but two patients who had "'walked off' with their forms." For the official record of that session Chabot had said nothing about a "misplaced" consent due to "a change in staffing."

His new explanation for patients approved in violation of the eight-week rule seemed simply incomprehensible to us:

> Several of these subjects were originally treated as part of the trial due to extenuating circumstances at the time of evaluation resulting in excessive elapsed time between diagnosis and therapy. Subjects often traveled great distances to be considered for this trial, and on several occasions, obtaining data at long

distance or the requirements for subject travel (eg, travel to New York around the time of September 11, 2001) resulted in excessive delay.

Dr. Isaacs and I have identified three patients admitted into the nutrition group beyond eight weeks from biopsy, Patient #14(129), Patient #16(133), and Patient #34(113). In its determination letter OHRP had included only Patient #14(129) and Patient #34(113), but not Patient #16(133), as entered in violation of this rule. For the two OHRP did consider inappropriate entries we know of no "extenuating circumstances," no delays due to travel or long distances, and in neither case could September 11, 2001 explain away the problem.

After learning about the trial, Patient #34(113) had forwarded copies of her records to Chabot in early August 2001, but when she did not hear back from him, in frustration she faxed the documents to us on August 24, 2001. When I realized that 57 days had already passed since her biopsy, the day I received her records I e-mailed Chabot expressing my belief she did not qualify. Nonetheless Chabot instructed us we set up our intake appointments. According to our records he subsequently approved her on September 6, 2001, some 71 days after her biopsy, and we consulted with her in our office on September 6 and September 7, 2001—several days *before* September 11, 2001. In this case the only extenuating circumstance we know of was Chabot's improper processing of the case.

Chabot approved Patient #14(129) on or about January 24, 2003, some 11 weeks after her biopsy. Once again we know of no "extenuating circumstances," no travel delays, and since she was entered a year and a half after September 11, 2001, I do not think that tragedy explains away the protocol misstep.

We first consulted with Patient #16(133), whom we considered the third patient admitted beyond eight weeks from diagnosis, the first week of February 2003, again well beyond 9/11. He too had experienced no "extenuating circumstances" or difficulties arranging travel to New York.

So for the nutrition patients qualified in violation of the eight-week rule, in no case did 9/11 play a role. We did meet with one trial subject, Patient #5(114), shortly after 9/11, on September 20 and September 21, 2001, but the biopsy in this case dated from August 28, 2001, less than four weeks earlier, so this entry *did not* violate the protocol requirements. Regardless, this individual reported no problems getting to New York despite the proximity of her visit with us to

9/11. Besides Patient #113, who came in just before 9/11, and Patient #114, who was admitted within eight weeks, none of the other 39 in the nutrition group were accepted "around" 9/11.

According to Chabot's last data chart, he did approve two chemotherapy patients in mid and late October 2001, one on October 19, 2001, the other on October 31, 2001. I know nothing about these two since Chabot told us nothing, but as Columbia patients I doubted either had to journey any "long distance" for their initial evaluation. And travel delays persisted for a week or two after the unfortunate 9/11 attack, not into October: Patient #5(114) discussed above and seen in our office only nine days after 9/11 reported no difficulties getting to New York. Most importantly, OHRP nowhere reported that any chemotherapy patients had begun treatment more than eight weeks from biopsy. Chabot's statements about "extenuating circumstances" and "travel to New York around the time of September 11, 2001" made no sense whatsoever.

After reading through the print version of the article, I decided not to contact *JCO* but instead wait to see how their editors would handle the situation with me. Days passed with no word. Finally on March 29, 2010, fourteen days after the Google alert, I received a letter from Ms. Van Schaik, cosigned by Dr. Haller, informing me that the Chabot article would be published in the April 20, 2010 issue of *JCO*:

> Dear Dr. Gonzalez:
>
> Journal of Clinical Oncology has completed its investigation into your concerns regarding *Pancreatic Proteolytic Enzyme Therapy Compared to Gemcitabine-Based Chemotherapy for the Treatment of Pancreatic Cancer* (J Clin Oncol 2009; JCO 2009.22.8428). We have tentatively scheduled the article for print publication on April 20, 2010.

I discussed the situation with Beth Clay, who thought it most peculiar that in their letter *JCO*'s editors neither denied nor disputed any of the allegations raised or facts presented in my various communications with them. The two only acknowledged that the article was to be published. After thinking about the issue, I decided I must respond for the record, so in an e-mail dated April 11, 2010 addressed to Ms. Van Schaik, I expressed my disappointment with *JCO*'s decision to publish the Chabot article with little change:

> Thank you for your March 29 letter. I found it odd since we had already been alerted via our publication alert system that the article was being or had been

published in the print version of JCO. So I gather you decided to publish it without alerting me.

According to your letter, your investigation is completed. But you do not tell me its results.

If you found anything I communicated regarding this article to be in any way inaccurate or misleading please tell me what, and why. I strongly urge you to consider the overwhelming evidence that the article is grossly inaccurate and misleading. I carefully documented much of that evidence, without refutation, during the study.

At best it would be scientifically irresponsible to publish that article.

The above is not meant to be a statement of my legal rights or remedies should you publish.

I am available to discuss, in a factual manner, any questions you have regarding anything I have communicated to you.

On another front, I had no idea what Mr. Melo of the Inspector General's Office finally did or did not do in regard to the clinical trial. The promised letter never came, nor did he respond to several voice mail messages I left for him after I first learned from our Google alert that the print version of the *JCO* article would soon appear. In late March 2010 I discussed the situation with Ms. Clay, who decided to call Melo herself. After several unsuccessful attempts, she finally connected with him but found his manner vague and non-committal.

The April 20, 2010 issue of *JCO* included not only the Chabot article, but an accompanying editorial written by Dr. Mark Levine of the Department of Oncology, McMaster University in Canada. Dr. Levine, whose analysis took up nearly two full pages, first addressed CAM (Complementary and Alternative Medicine) research in a general sense at some length, before finally turning his attention to Chabot's paper. In his statements, Dr. Levine seemed thoroughly unaware of any of the study's managerial and methodological shortcomings. Perhaps the *JCO* staff forgot or failed to send my complaint and documents to him, or he had the evidence in hand but chose to ignore the discrepancies between Chabot's claims and what we believed the truth to be. Nonetheless, without any apparent knowledge of my allegations, of Dr. Engel's letter or of the OHRP findings, he did astutely question the study's data and conclusions based on the internal evidence within the article itself.

Specifically, Dr. Levine wrote in part:

> *Is the study design valid?* I would like to focus the discussion on the validity of the use of a controlled observational design to establish efficacy in the Chabot et al study. Although 55 patients were enrolled onto the cohort study, nine more enzyme-treated patients than chemotherapy patients were analyzed. This imbalance is troubling. Fifteen patients were excluded, but one wonders whether they received treatment and were excluded after the analysis was performed. If this occurred, it could lead to bias. Second, in any observational study, there is the possibility of an imbalance in baseline prognostic factors between intervention groups that could confound analysis and potentially lead to bias. . . . One wonders whether there were more liver metastases in the enzyme-treated group than in the chemotherapy group, but this information is not provided.
>
> Chabot et al should be congratulated on their persistence and determination to compare pancreatic enzymes versus chemotherapy. Can it be concluded that their study proves that enzyme therapy is markedly inferior? On the basis of the study design, my answer is no. It is not possible to make a silk purse out of a sow's ear.[86]

Though I believed Dr. Chabot's article hardly warranted congratulations of any sort, at least someone in academia—seemingly unaware of the body of evidence that would have clinched the point—said the study, proving nothing, was little more than a pig's ear. I couldn't have agreed more.

As an interesting footnote, as I was preparing an earlier draft of this book, an article entitled "Studies Halted at Brain Lab Over Impure Injections" appeared in the *New York Times* on July 16, 2010, reporting a major scandal at Columbia University Medical Center. In this, the author Benedict Carey described an unfolding drama at Columbia's highly regarded Kreitchman Center, often lauded for its pioneering use of PET scans, a sophisticated imaging study, to assess mental illness as well as cancer.[87]

During this procedure, an intravenously injected radiotracer concentrates in highly active, or "hypermetabolic" cells, such as those found in malignant tumors or in abnormal regions of the brain. These areas of concentrated dye can then be visualized with a radiographic scan, the PET (Positron Emission Tomography). Staff scientists at Kreitchman, the recipient of millions in federal and drug company funding, allegedly routinely injected radiotracers containing toxic impurities into research subjects diagnosed with psychiatric disease such as schizophrenia and severe depression, putting these patients at significant risk.

According to the writer, the Food and Drug Administration began investigating the Center in 2006 when serious allegations of mismanagement first surfaced. After its preliminary assessment, the FDA wrote to Columbia in 2008, requiring that Center administrators correct a series of failings including, as the reporter stated, "lax internal quality control and sloppy procedures for formulating drug injections." However, during a follow-up visit to Columbia in January 2010, the FDA discovered the situation had not changed. To make matters worse, the FDA learned that Columbia staffers not only injected radiotracers with impurities far above allowable levels, but then tried to cover up the practice by altering Center records. Finally, with the problems uncorrected, the FDA subsequently conducted an unannounced raid, described in the article:

> F.D.A. investigators . . . cited a long list of specific violations, including one instance in which the staff hid impurities from auditors by falsifying documents.

> "They raided the place like it was a crime scene, seizing hard drives," said one former lab worker, who requested anonymity because he feared reprisals from the university.[87]

The author then cited evidence indicating that the dangerous practices and the cover-up were hardly isolated events but rather par for the course:

> Former employees . . . said those practices were not only commonplace but also condoned. . . .

> "These are not the actions of a rogue, but instead are systematic forgeries condoned and approved by the lab director," wrote one employee in a 2009 resignation letter. . . .[87]

I found the article most pertinent, for a number of reasons. First, I think it informative that in this case the FDA, yet another powerful federal office charged with protecting patients enrolled in clinical trials, initially turned its investigation over to Columbia—as had OHRP, and possibly *JCO,* in response to my own complaints. In this case Columbia seems to have done very little, to the point that the FDA, grabbing evidence off computers, raided the Kreitchman Center as if it were some criminal cartel.

The strong words of the former Kreitchman employee made the case not for an isolated careless error by an overworked stressed-out staff, but for deliberate failings at supervisory levels, a disregard by the Center's staff for the tenets of scientific research and the fundamentals of patient protection, and, of course, a disregard for the truth.

Our more recent review of this situation in November 2011, some sixteen months after the *Times* article, uncovered a "WARNING LETTER" issued by the FDA appearing on their website September 20, 2011, and addressed to G. Michael Purdy, Ph.D., Executive Vice President for Research, Columbia University. The lengthy document indicated ongoing serious shortcomings at the Columbia Radioactive Drug Research Committee (RDRC), the office presumably overseeing Kreitchman, that still had not been appropriately corrected. Below, I extract pertinent points (note: boldings are in the original):

> **The RDRC failed to assure the necessary conditions so that radioactive drugs used in research under their purview are considered safe and effective. . . .**
>
> 1. **The RDRC failed to assure the quality of radioactive drugs. . . .**
>
> 2. **The RDRC failed to assure that investigators immediately report all adverse events (effects) associated with the use of the radioactive drug in the research study. . . .**
>
> 3. **The RDRC failed to review and approve research at meetings at which a quorum, defined as more than 50% of the membership . . . is present. . . .**
>
> 4. **The RDRC failed to submit a special summary report to FDA immediately after approving research proposals which involve exposure of more than thirty research subjects. . . .**
>
> 5. **The RDRC failed to assure research was reviewed and approved by an institutional review board (IRB). . . .**
>
> Our inspection revealed that the RDRC failed to protect the safety and welfare of human subjects, including a potentially vulnerable subject population (i.e., subjects with psychiatric disorders), because the RDRC failed to assure the necessary conditions described above. . . .[88]

Columbia was given 15 days in which to respond with a serious plan "to prevent similar violations in the future." The letter was signed by none other than

Patrick J. McNeilly, Ph.D., Acting Branch Chief, Human Subject Protection Branch, Center for Drug Evaluation and Research, Food and Drug Administration, my old friend from OHRP. It seemed to me that this time around, for whatever reason, Columbia would not escape with just a gentle rap on the knuckles.

Just about the time I learned of the problems plaguing the Kreitchman Center in July 2010, from contacts in Washington I first heard inklings that the FDA might be looking into our clinical study. Though I had no confirmation of any such activity nor had the FDA approached me, I wasn't surprised the agency might become involved independently of any other government investigation. No federally sponsored clinical trial can begin without that office's approval, so after the NCI formally offered its support for our effort, Columbia submitted an Investigational New Drug (IND) application to the FDA for my therapy and for the project. Such requests can sometimes take years to process, but to our pleasant surprise, the FDA gave its blessing quite quickly, within several months, and we were free to proceed.

After the final OHRP findings became public information in mid-2008, it made sense to me that the FDA would itself show interest in probing the trial's management, since the agency had signed off on the project and I knew took its regulatory role very seriously. But as 2010 turned into 2011 and I still heard nothing from the FDA, I assumed either I had been given incorrect information, or the agency had decided against any further action. I myself never thought of approaching the FDA, since I was not sure the agency would do any more than OHRP or ORI, the two federal offices specifically set up to investigate mismanagement and malfeasance on the part of clinical trial personnel.

Then in early December 2011 I was contacted by a reporter working at a major Midwestern newspaper who told me she was writing a story about NCCAM, highlighting my clinical study and its problems. Though at this point in my life I respond to mainstream journalists as one might respond to a rabid rattlesnake (if one existed), cautiously, quietly, while quickly moving away as fast as possible, this woman seemed to have done her homework and at least from what she told me, believed the project had been mismanaged. I agreed to a formal interview to tell my side, at which point she informed me that the FDA had indeed conducted and completed its own assessment of Chabot's supervision of the trial, which they found sorely lacking. Though pleased to have such unexpected vindication from that federal office, I found myself somewhat dumbfounded by the turn of events, since I knew nothing about their involvement or any such report.

The reporter explained how I might locate the official findings on the FDA website, which I immediately scoured after completing the interview. Sure enough, there it all was, under "Center for Drug Evaluation and Research Clinical Investigator Inspection List." The FDA presents the information quite differently than the OHRP site, which provides the actual determination letters arranged by date and identified by the institution involved. In contrast, the FDA had arranged alphabetically the names of the various offending physicians and scientists targeted by their investigations, along with the date of the audit and the findings alongside presented in coded form. All the information appears on a single line in each case, with a link set up to a separate page explaining the codes in detail.

I located "Chabot, John A MD" easily enough, and learned the FDA had conducted its "Inspection" on September 2, 2009, more than a year after the last OHRP posting. The document categorized the purpose of the visit, or "Type" to use FDA terminology, by the term "FC," which I learned meant:

> **FC—For Cause:** An inspection in which the focus is on the conduct of the study by the Clinical Investigator.

Under the column "Deficiency Codes" I found four for Chabot, "03, 05, 06, 12." These translated to:

> 03 Inadequate informed consent form
> 05 Failure to follow investigational plan
> 06 Inadequate and inaccurate records
> 12 Failure to list additional investigators on 1572

I wasn't sure what the explanation for offense #12 meant, nor did I understand why the FDA reported Chabot had used an "inadequate consent form" but did not include as a violation category "02 Failure to obtain and/or document subject consent." Nonetheless, I felt vindicated that after all the denials reaching right to the offices of Dr. Zerhouni, the FDA, one of the most powerful agencies in Washington, had confirmed Chabot's mismanagement of the study.

In some respects, I thought the FDA findings, though certainly less detailed, more significant that those of OHRP. After all, the basic rules of any legitimate clinical trial require that the chief investigator perform appropriate informed consent, follow the "investigational plan," i.e., the protocol, and keep accurate records. Chabot, according to the FDA, had failed on all three points, as I had long claimed. OHRP had agreed Chabot mishandled informed consent in multiple patients and admitted two beyond eight weeks, but that office made no generalizations about Chabot's management, as had the FDA in their simple one-line analysis.

The FDA report also strongly contradicted Zerhouni's claim made in his December 2005 letter to Congressman Burton:

> It is our understanding that rules of clinical trial management were strictly adhered to by the Columbia research staff at every point in this process. The protocol was prospectively set and followed in order to avoid any insertion of bias. Dr. Chabot remained steadfast to the predetermined trial design and discussed with Dr. Gonzalez the critical nature of maintaining a predetermined trial design and assuring its ethical oversight by an impartial data and safety monitoring board, which is charged with deciding whether the evolving safety and efficacy data in any clinical study warrants continued patient enrollment, treatment, and follow up.

Despite the confirmation that Chabot had not supervised the study properly, I could find no evidence that the FDA had levied any penalty on him or limited his research activities. In the column headed "Classification," the site lists the final actions taken in response to the various offenses. On Chabot's data line, I found the code VAI, identified as:

> VAI—Voluntary Action Indicated. Objectionable conditions were found but the problems do not justify further regulatory action. Any corrective action is left to the investigator to take voluntarily.

As a footnote, I have learned that Dr. McNeilly, who has aggressively supervised the ongoing Kreitchman Center drama, works at the same FDA office that investigated Chabot's handling of our clinical study. I wonder if he was involved personally with this evaluation. If he was, I owe him thanks this time around.

Shortly after learning about the FDA investigation, in mid-December 2011 we discovered that at some point the editors of *JCO* had posted an online "Publisher's Note" identifying several "errors" in the initial August 2009 Chabot article appearing on their website:

> The article by Chabot et al, entitled, "Pancreatic Proteolytic Enzyme Therapy Compared With Gemcitabine-Based Chemotherapy for the Treatment of Pancreatic Cancer" . . . was published online August 17, 2009 with errors.
>
> In the Abstract, under Methods, the second sentence indicating that all patients met strict criteria for eligibility should have been omitted.[89]

Indeed. The editors then go on to state that the paragraph added in the final version of the paper that referenced "September 11, 2001" should have been included in the original 2009 posting. So I gather then that the *JCO* staff feel it appropriate for Chabot to revise his article repeatedly after its initial publication, and years after the study had come to a close.

In any event, the note ends stating:

> These corrections do not alter the study's conclusions, which were supported by the results of an investigation conducted by Columbia University Medical Center at the direction of the Department of Health and Human Services' Office for Human Research Protections. At the time of publication, there is an ongoing review of the study by the FDA.[89]

In my many conversations with the OHRP staff, never once did they even imply their office would address the validity of the data—I was told their concern was the study's management, not its outcome.

Nonetheless, despite *JCO* and the Chabot article, our offices have never been busier, the patients never more determined, the therapy never more effective. In many respects, I owe our continued survival and growing success to Suzanne Somers whose book continues to sell long after its initial publication. The sales of *Knockout,* currently available in paperback, have already topped one million copies.

And, our first two books are now available, *The Trophoblast and the Origins of Cancer,* the manuscript presenting Dr. Beard's theories from the perspective of contemporary molecular biology, and *One Man Alone,* my updated monograph describing my five-year investigation of Dr. Kelley. During the summer of 2010 we also released a replica of Dr. Beard's original 1911 monograph, *The Enzyme Treatment of Cancer,* with a lengthy foreword by me. So, despite the contempt and indifference of the academic community toward us, the enzyme treatment survives, and will hopefully continue to do so.

One final point, before I move on. During the preparation of this manuscript, as I reviewed the various official documents of the study, I reread the contracts Columbia required I sign. I found an interesting paragraph I had earlier overlooked, appearing in Article 19 of the May 2003 "Subaward" (subcontract) that read:

> It is understood that decisions concerning publication of this research at the Subgrantee will be made jointly by Karen Antman, Principal Investigator at CU [Columbia University], and Nicholas J. Gonzalez, MD prior to any such publication.

This provision does seem to indicate Columbia was required to consult with me before publishing any data about the study. Since Chabot succeeded Dr. Antman as "Principal Investigator" at Columbia, presumably this rule applied to him as well. I can find no evidence that it does not. Consequently, it would seem that Chabot, by placing his article in *JCO* without my approval, and Columbia for allowing him to do so, violated the very contract they all insisted I sign.

Conclusion

I had finished an earlier draft of this book prior to the unexpected appearance online of Chabot's first *JCO* article in late August 2009, and before publication of Ms. Somer's *Knockout*. Those events required that I extensively revamp the latter chapters, and of course, rewrite this conclusion. Then, the more recent April 2010 print version of the Chabot paper along with Dr. Levine's interesting editorial, and the FDA investigation, needed to be addressed.

My original "finale" started off quite dark and dreary, effusive with my disgust with those I've had to deal with over the years at Columbia, the IG's office, the NCI, the NIH, OHRP, and ORI—those bastions of scientific virtue, and its so-called guardians. But out of nowhere Suzanne Somers appeared with her wonderful best-selling book that told the truth about my therapy, and changed our lives for the better. In comparison, *JCO*, small journal that it seems to be, and its bewildering Chabot article, have had virtually no effect, except to fuel certain physician bloggers with too much time on their hands. I suppose Chabot's efforts might have sunk our practice, but with *Knockout* still selling well, with its enormous influence, it is as if the *JCO* piece never happened. So, it's hard to be negative, with such unexpected gifts on so many levels sent our way.

There have been other victories as well. Dr. Engel's official NIH letter to Chabot honestly reported the epidemic non-compliance affecting the nutrition arm, resulting, we believe, from the repeated admission of patients too ill, or too mentally or emotionally unsuited, to proceed with our self-administered treatment regimen. I will always have great respect for the integrity of that letter and its writer, who willingly stated the truth.

OHRP, as slow-paced as it seemed at times, as unsatisfactory as I may have found its investigation, did conclude that Chabot committed multiple serious protocol violations, entering 42 patients improperly and in our mind ultimately undermining the entire eight-year effort. In the process, Chabot finally admitted his failings for public consumption, so there can be no doubt who committed the management lapses. OHRP also required Columbia staff undergo training in research methodology—the ultimate insult, I suspect, for an academic institution.

In December 2006 *JAMA* responded honorably and incisively to the first Chabot attempt at publication. Dr. Pasche, the *JAMA* Oncology Editor, could have let the article pass, allow his journal to print it, but he did what was right, calling me to find the truth. For that action I remain forever grateful to him, even if Chabot subsequently managed to place the retooled paper somewhere else. Dr. Pasche's actions certainly helped me, but he also protected the reputation of *JAMA* and of its editor-in-chief, Dr. DeAngelis. This hard-working idealist hardly deserved to be dragged unknowingly into the middle of the scandal that might have resulted from that article's appearance in her journal.

Then there are the FDA findings about Chabot's management of the trial that came out of nowhere, just as I had finished what I thought was the last draft of this book in December 2011. That agency's report was, in some ways, the sweetest victory of all. In alternative medicine circles, the FDA strikes fear and dread because of its enormous regulatory power, and a long history of antagonism toward the free availability of nutritional supplements. In my case, I must report quite a different experience. First of all, the FDA approved the IND for our study promptly, with no delay despite the unusual and controversial nature of my treatment. Though the study did not turn out the way I would have wanted, that agency did everything it could to expedite the IND process, for which to this day I remain grateful. Once the study was up and running, they let us proceed with no interference, no opposition, and no "bias" that I ever saw.

Then, without my knowledge, the FDA team investigated Chabot's management, which they found, as had I, lacking. I don't know when, how, or why that agency got involved—maybe it was because of the earlier OHRP findings, maybe not. Yes, Chabot escaped again with no severe penalty, but the FDA did uphold my allegations that the trial was improperly supervised, undermining in the process Zerhouni's misguided defense of Chabot.

And despite the hostility of the oncology community toward us and the project, despite the entry of so many patients too sick or too unmotivated to follow our treatment, despite the indifference of the NCI to supervising this study properly, we did have responders among those few who complied. Our two longest survivors at the time of the *JAMA* submission outlived by far all 126 subjects entered into the gold standard Gemzar study, and outlived, one substantially, all those to that point who had been treated by Fine and Chabot. That fact, considering the obstacles we faced, the indifferent support given our patients by their local doctors and the aggressive care available to those receiving chemotherapy, represented a victory.

Though for *JCO* Chabot described two chemotherapy patients as the longest survivors, Dr. Isaacs and I still wonder how these subjects ended up in this study—were they hand-picked from other Columbia clinical trials running concurrently along with ours? Did they receive "neoadjuvant" radiation along with their GTX chemotherapy, perhaps even undergoing surgery with curative intent after chemotherapy and radiation, in violation of the purpose of our study? We do not know, and perhaps will never know, since Chabot operated with complete secrecy in terms of his approval process for these patients.

As for *JCO* and its staff, the online Chabot article of August 2009 sailed through the peer-review process with no one apparently questioning at any time why I was not a co-author, or even referenced other than in passing. In comparison to *JAMA* and Dr. Pasche, *JCO*'s handling of the situation will remain to me extraordinary. To make matters worse, despite my complaint and the evidence given them, the *JCO* editors eventually published the print version of Chabot et al, with some additional justifications, after a six-month investigation during which time I was not contacted. This time around, the article seemed to me only odder than the original *JCO* website report, with Chabot evoking 9/11 to defend his inappropriate admission of certain patients into the trial. I am grateful that in his editorial Dr. Levine obviously sensed trouble, concluding the study proved nothing, but in my opinion this paper should not have been published in the first place.

In retrospect, I am not at all surprised by Dr. Chabot's efforts to place the article in a peer-reviewed journal. He had admitted to us he had not before supervised a federal grant, so a well run, properly executed study would have been a major achievement for him, perhaps opening the doors for future government funding. On the other hand, I can think of no greater stain on one's resume than to have served as Principal Investigator of an NCI-NIH clinical trial that after eight years and $1.4 million of taxpayer money spent ended up mismanaged, with data the NIH itself identified as meaningless (as reported in Dr. Engel's 2005 letter).

A few weeks after the *JCO* online posting appeared in August 2009, one of my long-term patients, a man who has followed my regimen for twenty years with some dedication, came into my office very shaken, having learned of the article on the Internet. Several physician bloggers, he told me with some dismay, were using the report to attack me with irrational vitriol. Though he had seen my website response, I could sense at once how deeply the situation troubled him—not that he doubted the legitimacy of my treatment but because of what he perceived as terrible and undeserved damage to my credibility as a scientist. I talked to him about the situation, assuring him Dr. Isaacs and I would do just fine because of loyal patients like him, and we would survive regardless, though at the time I didn't realize just how right I was with Ms. Somers' book as yet unpublished. Nonetheless, that meeting put a very human face to the *JCO* article, in my mind making the editors' behavior even more appalling, proceeding as they did with such apparent disregard for its possible effect on patients like this.

Though we are indeed surviving despite the *JCO* fiasco, when I look back I can only think what a shame, what a tragedy, what an ultimate disappointment, what a waste of time, resources, and valuable taxpayer money all this has been. I began working with Dr. Antman on the first draft of the protocol in the summer of 1997, more than 14 long years ago, even before the NCI had committed its support to the project. Fourteen years represents a big chunk of my life as well as of the life of Dr. Isaacs, much of it devoted to a research study that ended up in our opinion as a total and complete disaster. One might think that as a saving grace we might all learn something of value from the shambles of this effort, but I suspect few will learn anything, as few learned from the HIV-Nevirapine trial.

I wonder what the star supervisors at the NCI and NCCAM took home from all this—less than nothing, I would say. We have Jeff White, who knew full well of the study's mismanagement under his watch, telling the NCI Cancer Bulletin that the project provided a "good strategy for other studies." A "good strategy"? Are you kidding, Dr. White? And Jack Killen, what did he learn from his earlier experiences with HIV-Nevirapine and now from our adventure? I do not know what the answer might be in his case, but he has earned yet another promotion within the strange universe of government science.

As for us, we had hoped to show the world that we can all work together, alternative and mainstream scientists alike, despite the prevailing irrational bias against nutritional treatments and therapies developed outside the academic world. But that dream of common goals for the benefit of cancer patients everywhere wasn't to be.

To our dismay, we have to report the same tired old refrain, that the mainstream institutions and the people who inhabit them appear to have little regard for new ideas developed outside of their universe, outside of their narrow realm of experience. Sinclair Lewis wrote all this in his Pulitzer Prize winning (though he declined the gift) novel *Arrowsmith*, first published in 1925. The book, the darling of generations of high school students and idealistic premeds, tells the story of a dedicated young physician, Martin Arrowsmith, who found himself battling the unyielding forces of convention, the power of the status quo, the stubborn prejudices and enormous egos of his colleagues, to gain acceptance for his new, life-saving scientific truth about infectious disease. Lewis, who wrote the book with the former Rockefeller Institute microbiologist Paul de Kruif, himself the author of the bestselling *The Microbe Hunters*, said it all 85 years ago, even down to the destructive temptations of fame, money, glory, and adulation, seductions that almost derailed Dr. Arrowsmith from his pristine, honorable path. I could hardly say it better than Sinclair Lewis, 85 years later, Nobel Laureate that he would eventually be.

Nonetheless, I still think it's tragic, this pervasive bias that infects so many scientists at the highest levels of achievement within the medical profession. Bias tarnished this study almost from the beginning, despite Zerhouni's denial in his letter to Congressman Burton. It was evident early on in the late Victor Herbert's attempt to derail the study, it was evident in the many physicians who discouraged their patients from entering our trial or continuing on it once they had joined, at times using words like "fraud" or "quack" to make the point.

If Zerhouni wanted proof of the bias against us and our treatment approach he denied existed, he need not have looked any further to find it than in the published words of his own NIH staff. In his *Science* interview from January 2000,[69] and in the *New York Times* story from April 2001,[67] Dr. Straus could not speak objectively or positively about the pilot study, or its impressive data. Instead he denigrated the effort, belittled the results, then expressed his support only "lukewarmly" for the NCI-NCCAM trial. Prior to the lengthy *Science* article, Straus had never spoken to me, had made no attempt to communicate with me, had made no effort to enquire about the rationale underlying my approach which I would have been more than happy to share with him. True, I did eventually meet Straus in October 2000 at the White House Commission conference, some months before the *Times* piece appeared. But after our very brief and unpleasant encounter, he still made no effort to learn from me the reasons why I chose to do what I do.

Nonetheless, Straus felt perfectly righteous expressing his opinions to these enormously influential media outlets, both of which the scientific community holds in great esteem. Unfortunately, his borderline pejorative comments about me, my therapy, my pilot study data, and the NCI trial itself I suspect helped make the work of this difficult project much more difficult, probably discouraged the cooperation of reasonable oncologists, and hampered the accrual of suitable patients. What sensible physician would refer a patient into this trial if the scientist heading the very agency providing the funds could only offer his support "lukewarmly"? Sadly, if Straus was the great scientist everyone at the NIH claimed him to be, we can assume he was intelligent enough to know exactly what he was doing, and understood perfectly well the ramifications of his words.

Within the *Science* article, in one sentence Straus clearly expressed his problem with my treatment:

> "I'm more comfortable and find it easier to approach and fund things that already make a lot more sense to me," he admits.[69]

Here, Straus summed up the nature of bias better than I ever could in ten thousand words. Bias, at its root, is always about feeling comfortable, secure and at ease with the familiar and as a corollary, uncomfortable, distrustful, and angry with the unfamiliar, however irrational the discomfort, distrust, and anger might be.

A good journalist would have immediately jumped on that comment, called Straus out for it, and in a just world Straus would have been moved out of NCCAM immediately when that quotation appeared in print. After all, he had been hired to run the one NIH Center deliberately set up to investigate treatments that did not fit within the comfort zone of the conventional, familiar medical model. If he lacked the makeup to deal with the unfamiliar, as he himself here admitted, he should have not been running NCCAM.

Dr. Zerhouni's December 22, 2005 letter to Congressman Burton nicely illustrated the prevailing attitude toward me and my work at the highest levels of the scientific establishment. In November 2005 Congressman Burton had written a very thoughtful letter to Dr. Zerhouni, cataloguing the various protocol violations and instances of mismanagement that had gradually undermined the entire multi-year effort. I had provided the Congressman's staff with ample documentation to substantiate these serious allegations. Six weeks later, Dr. Zerhouni responded, though no one from his staff had contacted me in any way, via e-mail, telephone, or letter, to learn what evidence I might actually have in my possession to support the Congressman's point that the study had been run badly. For example, I would have been willing to turn over the 2½ years worth of documents proving beyond any doubt that Dr. Chabot had sent to us for treatment three patients lacking proof of the required signed consent, in violation of the written protocol, Columbia IRB rules, and federal regulations. I could have even provided Dr. Chabot's own e-mails to us in which he finally admitted, after our many months of questioning, that no evidence of the required documents existed for patients #9 and #16.

But Dr. Zerhouni apparently saw no need to communicate with me, relying as he did on explanations offered by the NCI and NIH trial supervisors:

> I have consulted with the National Cancer Institute (NCI), which currently administers the grant for this project, and the National Center for Complementary and Alternative Medicine (NCCAM), which currently funds the grant, regarding the issues you raise and would like to take this opportunity to address all of your concerns.

Dr. Zerhouni, based on what the government staff reported, proceeded to deny forcefully each of my allegations about the study's management. He not only categorically repudiated each claim, but lauded Dr. Chabot as the defender of the study, a true scientific hero, his honorable resolve determinedly holding strong against my insidious attempts to sabotage the effort. Magically, Dr. Zerhouni thus turned me into the problem:

> Dr. Gonzalez has raised very serious allegations against Dr. Chabot in terms of the conduct of the trial. We have seen no evidence to support Dr. Gonza-

lez's assertions of scientific misconduct by Dr. Chabot or his staff. It is our understanding that rules of clinical trial management were strictly adhered to by the Columbia research staff at every point in this process. The protocol was prospectively set and followed in order to avoid any insertion of bias. Dr. Chabot remained steadfast to the predetermined trial design . . . and assuring its ethical oversight. . . .

I think it's sad for a man in Dr. Zerhouni's position to have believed, without the slightest hesitation, the misinformation fed him by his NCI and NIH colleagues.

The trial supervisors with whom he consulted knew Chabot had entered multiple patients without evidence of the required consent form, a serious oversight requiring no debate since he had admitted the violation himself in writing and for the official study record. By that point I had already accumulated documentation that in addition Chabot had approved patients beyond the eight-week cut-off from biopsy, patients who could not eat as required by the protocol, patients affected by significant mental illness, and so on. Dr. Zerhouni could say correctly "we have seen no evidence to support Dr. Gonzalez's assertions of scientific misconduct" because the government employees he trusted apparently didn't give it to him and he didn't ask me for it.

Dr. Zerhouni's approach led him down a tricky path, to the point of disregarding all caution and common sense. Before putting anything in writing regarding these serious complaints of mismanagement or worse, it seems to me Zerhouni should at least have instructed one of the underlings roaming the halls of the NIH to call me, just on the off chance I might actually have some evidence to justify my allegations. For goodness' sake, forget about justice, or righteousness, or scientific truth, he should have contacted me for his own protection. I must assume he was so convinced I could add nothing of importance that he instead ennobled Chabot's management of the study. As we have seen, the June 2, 2008 OHRP determination letter and the FDA report prove rather conclusively that Dr. Chabot did not "remain steadfast" in "maintaining a predetermined trial design and assuring its ethical oversight," and admitted as much.

During the earliest years of the study, I did not suspect in Chabot the typical knee-jerk view of many academicians toward us, that old institutional prejudice against our "strange" nutritional treatment, centering as it does on pancreatic enzymes, diet, and coffee enemas. But both Dr. Isaacs and I sensed a change in attitude as the controversies surrounding our therapy and this trial continued to swirl. Then his obvious enthusiasm for chemotherapy expressed during that December 13, 2004 group meeting convinced us he was no longer as dispassionate an observer as he needed to be in his role of Principal Investigator.

As for our friends at *JCO*, what were they thinking? I do not know of course what passed through their minds during their review of the Chabot paper, either initially or after my complaint about the online version. But even before the Chabot publication, I myself had long ago lost my respect for *JCO*, ever since it published one of the most fraudulent scientific articles in modern times, the October 13, 1995 report "High-dose chemotherapy with hematopoietic rescue as primary treatment for metastatic breast cancer: a randomized trial," authored by the now infamous WR Bezwoda of the University of the Witwatersrand, South Africa. In this expostulation, Bezwoda and colleagues described a significant treatment benefit for autologous bone marrow or peripheral blood stem cell transplantation after high dose chemotherapy, compared to standard chemotherapy, in the treatment of women with poor-prognosis breast cancer.

Bone marrow transplantation (BMT) or, as it is known today, stem cell transplantation, has proven most effective against diseases of the marrow cell lines, such as inherited immunodeficiency diseases, leukemia, and lymphoma.[90] For these conditions, during the treatment patients first undergo high-dose chemotherapy, often coupled with total body radiation, to obliterate, deliberately, the diseased bone marrow. Subsequently, hematopoietic (marrow) stem cells from a genetically compatible donor are infused intravenously into the patient. These foreign stem cells, by a very precise homing mechanism, make their way to the marrow where they restore the depleted cell lines. Theoretically, the process offers great promise, but the obstacles have been many. As a start, at the time of the Bezwoda publication most studies reported that at least 10% of patients undergoing the procedure died as a consequence of the treatment, with mortality rates described as high as 30–50% in cases of an unrelated but matched donor.[90-92] The transplant can also fail for any number of reasons, or the newly formed immune cells with the donor's genetic identity may start attacking the tissues of the host patient in the potentially deadly graft-versus-host disease. Even if the transplant does take hold without significant damage to the host, in cases of leukemia and lymphoma nests of cancerous cells can survive the induction therapy, allowing the disease to recur.[90]

During the 1980s, many oncologists and researchers—including my former boss, Dr. Robert Good, who performed the first bone marrow transplant in history in 1969—began suggesting that in addition to such immune or blood malignancies, BMT might prove useful against a host of difficult-to-treat recurrent or metastatic cancers, such as metastatic breast and ovarian cancer, that do not involve abnormalities in the bone marrow cell lines. For these diseases, the threat of significant toxicity, particularly life-threatening suppression of the bone marrow, limited the amount of chemotherapy that could be prescribed. With the tool of BMT at their disposal, oncologists theoretically could administer very high doses of chemotherapy to these patients, far higher than would previously be possible, then heroically infuse hematopoietic stem cells to salvage the destroyed marrow. As an underlying principle, oncologists assumed if chemotherapy provided some value at standard, tolerable levels against a particular cancer, extremely high doses would offer even greater benefit. Some researchers enthusiastically claimed BMT might even lead to a cure in many previously intractable cancers. It was a hypothesis that, at the time, few challenged.

However, the procedure cost anywhere from $75,000 to $450,000, a major obstacle to patients since many insurance companies refused to pay for what they perceived as an unproven, strictly experimental treatment. But during the early 1990s the media came to the rescue, nearly universally portraying insurance companies as heartless, money-hungry, cold-blooded tyrants, denying an obviously useful therapy to the most desperate of patients, these women with metastatic and poor-prognosis breast cancer. In 1993, even Congress got into the fray, with 54 of its members demanding insurance companies, in the case of women with breast cancer, be forced to cover this presumed life-saving but expensive procedure. Other than the insurance industry, virtually no one in the medical profession, no one in the media, and no one in Congress seemed to care too much that little if any evidence actually existed to indicate this potentially deadly treatment benefited women with the disease. Eventually, by 1994, the oncology profession, working with aggressive attorneys and patient advocacy groups, had forced insurance companies through a series of lawsuits to cover the therapy in women diagnosed with metastatic or poor-prognosis breast cancer, though no real evidence yet existed to support its use in this circumstance.

To make a long story short, eventually the National Cancer Institute decided that it might make sense to test the procedure in controlled clinical trials, to determine if this therapy—by the 1990s already in routine use—worked. By the mid to late 1990s, five such studies had been completed and the results were published in the peer-reviewed literature. Four of the trials showed no benefit at all, but in stark contrast to the negative findings, the data from the fifth, as described in the 1995 Bezwoda article published in *JCO*, indicated a significant advantage for bone marrow transplantation over conventional chemotherapy, with a complete response rate of 51% for BMT versus 4%—truly a remarkable difference. Although the results seemed far too good to be true, I remember so well the media, as well as the scientific establishment, lauding the one positive study.

Fortunately, a few honest researchers began to question the South African trial and its methodology, since its findings so strongly contrasted with those of the other four studies. Though approached by several concerned oncologists, the NCI refused to support an independent audit of the South African data, and *JCO* did not retract the article. Subsequently, when the author declined to open up his books to appropriate scrutiny by a team of skeptical oncologists, the data's legitimacy came into question. Eventually, a formal investigation into this miraculous Bezwoda trial concluded the whole affair was a fraud, the data essentially created out of thin air.

Tragically, the oncology profession at large ignored early warning signs, so desperate were doctors to believe this therapy—which conformed to their belief in the value of chemotherapy—must show benefit. In 1999, even after serious doubts had been raised, the American Society of Clinical Oncology, the publisher of *JCO*, invited Bezwoda to present the honored plenary session lecture at one of their international conferences. It wasn't until 2000, five years after the initial publication, when faced with indisputable evidence proving the article a fraud that *JCO* finally retracted the document. At that point, oncologists stopped promoting the procedure for patients with solid tumors, before seamlessly moving on to the next new therapeutic miracle—anti-angiogenesis as I remember—with no apology to the families of those women who had been victimized.

The May 4, 2002 issue of the *British Medical Journal* published a lengthy summary of the entire fiasco, written by physicians associated with the Brown University Medical School, and entitled "Presumed benefit: lessons from the American experience with marrow transplantation for breast cancer."[93] I suggest anyone naive enough to believe that conventional physicians in general, and oncologists in particular, are overall objective, unbiased scientific practitioners employing only proven methods of treatment as is often stated or implied, should read this article. The authors place the concept of unproven medicine where it rightly belongs, smack in the middle of the conventional academic world.

More recently, the insightful book *False Hope,* published in 2007 and written by two physicians along with a Ph.D. political scientist and a lawyer specializing in public health issues, chronicled the whole breast cancer-bone marrow transplantation affair from the beginning.[94] In great detail, the authors tell the incredible story of enthusiastic oncologists—among those named, Dr. Karen Antman, former ASCO President, early supervisor of my trial, and co-author on the current *JCO* Chabot article—advocating for bone marrow transplantation as if it were some grand solution, despite minimal positive evidence to support its use, and despite good data showing it did nothing for the disease.

The whole bone marrow transplantation-breast cancer travesty wasn't just a question of over-zealous scientists promoting some new harmless theoretical idea in the laboratory that subsequently proved to be nonsense. The bone marrow transplantation story is much darker than that, it's a story of oncologists manipulating the legal profession and the media to promote an expensive and potentially deadly procedure that killed anywhere from 10–30% of the women undergoing the treatment without any real documentation to support its use. At the time, even under the best of circumstances, the toxic and debilitating treatment often required long hospital stays, frequently involving battles with infection and bone marrow failure. Unfortunately, the false *JCO* article kept this worthless treatment alive, encouraged women with incurable and poor-prognosis breast cancer to line up, positive and optimistic, anxious to receive a therapy that at best did nothing and at worst killed many prematurely. It is estimated—though no one knows the exact number—that upwards of 40,000 women underwent the procedure.

Imagine the situation a little differently. Let's think what would happen if some alternative practitioner promoted a nutritional or herbal regimen that cost up to $450,000 for a year's worth of therapy, that was extremely toxic and in fact so toxic it killed 10–30% of those foolish to put down the money and undergo the treatment, that initially had no legitimate data to support its efficacy, and when tested in clinical trials under the supervision of its proponents, the extraordinarily positive data reported ultimately proved to be fabricated? That alternative practitioner not only would be the subject of intensive legal and media attack, but he or she would be in prison for fraud, for racketeering, you name it. But I know of no oncologist sent to jail for encouraging women, in the absence of legitimate data, to undergo bone marrow transplantation for breast cancer.

With bias around me on a seemingly regular basis, I've often thought about its origins, how it comes to be in men and women who would loudly proclaim their rationality and objectivity. I don't think it's that mysterious, when all is said and done. Dr. Straus and Dr. Zerhouni, the peer reviewers at *JCO*, and in truth all other physicians come to scientific maturity exposed to a particular reigning model of medicine, whose proponents believe that disease, all disease, whether degenerative, genetically-based, infectious, or malignant, requires for effective treatment the ingenious creations of the human mind, the high-tech approaches of pharmacology, genetic manipulation, and for cancer, additional powerful interventions such as radiation. To this way of medical thinking, something as seemingly simplistic as mere nutrition, that is, diet, food, and the nutrients from food, could never provide significant or lasting benefit against any of the major health threats we humans face. True, during their schooling all physicians learn the various syndromes associated with specific nutritional deficiencies such as beriberi, rickets, and scurvy, but only in these limited and assumed rare circumstances of overt depletion does nutrition provide a solution. Otherwise, for the vast majority of human diseases, we need to be aggressive, we need more than food and vitamins, we require pharmaceuticals like antibiotics for infection; anti-inflammatories with all their side effects; steroids and toxic immune modulators for arthritis; dozens of potent mood enhancers and mood stabilizers with multiple side effects for bipolar illness, depression, and schizophrenia; chemotherapy, radiation, and targeted therapies for cancer; tranquilizers for insomnia; the various bisphosphonates for osteoporosis, etc., etc., etc. Even for those illnesses in which conventional researchers admit to a lifestyle and dietary component such as diabetes, heart disease, hypertension, and stroke, most physicians still emphasize the pharmaceutical option as primary treatment; the myriad of hypoglycemic agents for Type II diabetes, the statins by the handful for coronary artery disease and high cholesterol, the literally dozens of drugs, the angiotensin inhibitors, the beta blockers, the calcium channel blockers, and diuretics for hypertension and its often devastating partner in misery, stroke.

This particular model of medicine—and it is just that, a model—lauds these synthetic and high-tech creations as it relegates diet, food, and nutrition to a very minor role in any consideration of human health and disease. This cosmology dominates academic medical thinking, and certainly dominates all teaching in medical schools. Aspiring physicians scientifically mature in their education exposed only to this worldview, with hundreds of hours of their schooling, for example, devoted to pharmacology, and minimal time—if any time at all—allocated to nutritionally related subjects. Not surprisingly, the pharmaceutical, high-tech view becomes imprinted in their minds, becoming part of their scientific identity, their very scientific being.

I remember reading the works of Konrad Lorenz, the great Austrian animal behaviorist who popularized the term "imprinting" some four decades ago. In experiments with goose hatchlings, Lorenz showed that if the little birds were exposed to his bearded grizzled face after entering the world, rather than their true goose mother, they would accept him in that role. I remember so well the humorous photographs of Lorenz's geese marching in a line behind this distinctly non-goose eccentric human scientist, treating him for all intents and purposes as if he were indeed Mother Goose. To their graves, these geese considered him mom, so strongly had the idea been instilled in their neurological circuitry.

To little medical student goslings, the aggressive, high-tech approach to disease becomes imprinted, perhaps in a more sophisticated way than the Mother Goose scenario with the razzle-dazzle of biochemistry and molecular genetics and pharmacology, but imprinted nonetheless it is, following them right into their respective graves. It's a tough thing to overcome, this imprinting.

But there is another medical model, one that developed outside the academic mainstream, one never taught in the bastions of medical schools, one not even largely known there. In this case, in something as basic as diet, as foodstuffs, as the nutrients nature provides, and not in the synthetic creations of the human mind, lies protection against, and solutions for, most human disease.

I came to that conclusion myself only after a circuitous route. I've always had a great interest in natural history, and during my journalism days, long before I decided to change careers and attend medical school, I read extensively in ecological science and ecosystem modeling. As I delved into the technical aspects of natural history, I remember feeling amazed by the inherent stability of earth's complex and varied ecosystems—the Amazon rain forest, for example, with its nearly 150 different species of trees per acre, the great savannah of Africa, supporting huge migrating herds of grazers and a variety of ingenious predators, the American plains that once sustained millions of buffalo, the Pacific Northwest, with its majestic, towering forests. I was struck that these systems, as diverse as they might be, matured into highly productive entities, both in terms of plant and animal biomass, without man's ingenuity, without the use of antimicrobials, or synthetic fertilizers, or herbicides, or pesticides. They did just fine without any human tinkering.

In my studies, I learned that much ecologic science dealt with the cycling of nutrients, the movement of essential elements of life from the rock and soil into the plants, into the animals that eat the plants, into the animals that eat those animals, then back into the soil. I remember reading a very erudite but wonderfully written essay about the biochemistry of the dogwood tree, which we appreciate for the beauty of its flowers but which ecologists respect for its extraordinary ability to turn the calcium in underlying rock into a usable organic mineral, available for other plants and for the animals that live off those plants, and the animals that live off the animals that live off the plants. The dogwood, whatever a poet might think of it, serves, ecologically speaking, as an extremely important calcium pump in any field or forest in which it resides, fulfilling a most critical function.

The health of any ecosystem, and of any species of plant or animal living within, I discovered, depended as a first principle on the efficient cycling of many different nutrients. Should the process break down for even one critical element—such as calcium—the entire system, including its plant and animal populations, collapses, with the failure usually expressed initially as disease. To an ecologist, disease, whether in plant or animal, represented not a normal or inevitable state of affairs but rather the end result of unusual biologic stress, most often a deficit in nutrient cycling. Botanists and wildlife biologists accepted this premise as fact.

During this period of my life I also happened to read the works of the great English agronomist, Sir Albert Howard (1873–1947), the father of the organic farming movement and author of numerous books including *Agricultural Testament*. Howard, who spent much of his life working in India, observed that farmers following traditional composting techniques without the use of any synthetic chemicals maintained a very nutrient-rich and stable soil that in turn produced high-yield, nutrient-dense crops. Not only were the harvests substantially larger and the produce more nutritious than from farms tended according to modern practices, but the plants effectively resisted most insect attacks as well as the infectious diseases common in crops grown according to Westernized scientific principles. Furthermore, the livestock that lived off these plants seemed healthy and largely disease-free.

As an agricultural scientist, Howard's main interest may have been the soil and the plants that grew on it, but Sir Albert also noted that the farmers and local villagers living off these high-nutrient crops and vigorous livestock themselves tended to be extremely healthy, largely free of the degenerative and infectious disease already so common in the Western world. Howard concluded that healthy soil produced nutritious crops and livestock, and in turn healthy humans. It is a simple lesson but one ignored today in most of the world, enamored as our experts are by the wonders of chemistry, and ignorant as they seem to be of traditional agricultural techniques. Nonetheless, the lesson observed and taught by Howard still holds true—healthy soil yields healthy food that in turn produces healthy humans.

I found Howard's conclusions quite extraordinary. To a large extent, the dreaded diseases of mankind we fear so much may not be so mysterious, frightening and inevitable as they appear on the surface, but instead simple problems in nutrient cycling, that is, problems in nutrition.

Spurred on by Howard's writings, I began searching for other evidence that human disease might be largely a problem in nutritional ecology. Quite by chance, shortly after I read Howard's book I came across the works of the famed Rockefeller University microbiologist René Dubos, who spent his career challenging the typical twentieth century American ideas about infection, that if you should be unfortunately exposed to some pathogenic micro-organism, you're going to get sick. In this conventional model, the dedicated men and women of the pharmaceutical industry had discovered penicillin and related antibiotics that alone would save us from the plagues threatening us every day and everywhere. This popular view had been imprinted in my own mind when I was growing up in the 1950s via the media and also by our family doctor who injected penicillin at the hint of a runny nose without considering that most runny noses are viral in origin and do not respond to penicillin, that we need to be concerned about drug resistance and the destruction of our healthy intestinal flora by the overuse of such pharmaceuticals. For him, a runny nose meant a penicillin injection, which elicited much fear and dread in my young mind.

Dr. Dubos had a somewhat different take on infectious disease. He demonstrated rather eloquently, microbiologist that he was, that the susceptibility to infection and the severity of infection really depended not only on exposure to a pathogen, but on the underlying health and nutritional status of the individual. Of two people exposed to the same microorganism, one might die in terrible distress, and the other might go about his or her business symptomless, as if nothing had happened.

I remember reading a reference to polio, in my childhood the most threatening, most frightening, penultimately evil infection that a human could suffer, causing children to be taken from the families, forced into iron lungs for years at a time, leaving its victims paralyzed, deformed, their lives forever impacted. It was quite a scary concern for a child growing up in the 1950s, almost as terrifying as the Russian arsenal of nuclear A-bombs aimed at our little heads. However, I learned from Dubos and his colleagues that prior to the development of the Salk vaccine in the early 1950s, researchers had studied the incidence of polio infection in various locales including population-dense urban areas. To their very great surprise, they discovered that up to 90% of all children and adults living in crowded cities tested positive for polio antibodies, meaning they had been exposed to the virus, but very few had developed overt disease and its devastating sequelae. For most, the infection passed unnoticed, with symptoms no more serious than a common cold. Only rarely did flagrant illness develop.

Apparently this horrific deadly virus as it had been portrayed perhaps was not so debilitating nor so deadly. Some researchers believed that the underlying nutritional state determined who survived polio infection intact and those who did not; in the well-nourished, the virus did little, in those inadequately supplied with basic nutrition, the virus flourished unchecked. I remember reading all this with some astonishment, struggling against my own neurological imprinting. I previously thought that if a single polio virus came within a hundred feet of your body, you're done, but scientists like Dubos said that is not quite the case.

Not long after I read through Dubos' various books, I came upon the classic text *Nutrition and Physical Degeneration*, written by the dentist Weston Price and published in 1945.[95] It was this tome that finally helped tie together my earlier readings in ecosystems dynamics, wildlife biology, organic farming, and Dubos. Though within the alternative medical world this text is well known and often read, in the academic medical universe the book is unknown and never read, as if it just didn't exist.

For some seven years beginning in the early 1930s, Dr. Price traveled the world studying isolated groups of humans still following a way of life largely untouched by Western industrialization, modern agricultural science, and modern food technology. Price's journey took him from the Arctic of the Eskimos, to the high Andes of the Inca descendents, to the African savannah of the Masai, to high mountain valleys of Swiss Alpine herders, to Polynesia and its fisherman culture, and just about everywhere else in between. Though he evaluated many aspects of each indigenous group in the many regions he visited, Price focused his attention on the diet and the health of the people living according to time-honored, centuries-old wisdom about food and eating. Then he investigated the dietary habits and health of those people in each area who had migrated to regional towns and adopted a more Westernized lifestyle and eating pattern, consisting primarily of canned, chemicalized, processed, refined, overcooked and highly sweetened foodstuffs shipped from long distances. He compared the incidence of various diseases, such as cancer, dental caries, and tuberculosis among those living a traditional life to those eating "Western."

Wherever Dr. Price journeyed, tribes and communities of humans still following a traditional locally and freshly obtained, whole, unprocessed, unrefined, often largely raw foods diet enjoyed enduring superb health. These peoples seemed remarkably immune not only to infectious disease such as tuberculosis, but also to degenerative illnesses already reaching epidemic and near-epidemic proportions in Price's day such as arthritis, cancer, dental disease, diabetes, heart disease, and stroke. Even those groups following what we might consider extreme eating practices, such as the Eskimos living on nothing but fatty meat and fish or the Masai surviving on raw fermented milk, meat, and raw blood, seemed to Price in extraordinary physical condition, not only largely disease-free but capable of enormous prolonged exertion and strength in often difficult and trying circumstances.

Among those who had migrated from their traditional communities to take up residence in Westernized towns, Price recorded along with a drastic change in diet, a catastrophic deterioration in their health. Living among the "civilized," these folk consumed not the wholesome fruits and foods from the land but the fruits and foods of modern industry, canned, chemicalized, heavily cooked, processed, refined goods—with large amounts of white flour and white sugar thrown in for good measure. Those who might have only recently abandoned the traditions of their ancestors, perhaps raised as children on locally obtained whole foods, still enjoyed fairly good health, though not as vibrant or as disease-free as their cohorts who as adults still lived and ate as did their ancestors.

But among the offspring of the citified migrants, living from infancy on the in-dustrialized foods favored by their parents, Price documented an extraordinary surge in various illnesses, an avalanche of arthritis, cancer, dental disease, heart disease, infectious disease such as tuberculosis, often vaguer but debilitating chronic problems, described as persistent fatigue, malaise, even depression and mental illness, the latter rarely seen among the more traditional groups.

Price believed only the industrialized diet could explain this profound and rapid fall from good health, this remarkable rise in disease and disability among the children descended from healthy, traditional peoples now eating modern. I remember distinctly how in several instances to illustrate his case, Price compared the health of families he had encountered in which some of the siblings still ate by tradition while others had adopted a largely Westernized diet. Those eating whole unprocessed unrefined locally obtained foods enjoyed excellent health throughout their lives as did their offspring, while the children of their brothers and sisters who had moved into town and succumbed to Western eating habits suffered chronic ill health along with a plethora of serious diseases.

In Price's worldview, appropriate diet and nutrition provide us with the tools we need to allow for healthy and long lives, free of the majority of diseases we so fear in the civilized West—degenerative, infectious, malignant, perhaps even what we call genetically-based illness. Far from some inevitable process, these assaults largely develop because of our own doing, as we live and eat indifferent to cultural traditions, ignorant of the nutritional wisdom of our forefathers, enamored of a technology and industrialized agriculture that may ultimately be more of a problem for us than a solution.

Critics of Price, most of whom in my experience have never read the book, belittle him as some type of dangerous latter-day Druid, with some perverse aversion to the wonders of modern life. Quite the contrary, he was a most careful scientist, whose facts cannot be objectively or rationally countered, only emotionally and irrationally denied. And though his study could never be repeated today—few isolated cultures currently exist—the lessons remain certainly valid.

Our own approach to disease aligns more closely with the teachings of Price than with the "better living through chemistry" high-tech model. Though in practice what we do is complex, simply put we prescribe diet and nutrients, that is, natural substances in their most optimal form, to restore the metabolic efficiency of our physiologically ravaged patients without resorting to toxic interventions. For those diagnosed with cancer, we do recommend large doses of specially processed pancreatic enzymes that we believe provide a direct anti-cancer effect, but even this supplement is a naturally occurring product, not a synthetic creation. To those believing disease must always be outsmarted with human ingenuity, my use of something so primitive as a nutrient-dense whole-foods diet, nutritional supplements, and enzymes must seem preposterous at best. How could I, with the gifts of an Ivy League education, possibly believe that food and nutrients could be effective against a disease as complex and deadly as cancer? I was trained like one of them, to make my defection to the dark side all the more unconscionable.

Bias is a double-edged sword, or a two-sided coin, choose the analogy you like best. On the one hand, bias, as I have experienced it, is a fundamental, irrational, often fanatical disdain for someone or something not conforming to the accepted, perhaps a better word is "imprinted," model, regardless of fact or reason.

As its corollary, bias is at the same time a basic irrational belief, even a fanatical belief, in the goodness of someone or something, despite all evidence to the contrary. I could provide any number of examples in medicine to illustrate this second side of bias: the breast cancer/bone marrow transplantation tragedy certainly qualifies, and then there is my favorite of all time, the HIV-Nevirapine study. In this latter case we have scientists at the highest level of government turning a chaotic, mismanaged clinical trial in which researchers couldn't even be sure which patients received the medication, in which they ignored then covered-up patient deaths and serious side effects, into a gold standard for HIV treatment. Here we've seen how academic physicians and scientists right up and down the line can work hard to promote the value of a treatment that fits their model even when the data of a bungled study could not be trusted, we have seen how these folks can ignore gross and rampant mismanagement, violations of federal regulations, and the patients whose lives were put at risk. And they might have gotten away with it all, had not the "team" run into one stubborn obstacle in the form of Jonathan Fishbein, who most curiously would not bend the truth for the sake of science. They almost did escape unscathed, but for Dr. Fishbein. True to form they tried to demolish Dr. Fishbein, belittling his character, firing him, hoping to insure he never worked in science again.

But why would they try and squash the truth, these highly trained M.D.s and Ph.Ds? Well, HIV is the ultimate medical drama of our time, a drama played out on an international scale involving this insidious unseen virus that destroys immunity even in the strongest. This illness has been responsible for millions of deaths, striking down the helpless, mothers and their innocent babies, devastating economies in Africa, leaving hordes of street orphans across the continent, the focus of desperate research by our best and brightest, the topic of international conferences, a plague provoking UN intervention, Presidential press conferences, even mention in more than one State of the Union Address. The stakes are indeed high for the scientific community.

In the HIV crisis, the vast majority of scientists knew that their drugs and only their drugs could offer a solution. So completely did the HIV-Nevirapine team believe in the righteousness of their cause that they would do anything to prove the point, even alter the facts of a catastrophically bungled study, glorify meaningless data, cover up 14 deaths and more than 1000 side effects. So totally did they believe in the righteousness of their cause that they suppressed the truth, lied to colleagues, lied even to the President, and tried to destroy the reputation and career of the one man who believed the truth should be told. This is fanaticism, pure and simple, immune to fact, reason or reality.

While scientific bias in high places hardly heralds some new revelation, I must say both Dr. Isaacs and I were astonished, perhaps flabbergasted is the word, at the handling of our study by the managers from the various institutions assigned to the task. It isn't that difficult to obtain informed consent, and had we been allowed to participate in the entry of study patients as we had asked, we promise every one qualified would have signed the required forms. Once we realized no evidence of these documents existed for two patients, why did Dr. Chabot get annoyed with us for insisting he explain what had happened? Had he simply said, "I screwed up, I'm sorry," at least with such an honest response we could have begun dealing with a difficult problem. Instead, Dr. Chabot's office offered no reasonable explanation for nearly 30 months, before he admitted that the forms were missing but that their absence made no difference anyway.

We will always be troubled by his approval for the nutrition arm of so many patients, we still believe the great majority, who were clearly too ill, or were emotionally or mentally unsuited to adhere to our self-administered nutritional therapy, patients we would never have accepted into our private practice. And we will always be particularly troubled by those desperate trial candidates facing death, waiting four and five weeks for Dr. Chabot's decision about their eligibility, while they received no treatment of any kind as their aggressive disease progressed relentlessly.

So what advice can we give, after all of this? Well, as a general suggestion to all, forget about a new dawn of cooperation, a new era in medical history, the new millennium when everyone comes together, alternative and conventional scientists alike, proponents of a new idea and defenders of the old, for the benefit of science and truth. Forget it, that assuredly isn't going to happen. The academic institutions are simply too entrenched in their ways to allow for fair evaluations of treatment methods that in their very heart they abhor.

As for NCCAM, I hear rumors that many activists within the alternative medical world still cling dearly to the hope that the Center will get back on course with its new director and will fulfill its mission of funding promising new therapies developed outside of the academic mainstream, that NCCAM-supervised clinical trials of alternative approaches will be done fairly and honorably. My advice—forget it. I have been hearing the same rumors now for 20 years. The NIH resisted tooth and nail OAM's creation, they resisted its Congressionally mandated mission in 1991 and continue to resist only more strongly today. I will say that under Straus' creative and brilliant leadership, the NIH hierarchy did find a way to outsmart Congress, a coup for which Straus should be long remembered. The NIH cabal realized some time ago they couldn't shut NCCAM down, but they could turn the place to their own advantage by funneling multi-million dollar grants to their conventional academic friends inhabiting mainstream academic medical centers, the very scientists who for a generation have scoffed at any form of alternative medicine. So there, take that, Senator Harkin! Who gets the last laugh, after all?

I read somewhere on the Internet that Dr. Briggs, the current NCCAM director, apparently with no prior interest in, experience with, or knowledge of any form of unconventional medicine, intends to "reach out" to the alternative world, as she "reached out" to me, and I have heard that certain activists are in an absolute tizzy of excitement over the prospect. Are you kidding? I heard the same thing 19 years ago, when the NCI and NIH, realizing they had to accept OAM, started "reaching out," convened meetings, and brought certain well-known alternative personages to Washington to have lunch at taxpayers' expense. But all of the talkathons and titillation about having lunch with semi-important bureaucrats in Washington led nowhere, to nothing, it's all public relations and nothing more. My meeting with Dr. Briggs in December of 2008 led nowhere, to nothing, she didn't even respond to my letter after Chabot succeeded in publishing his *JCO* article.

The problem is the bias, it's in the very DNA of these academic scientists, the bias against treatments developed outside the esteemed centers they trust and outside the medical model that makes them feel safe. Straus said it so clearly, in the January 2000 *Science* interview, admitting that for him it was about feeling comfortable and feeling at ease. You can't beat an attitude like that, ever, and they won't change, one might as well ask a dog to be a bird, they can't help themselves, it's just biologically impossible. No one can tell me otherwise because I was there for 12 years, I didn't read about it in some fringe alternative journal or hear about it on some late night radio show. I lived it, I saw first hand the poisonous, pernicious effects of bias, I witnessed Straus, the director of the very Center funding and supervising our trial repeatedly denigrating my treatment, my pilot study data, and the NCCAM project itself in the influential media just as we were struggling to convince oncologists to cooperate. How can you beat that?

I didn't read about it, I lived with it. I earned the big NCI grant, I worked with the fancy Ivy League medical center, the big powerful NCI and NCCAM and the NIH right up to the Director's offices of each, and it led—in my opinion—to a shambles. And despite official government findings of significant mismanagement under Chabot's supervision, he still succeeded in publishing the article in one of the so-called pre-eminent oncology journals in the U.S., without even an e-mail or phone call to me first.

So, what to do? In terms of practical advice, as a start I would shut down NCCAM immediately, just send everyone packing. The American taxpayer doesn't need yet another bloated bureaucracy distributing huge sums of money to the same people who already receive huge sums from other bloated bureaucracies. We don't need that, save the money, send out taxpayer rebates.

I would even be bolder, and suggest that the entire NIH kingdom with its 27 vassal Centers and Institutes be dismantled as soon as practically possible, to end this system of welfare science and welfare scientists who in the NIH welfare state spend enormous amounts of time doing very little of anything, all at taxpayers' expense. Forget the impressive sounding titles and the important sounding conferences at exotic locales, close the place down for good.

Yes I know, I know, some serious employees at the NIH and its 27 Centers and Institutes do actually care about science *and* work hard, an unusual combination for a government researcher, but based on my experience such men and women are rare birds indeed. I run a full-time medical practice, spend 10–12 hours a day in direct patient care tending to the very sick who come to me from around the country and around the world. I also continue refining the therapy, keep up with the medical literature, and pursue my various difficult writing projects. It is a very demanding, very time-intensive way to spend one's life. Yet despite the commitments required by my day job, in past years Dr. Isaacs and I, in our spare time with no other help, wrote two lengthy manuscripts about the clinical trial for the NIH in addition to this book, accompanied by hundreds of pages of documents we reviewed, collected, collated, and organized. Numerous government personnel have seen at least one of these manuscripts, many have seen both, and to date they have pointed out only one rather minor factual error.

Over a period of 21 months, the OHRP with its full time staff of dozens of M.D.'s and Ph.D.'s conducted their investigation into this clinical trial, finally producing an initial determination letter of less than a single page of text. The document was not even accurate regarding basic, easily verifiable issues, such as the number of patients beginning therapy beyond the eight-week cut-off from diagnosis and the lack of signed consent in three patients. Though I gave them everything on a silver platter, they still couldn't get it right. What is this, some sort of inside joke that I, the outsider, just missed? Yes, the second determination reads better, they reported as a protocol violation the *second* patient Chabot entered beyond eight weeks, they now included a statement essentially confirming that the Principal Investigator (Dr. Chabot) "acknowledged" his faulty management of the study. But why couldn't they get it right the first time, with all the data I had given them? And what about the remaining issues they still have not properly addressed?

Without all these bureaucracies, I have no doubt that good science would survive and I believe do much better. Remember, James Lind figured out scurvy without government grants and despite the prevailing academic oligarchy which fought him tooth and nail. Edward Jenner discovered a solution to smallpox without government help and despite the fact that the academic authorities tried to kill him. Pasteur did much of his great work in defiance of the French Academy whose eminent members knew rabies could not possibly be successfully treated with his nonsensical vaccine. Then there's poor Semmelweis, the Austrian obstetrician who proved the value of aseptic technique in preventing puerperal fever of childbirth, but ended up dying in a mental hospital because of the constant scorn of his ignorant but powerful colleagues. And Gregor Mendel, the true father of all molecular biology and an example for all time, did not need a fancy degree or highly financed laboratories at prestigious institutions, only a plot of land in the countryside and some pea plants to prove his point. No, creative thinking and creative thinkers don't need bureaucracy, they do best without it as Sinclair Lewis suggested eighty plus years ago when at the end of his novel he sent his hero Dr. Arrowsmith packing off to Vermont to continue his research unhampered by the accoutrements and seductions of a successful academic life. No, creative thinkers are best off as far from bureaucracies as humanly possible. If you want to do creative work, run as fast as you can, run from the impressive sounding titles and the important sounding conferences in exotic locales, flee as far as your legs can take you from the turf wars and egos and "prevailing paradigms."

As a final response to all this corruption of science in the highest of places, for sanity's sake we suggest the approach we have long had for ourselves, fancy NCI grant or not, official academic recognition or not, positive *New Yorker* profile or not. We, Dr. Isaacs and I, keep working, as hard as we can work, day in and day out, concentrating on the science of what we do, the science which we find so wondrous and intriguing, concentrating on the patients, whose victories over terrible disease make all the struggles worthwhile and invigorate us both to keep trying, whatever the world ultimately thinks of what we do. That's the solution, always—the work, the science and the patients. There is, I promise, no better answer.

Reference List

(1) Specter M. The outlaw doctor. *The New Yorker*. 2–5–2001;48–61.

(2) Bedside procedures. In: Lyght CE, Keefer CS, Lukens FDW, Richards DW, Sebrell WH, Trapnell JM, eds. *The Merck Manual of Diagnosis and Therapy*. 11th ed. Rahway, NJ: Merck Sharp & Dohme Research Laboratories; 1966:1682–1683.

(3) McClain ME. The patient's needs: Enemas. *Scientific Principles in Nursing*. St. Louis, MO: The C.V. Mosby Company; 1950:168.

(4) Stajano C. The concentrated coffee enema in the therapeutics of shock. *Uruguayan Med Surg Special Arch*. 1941;29:1–27.

(5) Beard J. The action of trypsin upon the living cells of Jensen's mouse-tumour. *Br Med J*. 1906;1:140–141.

(6) Beard J. Trypsin and amylopsin in cancer. *Med Rec*. 1906;69:1020.

(7) Beard J. The scientific criterion of a malignant tumor. *Med Rec*. 1907;71:24–25.

(8) Beard J. The system of branchial sense organs and their associated ganglia in Ichthyopsida. *Quart J Microsc Soc*. 1885;11:52–90.

(9) Beard J. *The Enzyme Treatment of Cancer and Its Scientific Basis*. London: Chatto and Windus; 1911.

(10) Campbell JT. Trypsin Treatment of a Case of Malignant Disease. *J Am Med Assoc*. 1907;48:225–226.

(11) Cutfield A. Trypsin Treatment in Malignant Disease. *Br Med J*. 1907;2:525.

(12) Cleaves MA. Pancreatic Ferments in the Treatment of Cancer and Their Role in Prophylaxis. *Med Rec*. 1906;70:918.

(13) Golley FB. Two Cases of Cancer Treated by the Injection of Pancreatic Extract. *Med Rec*. 1906;70:918–919.

(14) Lewis JJ. Marie Curie. http://womenshistory.about.com/od/mariecurie/p/marie_curie.htm. Accessed October 29, 2008.

(15) Marie Curie. http://en.wikipedia.org/wiki/Marie_Curie. Accessed June 26, 2008.

(16) Morse FL. Treatment of Cancer with Pancreatic Extract. *Wkly Bull St Louis Med Soc.* 1934;28:599–603.

(17) Shively FL. *Multiple Proteolytic Enzyme Therapy of Cancer.* Dayton, OH: John-Watson Printing and Bookbinding Co.; 1969.

(18) Gonzalez NJ, Isaacs LL. Evaluation of pancreatic proteolytic enzyme treatment of adenocarcinoma of the pancreas, with nutrition and detoxification support. *Nutr Cancer.* 1999;33:117–124.

(19) Burris HA, Moore MJ, Andersen J et al. Improvements in survival and clinical benefit with gemcitabine as first-line therapy for patients with advanced pancreas cancer: a randomized trial. *J Clin Oncol.* 1997;15:2403–2413.

(20) Burris H, Storniolo AM. Assessing clinical benefit in the treatment of pancreas cancer: gemcitabine compared to 5-fluorouracil. *Eur J Cancer.* 1997;33 Suppl 1:S18–22.

(21) Gori GB, Wynder EL. In search of hypotheses. *Nutr Cancer.* 1999;33:115–116.

(22) Okie S. The clout behind a cancer maverick. *The Washington Post* January 18, 2000;A1.

(23) Saruc M, Standop S, Standop J et al. Pancreatic enzyme extract improves survival in murine pancreatic cancer. *Pancreas.* 2004;28:401–412.

(24) Burke LE, Ockene IS, editors. *Compliance in Healthcare and Research.* Armonk, NY: Futura Publishing Company, Inc.; 2001.

(25) Friedman LM, Furberg CD, DeMets DL. *Fundamentals of Clinical Trials.* 3rd ed. New York, NY: Springer-Verlag New York, Inc; 1998.

(26) Ahern JA, Kruger DF, Gatcomb PM, Petit WA, Jr., Tamborlane WV. The diabetes control and complications trial (DCCT): the trial coordinator perspective. Report by the DCCT Research Group. *Diabetes Educ.* 1989;15:236–241.

(27) The Diabetes Control and Complications Trial (DCCT). Design and methodologic considerations for the feasibility phase. The DCCT Research Group. *Diabetes.* 1986;35:530–545.

(28) Ornish D, Weidner G, Fair WR et al. Intensive lifestyle changes may affect the progression of prostate cancer. *J Urol.* 2005;174:1065–1069.

(29) DeVita VT, Jr., Hellman S, Rosenberg SA, editors. *Cancer: Principles & Practice of Oncology.* 6th ed. Philadelphia, PA: Lippincott Williams & Wilkins; 2001.

(30) Allendorf JD, Lauerman M, Bill A et al. Neoadjuvant chemotherapy and radiation for patients with locally unresectable pancreatic adenocarcinoma: feasibility, efficacy, and survival. *J Gastrointest Surg.* 2008;12:91–100.

(31) Fogelman DR, Chen J, Chabot JA et al. The evolution of adjuvant and neoadjuvant chemotherapy and radiation for advanced pancreatic cancer: from 5-fluorouracil to GTX. *Surg Oncol Clin N Am.* 2004;13:711–735.

(32) GTX effective in advanced pancreatic ca with reduced toxicity. *Oncol News Int.* 2004;13:44–45.

(33) Frucht H, Stevens PD, Fogelman DR et al. Advances in the Genetic Screening, Work-up, and Treatment of Pancreatic Cancer. *Curr Treat Options Gastroenterol.* 2004;7:343–354.

(34) Simplification of informed consent documents. http://www.cancer.gov/clinicaltrials/under standing/simplification-of-informed-consent-docs/page4. Accessed October 28, 2008.

(35) Bhutta ZA. Beyond informed consent. *Bull World Health Organ.* 2004;82:771–777.

(36) Hays J, Hunt JR, Hubbell FA et al. The Women's Health Initiative recruitment methods and results. *Ann Epidemiol.* 2003;13:S18–S77.

(37) Lo R. Correlates of expected success at adherence to health regimen of people with IDDM. *J Adv Nurs.* 1999;30:418–424.

(38) Office for Human Research Protections. http://www.hhs.gov/ohrp/about/ohrpfactsheet.pdf. Accessed October 29, 2008.

(39) Office of Research Integrity. http://ori.hhs.gov/. Accessed October 29, 2008.

(40) Dr. Catherine D. DeAngelis. http://www.nlm.nih.gov/changingthefaceofmedicine/physicians /biography_77.html. Accessed October 28, 2008.

(41) Guay LA, Musoke P, Fleming T et al. Intrapartum and neonatal single-dose nevirapine com-pared with zidovudine for prevention of mother-to-child transmission of HIV-1 in Kampala, Uganda: HIVNET 012 randomised trial. *Lancet.* 1999;354:795–802.

(42) Timeline for the HIVNET 012 clinical trial, audits and investigation. http://www.honestdoctor .org/images/media/TimelineHIVNET012.pdf. Accessed October 28, 2008.

(43) U.S. officials knew of concerns with AIDS drug. http://www.usatoday.com/news/health/2004 -12-13-aids_x.htm?loc=interstitialskip. Accessed October 28, 2008.

(44) Jackson JB, Musoke P, Fleming T et al. Intrapartum and neonatal single-dose nevirapine com-pared with zidovudine for prevention of mother-to-child transmission of HIV-1 in Kampala, Uganda: 18-month follow-up of the HIVNET 012 randomised trial. *Lancet.* 2003;362:859–868.

(45) Solomon J, The Associated Press. Review substantiates concerns at AIDS research agency. http://www.boston.com/news/nation/articles/2005/07/04/review_substantiates_concerns_at _aids_research_agency?mode=PF. Accessed October 28, 2008.

(46) The Associated Press. NIH whistleblower returns to office. http://www.foxnews.com /story/0,2933,179712,00.html. Accessed October 28, 2008.

(47) Gonzalez NJ. Showdown at Sands Point. *New York Magazine.* 7–31–1972;36–43.

(48) Dr. Jeffrey D. White, M.D., Director, Office of Cancer Complementary and Alternative Medi-cine. http://dctd.cancer.gov/ProgramPages/OCCAM-ADBio.htm. Accessed October 29, 2008.

(49) Richardson MA, White JD. Complementary/alternative medicine and cancer research. A na-tional initiative. *Cancer Pract.* 2000;8:45–48.

(50) White JD. Comprehensive cancer care: integrating alternative, complementary and conven-tional therapies. *J Natl Cancer Inst.* 2000;92:1945–1946.

579

(51) Smith WB, White JD. Complementary and alternative medicine in cancer: a National Cancer Institute perspective. *Expert Opin Biol Ther.* 2001;1:339–341.

(52) White JD. Cancer: current research in alternative therapies. *Prim Care.* 2002;29:379–392.

(53) White JD. The National Cancer Institute's perspective and agenda for promoting awareness and research on alternative therapies for cancer. *J Altern Complement Med.* 2002;8:545–550.

(54) White JD. Complementary and alternative medicine research: a National Cancer Institute perspective. *Semin Oncol.* 2002;29:546–551.

(55) Buchanan DR, White JD, O'Mara AM, Kelaghan JW, Smith WB, Minasian LM. Research-design issues in cancer-symptom-management trials using complementary and alternative medicine: lessons from the National Cancer Institute Community Clinical Oncology Program experience. *J Clin Oncol.* 2005;23:6682–6689.

(56) Launso L, Drageset BJ, Fonnebo V et al. Exceptional disease courses after the use of CAM: selection, registration, medical assessment, and research. an international perspective. *J Altern Complement Med.* 2006;12:607–613.

(57) Smith WB, Olaku O, Michie J, White JD. Survey of cancer researchers regarding complementary and alternative medicine. *J Soc Integr Oncol.* 2008;6:2–12.

(58) Colleen Lee CD, Zia F, Olaku O, Michie J, White JD. Survey of complementary and alternative medicine practitioners regarding cancer management and research. *J Soc Integr Oncol.* 2009;7:26–34.

(59) Zia FZ, White JD. National Cancer Institute Best Case Series program. *Integr Cancer Ther.* 2009;8:113–114.

(60) Olaku O, White JD. Herbal therapy use by cancer patients: A literature review on case reports. *Eur J Cancer.* 2010.

(61) What is OCCAM? http://www.cancer.gov/cam/newsletter/2006-winter/1.html. Accessed October 28, 2008.

(62) Smith WB. Biofeedback and relaxation training: the effect on headache and associated symptoms. *Headache.* 1987;27:511–514.

(63) Smith WB, Weisner C. Women and alcohol problems: a critical analysis of the literature and unanswered questions. *Alcohol Clin Exp Res.* 2000;24:1320–1321.

(64) NCCAM appoints Dr. John Killen, Jr., to direct the office of International Health Research. http://nccam.nih.gov/news/2003/090803-1.htm. Accessed October 28, 2008.

(65) Chat transcript: Dr. Jack Killen on AIDS treatment. http://www.cnn.com/HEALTH/AIDS/9907/15/chat.killen/index.html. Accessed October 3, 2010.

(66) NIAID's Stephen Straus to direct NCCAM. http://www.nih.gov/news/NIH-Record/11_02_99/story05.htm. Accessed April 5, 2008.

(67) Dreifus C. A conversation with: Stephen Straus; Separating remedies from snake oil. http://query.nytimes.com/gst/fullpage.html?res=9800EEDA113FF930A35757C0A9679C8B63. Accessed October 28, 2008.

(68) National Center for Complementary and Alternative Medicine. http://www.nih.gov/about /almanac/organization/NCCAM.htm. Accessed October 28, 2008.

(69) Stokstad E. Alternative medicine. Stephen Straus's impossible job. *Science*. 2000;288:1568–1570.

(70) Marshall HK, Thompson CE. Colon irrigation in the treatment of mental disease. *N Engl J Med*. 1932;207:454–457.

(71) King LS. Prevention of virus-induced mammary tumors by an orally active pancreas factor. *Exp Med Surg*. 1965;23:345–347.

(72) Eisele JW, Reay DT. Deaths related to coffee enemas. *J Am Med Assoc*. 1980;244:1608–1609.

(73) Margolin KA, Green MR. Polymicrobial enteric septicemia from coffee enemas. *West J Med*. 1984;140:460.

(74) Gonzalez NJ. *One Man Alone; An Investigation of Nutrition, Cancer, and William Donald Kelley*. New York, NY: New Spring Press; 2010.

(75) George Gasparis Biosketch. http://www.columbia.edu/itc/hs/medical/bioethics/egir/cv/Gasparis .pdf. Accessed October 28, 2008.

(76) Josephine P. Briggs, M.D., named Director of NCCAM. http://nccam.nih.gov/news/newsletter /2008_april/briggs.htm.

(77) About the Director. http://www3.niaid.nih.gov/about/directors/biography/biography.htm. Accessed October 29, 2008.

(78) Dr. John E. Niederhuber, Director, NCI. http://www.cancer.gov/aboutnci/directorscorner/jen. Accessed October 29, 2008.

(79) Elizabeth G. Nabel, M.D., named new Director of the National Heart, Lung, and Blood Institute. http://www.nih.gov/news/pr/jan2005/nhlbi-26.htm. Accessed October 29, 2008.

(80) NIH AIDS Research Program Evaluation Ad Hoc Panel on Complementary and Alternative Medicine Therapies Research. http://www.nih.gov/news/AIDS-panel/ALTMED3.HTML. Accessed October 28, 2008.

(81) Jaroff L. Wasting Big Bucks On Alternative Medicine. http://www.time.com/time/columnist /jaroff/article/0,9565,237613,00.html. Accessed October 28, 2008.

(82) History of cancer chemotherapy. http://en.wikipedia.org/wiki/History_of_cancer_chemotherapy. Accessed October 24, 2008.

(83) Gonzalez NJ, Isaacs LL. *The Trophoblast and the Origins of Cancer: One solution to the medical enigma of our time*. New York, NY: New Spring Press; 2009.

(84) Chemotherapy Provides Longer Survival than Enzyme Therapy for Pancreatic Cancer. http:// www.cancer.gov/ncicancerbulletin/090809/page3#b. Accessed December 30, 2010.

(85) Questions & Answers: The Phase III Gonzalez Protocol Trial. http://nccam.nih.gov/news /19972000/121599.htm. Accessed December 30, 2010.

(86) Levine MN. Conventional and complementary therapies: a tale of two research standards? *J Clin Oncol*. 2010;28:1979–1981.

(87) Carey B. Studies Halted at Brain Lab Over Impure Injections. http://www.nytimes.com/2010/07/17/health/17columbia.html. Accessed August 11, 2010.

(88) McNeilly P. Columbia University Medical Center RDRC 9/20/11. http://www.fda.gov/ICECI/EnforcementActions/WarningLetters/ucm273526.htm. Accessed November 30, 2011.

(89) Publisher's Note. http://www.ncbi.nlm.nih.gov/pmc/articles/PMC2860407/bin/JCO.2009.22.8429_index.html.

(90) Leger CS, Nevill TJ. Hematopoietic stem cell transplantation: a primer for the primary care physician. *CMAJ*. 2004;170:1569–1577.

(91) Zikos P, Van Lint MT, Frassoni F et al. Low transplant mortality in allogeneic bone marrow transplantation for acute myeloid leukemia: a randomized study of low-dose cyclosporin versus low-dose cyclosporin and low-dose methotrexate. *Blood*. 1998;91:3503–3508.

(92) Hematopoietic stem cell transplantation. http://en.wikipedia.org/wiki/Stem_cell_transplant. Accessed June 18, 2008.

(93) Welch HG, Mogielnicki J. Presumed benefit: lessons from the American experience with marrow transplantation for breast cancer. *BMJ*. 2002;324:1088–1092.

(94) Rettig RR, Jacobson PD, Farquhar CM, Aubry WM. *False hope: bone marrow transplantation for breast cancer*. New York, NY: Oxford University Press; 2007.

(95) Price WA. *Nutrition and Physical Degeneration*. La Mesa, CA: Price-Pottenger Nutrition Foundation; 1938.

About the Author

Nicholas J. Gonzalez, M.D., graduated from Brown University, Phi Beta Kappa, magna cum laude with a degree in English Literature. He worked as a journalist, first at Time Inc., before pursuing premedical studies at Columbia University. He received his medical degree from Cornell University Medical College in 1983. During a postgraduate immunology fellowship under Dr. Robert A. Good, considered the father of modern immunology, Dr. Gonzalez investigated the nutritional cancer treatment developed by the dentist Dr. William Donald Kelley. Dr. Gonzalez's subsequent research has been funded by The Procter & Gamble Company, Nestlé, and the National Cancer Institute/National Institutes of Health. Since 1987, Dr. Gonzalez has been in private practice in New York City, treating cancer and other degenerative diseases with an enzyme-based nutritional regimen. He is in the process of publishing a series of books, of which *What Went Wrong* is the third. For more information on his practice or his books, see his website at www.dr-gonzalez.com.

To learn more about Dr. Nicholas Gonzalez's research and medical practice, please visit:

www.dr-gonzalez.com
or call 212–213–3337

For other published works and recordings by Dr. Gonzalez, please contact New Spring Press.

Thank you for your interest!

NEW SPRING PRESS
PO Box 200
New York, NY 10156

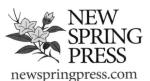

NEW
SPRING
PRESS
newspringpress.com